Current Clinical Strategies

Gynecology and Obstetrics

2008 Edition

New Treatment Guidelines

Paul D. Chan, M.D.

Susan M. Johnson, M.D.

Current Clinical Strategies Publishing

www.ccspublishing.com/ccs

Current Clinical Strategies Publishing
PO Box 1753
Blue Jay, CA 92317
Phone: 800-331-8227
Fax: 800-965-9420
www.ccspublishing.com/ccs
info@ccspublishing.com

Printed in USA   ISBN 978-1-934323-08-3

Contents

Surgical Documentation for Gynecology

Gynecologic History

Identifying Data. Age, gravida (number of pregnancies), para (number of deliveries).

Chief Complaint. Reason given by patient for seeking surgical care.

History of Present Illness (HPI). Describe the course of the patient's illness, including when it began, character of the symptoms; pain onset (gradual or rapid), character of pain (constant, intermittent, cramping, radiating); other factors associated with pain (urination, eating, strenuous activities); aggravating or relieving factors. Other related diseases; past diagnostic testing.

Obstetrical History. Past pregnancies, durations and outcomes, preterm deliveries, operative deliveries.

Gynecologic History: Last menstrual period, length of regular cycle.

Past Medical History (PMH). Past medical problems, previous surgeries, hospitalizations, diabetes, hypertension, asthma, heart disease.

Medications. Cardiac medications, oral contraceptives, estrogen.

Allergies. Penicillin, codeine.

Family History. Medical problems in relatives.

Social History. Alcohol, smoking, drug usage, occupation.

Review of Systems (ROS):
    General: Fever, fatigue, night sweats.
    HEENT: Headaches, masses, dizziness.
    Respiratory: Cough, sputum, dyspnea.
    Cardiovascular: Chest pain, extremity edema.
    Gastrointestinal: Vomiting, abdominal pain, melena (black tarry stools), hematochezia (bright red blood per rectum).
    Genitourinary: Dysuria, hematuria, discharge.
    Skin: Easy bruising, bleeding tendencies.

Gynecologic Physical Examination

General:
Vital Signs: Temperature, respirations, heart rate, blood pressure.
Eyes: Pupils equally round and react to light and accommodation (PERRLA); extraocular movements intact (EOMI).
Neck: Jugular venous distention (JVD), thyromegaly, masses, lymphadenopathy.
Chest: Equal expansion, rales, breath sounds.
Heart: Regular rate and rhythm (RRR), first and second heart sounds, murmurs.
Breast: Skin retractions, masses (mobile, fixed), erythema, axillary or supraclavicular node enlargement.
Abdomen: Scars, bowel sounds, masses, hepatosplenomegaly, guarding, rebound, costovertebral angle tenderness, hernias.
Genitourinary: Urethral discharge, uterus, adnexa, ovaries, cervix.
Extremities: Cyanosis, clubbing, edema.
Neurological: Mental status, strength, tendon reflexes, sensory testing.
Laboratory Evaluation: Electrolytes, glucose, liver function tests, INR/PTT, CBC with differential; X-rays, ECG (if >35 yrs or cardiovascular disease), urinalysis.
Assessment and Plan: Assign a number to each problem. Discuss each problem, and describe surgical plans for each numbered problem, including

preoperative testing, laboratory studies, medications, and antibiotics.

Discharge Summary

Patient's Name:
Chart Number:
Date of Admission:
Date of Discharge:
Admitting Diagnosis:
Discharge Diagnosis:
Name of Attending or Ward Service:
Surgical Procedures:
History and Physical Examination and Laboratory Data: Describe the course of the disease up to the time the patient came to the hospital, and describe the physical exam and laboratory data on admission.
Hospital Course: Describe the course of the patient's illness while in the hospital, including evaluation, treatment, outcome of treatment, and medications given.
Discharged Condition: Describe improvement or deterioration in condition.
Disposition: Describe the situation to which the patient will be discharged (home, nursing home).
Discharged Medications: List medications and instructions.
Discharged Instructions and Follow-up Care: Date of return for follow-up care at clinic; diet, exercise instructions.
Problem List: List all active and past problems.
Copies: Send copies to attending physician, clinic, consultants and referring physician.

Surgical Progress Note

Surgical progress notes are written in "SOAP" format.

Date/Time:
Post-operative Day Number:
Problem List: Antibiotic day number and hyperalimentation day number if applicable. List each surgical problem separately (eg, status-post appendectomy, hypokalemia).
Subjective: Describe how the patient feels in the patient's own words, and give observations about the patient. Indicate any new patient complaints, note the adequacy of pain relief, and passing of flatus or bowel movements. Type of food the patient is tolerating (eg, nothing, clear liquids, regular diet).
Objective:
    Vital Signs: Maximum temperature (T_{max}) over the past 24 hours. Current temperature, vital signs.
    Intake and Output: Volume of oral and intravenous fluids, volume of urine, stools, drains, and nasogastric output.
    Physical Exam:
        General appearance: Alert, ambulating.
        Heart: Regular rate and rhythm, no murmurs.
        Chest: Clear to auscultation.
        Abdomen: Bowel sounds present, soft, nontender.
        Wound Condition: Comment on the wound condition (eg, clean and dry, good granulation, serosanguinous drainage). Condition of dressings, purulent drainage, granulation tissue, erythema; condition of sutures, dehiscence. Amount and color of drainage
        Lab results: White count, hematocrit, and electrolytes, chest x-ray
Assessment and Plan: Evaluate each numbered problem separately. Note the patient's general condition (eg, improving), pertinent developments, and plans (eg, advance diet to regular, chest x-ray). For each numbered problem, discuss any additional orders and plans for discharge or transfer.

Procedure Note

A procedure note should be written in the chart when a procedure is performed. Procedure notes are brief operative notes.

Procedure Note

Date and time:
Procedure:
Indications:
Patient Consent: Document that the indications, risks and alternatives to the procedure were explained to the patient. Note that the patient was given the opportunity to ask questions and that the patient consented to the procedure in writing.
Lab tests: Electrolytes, INR, CBC
Anesthesia: Local with 2% lidocaine
Description of Procedure: Briefly describe the procedure, including sterile prep, anesthesia method, patient position, devices used, anatomic location of procedure, and outcome.
Complications and Estimated Blood Loss (EBL):
Disposition: Describe how the patient tolerated the procedure.
Specimens: Describe any specimens obtained and laboratory tests which were ordered.

Discharge Note

The discharge note should be written in the patient's chart prior to discharge.

Discharge Note

Date/time:
Diagnoses:
Treatment: Briefly describe treatment provided during hospitalization, including surgical procedures and antibiotic therapy.
Studies Performed: Electrocardiograms, CT scans.
Discharge Medications:
Follow-up Arrangements:

Postoperative Check

A postoperative check should be completed on the evening after surgery.
This check is similar to a daily progress note.

Example Postoperative Check

Date/time:
Postoperative Check
Subjective: Note any patient complaints, and note the adequacy of pain relief.
Objective:
  General appearance:
  Vitals: Maximum temperature in the last 24 hours (T_{max}), current temperature, pulse, respiratory rate, blood pressure.
  Urine Output: If urine output is less than 30 cc per hour, more fluids should be infused if the patient is hypovolemic.
  Physical Exam:
  Chest and lungs:
  Abdomen:
  Wound Examination: The wound should be examined for excessive drainage or bleeding, skin necrosis, condition of drains.
  Drainage Volume: Note the volume and characteristics of drainage from Jackson-Pratt drain or other drains.
  Labs: Post-operative hematocrit value and other labs.
Assessment and Plan: Assess the patient's overall condition and status of wound. Comment on abnormal labs, and discuss treatment and discharge plans.

Total Abdominal Hysterectomy and Bilateral Salpingo-oophorectomy Operative Report

Preoperative Diagnosis: 45 year old female, gravida 3 para 3, with menometrorrhagia unresponsive to medical therapy
Postoperative Diagnosis: Same as above
Operation: Total abdominal hysterectomy and bilateral salpingo oophorectomy
Surgeon:
Assistant:
Anesthesia: General endotracheal
Findings At Surgery: Enlarged 10 x 12 cm uterus with multiple fibroids. Normal tubes and ovaries bilaterally. Frozen section revealed benign tissue. All specimens sent to pathology.
Description of Operative Procedure: After obtaining informed consent, the patient was taken to the operating room and placed in the supine position, given general anesthesia, and prepped and draped in sterile fashion.

    A Pfannenstiel incision was made 2 cm above the symphysis pubis and extended sharply to the rectus fascia. The fascial incision was bilaterally incised with curved Mayo scissors, and the rectus sheath was separated superiorly and inferiorly by sharp and blunt dissection. The peritoneum was grasped between two Kelly clamps, elevated, and incised with a scalpel. The pelvis was examined with the findings noted above. A Balfour retractor was placed into the incision, and the bowel was packed away with moist laparotomy sponges. Two Kocher clamps were placed on the cornua of the uterus and used for retraction.

    The round ligaments on both sides were clamped, sutured with #0 Vicryl, and transected. The anterior leaf of the broad ligament was incised along the bladder reflection to the midline from both sides, and the bladder was gently dissected off the lower uterine segment and cervix with a sponge stick.

The retroperitoneal space was opened and the ureters were identified bilaterally. The infundibulopelvic ligaments on both sides were then doubly clamped, transected, and doubly ligated with #O Vicryl. Excellent hemostasis was observed. The uterine arteries were skeletonized bilaterally, clamped with Heaney clamps, transected, and sutured with #O Vicryl. The uterosacral ligaments were clamped bilaterally, transected, and suture ligated in a similar fashion.

The cervix and uterus was amputated, and the vaginal cuff angles were closed with figure-of-eight stitches of #O Vicryl, and then were transfixed to the ipsilateral cardinal and uterosacral ligament. The vaginal cuff was closed with a series of interrupted #O Vicryl, figure-of-eight sutures. Excellent hemostasis was obtained.

The pelvis was copiously irrigated with warm normal saline, and all sponges and instruments were removed. The parietal peritoneum was closed with running #2-O Vicryl. The fascia was closed with running #O Vicryl. The skin was closed with stables. Sponge, lap, needle, and instrument counts were correct times two. The patient was taken to the recovery room, awake and in stable condition.

Estimated Blood Loss (EBL): 150 cc
Specimens: Uterus, tubes, and ovaries
Drains: Foley to gravity
Fluids: Urine output - 100 cc of clear urine
Complications: None
Disposition: The patient was taken to the recovery room in stable condition.

Vaginal Hysterectomy

Hysterectomy is the most common major operation performed on nonpregnant women. More than one-third of American women will undergo this procedure. The surgery may be approached abdominally, vaginally, or as a laparoscopically assisted vaginal procedure. The ratio of abdominal to vaginal hysterectomy is approximately 3:1.

I. **Indications for hysterectomy**
A. Pelvic relaxation
B. Leiomyomata
C. Pelvic pain (eg, endometriosis)
D. Abnormal uterine bleeding
E. Adnexal mass
F. Cervical intraepithelial neoplasia
G. Endometrial hyperplasia
H. Malignancy
I. Pelvic relaxation is the most common indication and accounts for 45% of vaginal hysterectomies, while leiomyomata are the most common indication (40%) for the abdominal procedure.

II. **Route of hysterectomy**
A. Vaginal hysterectomy is usually recommended for women with benign disease confined to the uterus when the uterine weight is estimated at less than 280 g. It is the preferred approach when pelvic floor repair is to be corrected concurrently.
B. Contraindications to hysterectomy:
  1. Lack of uterine mobility
  2. Presence of an adnexal mass requiring removal
  3. Contracted bony pelvis
  4. Need to explore the upper abdomen
  5. Lack of surgical expertise
C. Vaginal hysterectomy is associated with fewer complications, shorter length of hospitalization, and lower hospital charges than abdominal hysterectomy.

III. **Vaginal hysterectomy operative procedure**
  A. A prophylactic antibiotic agent (eg, cefazolin [Ancef] 1g IV) should be given as a single dose 30 minutes prior to the first incision for vaginal or abdominal hysterectomy.
  B. The patient should be placed in the dorsal lithotomy position. When adequate anesthesia is obtained, a bimanual pelvic examination is performed to assess uterine mobility and descent and to confirm that no unsuspected adnexal disease is found. A final decision can then be made whether to proceed with a vaginal or abdominal approach.
  C. The patient is prepared and draped, and bladder catheter may be inserted. A weighted speculum is placed into the posterior vagina, a Deaver or right angle retractor is positioned anterior to the cervix, and then the anterior and posterior lips of the cervix are grasped with a single- or double-toothed tenaculum.
  D. Traction is placed on the cervix to expose the posterior vaginal mucosa. Using Mayo scissors, the posterior cul-de-sac is entered sharply, and the peritoneum identified. A figure-of-eight suture is then used to attach the peritoneum to the posterior vaginal mucosa.
  E. A Steiner-Anvard weighted speculum is inserted into the posterior cul-de-sac after this space is opened. The uterosacral ligaments are clamped, with the tip of the clamp incorporating the lower portion of the cardinal ligaments. The clamp is placed perpendicular to the uterine axis, and the pedicle cut so that there is 0.5 cm of tissue distal to the clamp. A transfixion suture is then placed at the tip of the clamp. Once ligated, the uterosacral ligaments are transfixed to the posterior lateral vaginal mucosa. This suture is held with a hemostat.
  F. Downward traction is placed on the cervix to provide countertraction for the vaginal mucosa and the anterior vaginal mucosa is incised at the level of the cervicovaginal junction. The bladder is advanced upward using an open, moistened gauze sponge. At this point, the vesicovaginal peritoneal reflection is usually identified and can be entered sharply using scissors. A Deaver or Heaney retractor is placed in the midline to keep the bladder out of the operative field. Blunt or sharp advancement of the bladder should precede each clamp placement until the vesicovaginal space is entered.
  G. The cardinal ligaments are identified, clamped, cut, and suture ligated. The bladder is advanced out of the operative field using blunt dissection technique. The uterine vessels are clamped to incorporate the anterior and posterior leaves of the visceral peritoneum.
  H. The anterior peritoneal fold is now visualized, and the anterior cul-de-sac can be entered. The peritoneal reflection is grasped with smooth forceps, tented, and opened with scissors with the tips pointed toward the uterus. A Heaney or Deaver retractor is placed into this space to protect the bladder.
  I. The uterine fundus is delivered posteriorly by placing a tenaculum on the uterine fundus in successive bites. An index finger is used to identify the utero-ovarian ligament and aid in clamp placement. The remainder of the utero-ovarian ligaments are clamped and cut. The pedicles are double-ligated first with a suture tie and followed by a suture ligature medial to the first tie.

IV. **Discharge instructions**
  A. The woman is encouraged to resume her normal daily activities as quickly as is comfortable. Walking and stair climbing are encouraged; tub baths or showers are permissible.
  B. The patient should avoid lifting over 20 lb of weight for four to six weeks after surgery to minimize stress on the healing fascia. Vaginal intercourse is discouraged during this period. Driving should be avoided until full mobility returns and narcotic analgesia is no longer required.

Endometrial Sampling and Dilation and Curettage

The endometrial cavity is frequently evaluated because of abnormal uterine bleeding, pelvic pain, infertility, or pregnancy complications. The most common diagnostic indications for obtaining endometrial tissue include abnormal uterine bleeding, postmenopausal bleeding, endometrial dating, endometrial cells on Papanicolaou smear, and follow-up of women undergoing medical therapy for endometrial hyperplasia.

I. Endometrial biopsy

   A. The office endometrial biopsy offers a number of advantages to D&C because it can be done with minimal to no cervical dilation, anesthesia is not required, and the cost is approximately one-tenth of a hospital D&C.
   B. Numerous studies have shown that the endometrium is adequately sampled with these techniques.
   C. **Pipelle endometrial sampling device** is the most popular method for sampling the endometrial lining. The device is constructed of flexible polypropylene with an outer sheath measuring 3.1 mm in diameter.
   D. The device is placed in the uterus through an undilated cervix. The piston is fully withdrawn to create suction and, while the device is rotated 360 degrees, the distal port is brought from the fundus to the internal os to withdraw a sample. The device is removed and the distal aspect of the instrument is severed, allowing for the expulsion of the sample into formalin.
   E. The detection rates for endometrial cancer by Pipelle in postmenopausal and premenopausal women are 99.6 and 91%, respectively.
   F. D&C should be considered when the endometrial biopsy is nondiagnostic, but a high suspicion of cancer remains (eg, hyperplasia with atypia, presence of necrosis, or pyometra).

II. Dilation and curettage

   A. Dilation and curettage is performed as either a diagnostic or therapeutic procedure. Indications for diagnostic D&C include:
      1. A nondiagnostic office biopsy in women who are at high risk of endometrial carcinoma.
      2. Insufficient tissue for analysis on office biopsy.
      3. Cervical stenosis prevents the completion of an office biopsy.
   B. Diagnostic D&Cs are usually performed with hysteroscopy to obtain a visual image of the endometrial cavity, exclude focal disease, and prevent missing unsuspected polyps.
   C. **Examination under anesthesia**. After anesthesia has been administered, the size, shape, and position of the uterus are noted, with particular attention to the axis of the cervix and flexion of the fundus. The size, shape, and consistency of the adnexa are determined. The perineum, vagina, and cervix are then prepared with an aseptic solution and vaginal retractors are inserted into the vagina.
   D. **Operative technique**. A D&C is performed with the woman in the dorsal lithotomy position.
      1. **Endocervical curettage** (ECC) is performed before dilation of the cervix. A Kevorkian-Younge curette is introduced into the cervical canal up to the internal os. Curetting of all four quadrants of the canal should be conducted and the specimen placed on a Telfa pad.
      2. **Sounding and dilation.** Traction is applied to align the axis of the cervix and the uterine canal. The uterus should be sounded to document the size and confirm the position. The sound should be held between the thumb and the index finger to avoid excessive pressure.
      3. **Cervical dilation** is then performed. The dilator is grasped in the middle of the instrument with the thumb and index finger. The cervix

is gradually dilated beginning with the #13 French Pratt dilator. The dilator should be inserted through the internal os, without excessively entering the uterine cavity.

4. **Sharp curettage** is performed systematically beginning at the fundus and applying even pressure on the endometrial surface along the entire length of the uterus to the internal cervical os. The endometrial tissue is placed on a Telfa pad placed in the vagina. Moving around the uterus in a systematic fashion, the entire surface of the endometrium is sampled. The curettage procedure is completed when the "uterine cry" (grittiness to palpation) is appreciated on all surfaces of the uterus. Curettage is followed by blind extraction with Randall polyp forceps to improve the rate of detection of polyps.

General Gynecology

Screening for Cervical Cancer

Cervical cancer screening should be started three years after the onset of sexual activity, but no later than age 21. The basis of this recommendation is that high grade cervical intraepithelial lesions (HSIL) are almost entirely related to acquisition of human papillomavirus (HPV) infection through genital skin to skin contact and these lesions usually do not occur until three to five years after exposure to HPV. HSIL is a precursor to cervical cancer.

I. **Screening interval**
    A. Cervical cancer screening should be started three years after the onset of sexual activity, but no later than age 21.
    B. The American Cancer Society recommends that initial cervical screening should be performed annually if conventional cervical cytology smears (Pap) are used and every two years with liquid-based cytology tests until age 30. The screening interval can then be increased to every two to three years in women with three or more consecutive normal cytology results who are $\geq$30 years old.
    C. The American College of Obstetricians and Gynecologists recommends annual screening for women younger than 30 years of age regardless of testing method (conventional or liquid-based cytology). Women aged 30 and over who have had three negative smears, no history of CIN II/III, and are not immunocompromised or DES exposed in utero may extend the interval between tests to two to three years. Women aged 30 and over may also consider the option of a combined cervical cytology and HPV test. Women who test negative by both tests should not be screened more frequently than every three years.
    D. Exceptions. Women at increased risk of CIN, such as those with in utero DES exposure, immunocompromise, or a history of CIN II/III or cancer, should continue to be screened at least annually. More frequent surveillance should also be considered in women whose smears do not contain endocervical cells or are partially obscured.
    E. **Discontinuing screening**
        1. The United States Preventive Services Task Force stated screening may stop at age 65 if the woman has had recent normal smears and is not at high risk for cervical cancer.
        2. The American Cancer Society guideline stated that women age 70 or older may elect to stop cervical cancer screening if they have had three consecutive satisfactory, normal/negative test results and no abnormal test results within the prior 10 years.
        3. Cervical cancer screening is not recommended in women who have had total hysterectomies for benign indications (presence of CIN II or III excludes benign categorization). Screening of women with CIN II/III who undergo hysterectomy may be discontinued after three consecutive negative results have been obtained. However, screening should be performed if the woman acquires risk factors for intraepithelial neoplasia, such as new sexual partners or immunosuppression.

Bethesda 2001 Pap Smear Report

Interpretation Result
Negative for intraepithelial lesion or malignancy
Infection (Trichomonas vaginalis, Candida spp., shift in flora suggestive of bacterial vaginosis, Actinomyces spp., cellular changes consistent with Herpes simplex virus)
Other Non-neoplastic Findings:
    Reactive cellular changes associated with inflammation (includes typical repair) radiation, intrauterine contraceptive device (IUD)
    Glandular cells status post-hysterectomy
    Atrophy
Other
    Endometrial cells (in a woman $\geq$40 years of age)
Epithelial Cell Abnormalities
  Squamous Cell
    Atypical squamous cells
        of undetermined significance (ASC-US)
        -cannot exclude HSIL (ASC-H)
    Low-grade squamous intraepithelial lesion (LSIL) encompassing: HPV/mild dysplasia/CIN 1
    High-grade squamous intraepithelial lesion (HSIL) encompassing: moderate and severe dysplasia, CIS/CIN 2 and CIN 3 with features suspicious for invasion (if invasion is suspected)
    Squamous cell carcinoma
  Glandular Cell
    Atypical
      -Endocervical cells (not otherwise specified or specify in comments)
      -Glandular cell (not otherwise specified or specify in comments)
      -Endometrial cells (not otherwise specified or specify in comments)
      -Glandular cells (not otherwise specified or specify in comments)
    Atypical
      -Endocervical cells, favor neoplastic
      -Glandular cells, favor neoplastic
    Endocervical adenocarcinoma in situ
    Adenocarcinoma (endocervical, endometrial, extrauterine, not otherwise specified (not otherwise specified)
Other Malignant Neoplasms (specify)

Management of the Abnormal Papanicolaou Smear

Result	Action
Specimen adequacy	
Satisfactory for evaluation	Routine follow-up
Unsatisfactory for evaluation	Repeat smear
No endocervical cells	Follow-up in one year for low-risk women with a previously normal smear; repeat in 4-6 months for high-risk women
Atypical cells	
Atypical squamous cells of undetermined significance (ASC-US)	HPV testing with referral to colposcopy if positive for high-risk HPV type; if negative for high-risk HPV type, then repeat cytology in 12 months

Result	Action
Special circumstances	Postmenopausal women with atrophic epithelium may be treated with topical estrogen followed by repeat cervical cytology one week after completing treatment
ASC-H	Immediate referral to colposcopy
Atypical glandular cells (AGS)	Immediate referral to colposcopy with sampling of the endocervical canal. Women over age 35 and any woman with unexplained vaginal bleeding should also have an endometrial biopsy
Intraepithelial neoplasia	
High grade	Immediate referral for colposcopy
Low grade	Immediate referral for colposcopy, except adolescents and postmenopausal women
Endometrial cells	Endometrial biopsy in selected cases
Other malignant cells	Referral to a gynecologic oncologist

References: See page 208.

Cervical Intraepithelial Neoplasia

Cervical intraepithelial neoplasia (CIN) refers to a preinvasive pathological intermediate of cervical cancer, which progresses slowly and can be easily detected and treated.

I. Nomenclature
   A. Histologic definitions of cervical intraepithelial neoplasia (CIN):
   CIN I refers to cellular dysplasia confined to the basal third of the epithelium
   CIN II refers to lesions confined to the basal two-thirds of the epithelium
   CIN III refers to cellular dysplasia encompassing greater than two-thirds of the epithelial thickness, including full-thickness lesions
   B. **Cytologic definitions.** Cytologic Pap smears are classified according to the Bethesda system. In this system, mild dysplasia/CIN I was combined with koilocytic or condylomatous atypia to create the category low-grade squamous intraepithelial lesion (LSIL or LGSIL). Moderate and severe dysplasia/CIS/CIN II/CIN III were merged to form the category of high-grade squamous intraepithelial lesion (HSIL or HGSIL) because of similarities in both the cytologic features and prognosis of these groups.
   C. Other new terms, such as atypical squamous cells of undetermined significance (ASCUS) and atypical glandular cells (AGC), were introduced to express equivocal findings.
II. Risk factors
   A. Sexual activity is a key factor in the etiology of cervical neoplasia. The incidence of squamous cell cancer of the cervix in women who have not had any sexual relationships is almost nonexistent. Sexual risk

factors for CIN include sexual activity at an early age, history of sexually transmitted infections (chlamydia, herpes simplex virus), multiple sexual partners, or sexual activity with promiscuous men. The major causal factor is infection with the human papillomavirus (HPV).

B. Other risk factors include cigarette smoking, multiparity, and exogenous or endogenous immunodeficiency.

C. Human papillomavirus infection is endemic among sexually experienced individuals. 80% of sexually active women will have acquired a genital HPV infection by age 50. Most HPV infections are transient, resolving spontaneously in six to 18 months.

D. **Diagnosis**
   1. **Cervical cytology.** Women are screened for CIN by cervical cytology (eg, conventional Papanicolaou smear or liquid based, such as ThinPrep or SurePath). Abnormal cytology results should be further evaluated.
   2. **Colposcopy** is used to evaluate abnormal cervical cytology. Abnormal areas of the epithelium turn white with dilute acetic acid. Capillaries may be identified within the abnormal epithelium. Capillary thickness and the intercapillary distances correlate with the severity of the lesion; high-grade lesions have a coarser vessel pattern and larger intercapillary distance. Abnormal areas can be targeted for biopsy.

III. **Management of cervical intraepithelial neoplasia**

A. Treatment of cervical intraepithelial abnormalities is undertaken after a histologic abnormality has been proven by tissue biopsy. Treatment is never performed based upon a cytologic diagnosis alone; but is sometimes initiated at the time of colposcopy/biopsy in women who are at high risk of loss to follow-up ("see-and-treat" protocols).

B. Atypical squamous cells (ASC, subcategories ASC-US and ASC-H) is a cytological screening diagnosis that does not justify treatment because it is not diagnostic of a cancerous or precancerous lesion. ASC does require further evaluation to exclude the presence of histologically confirmed high grade disease, which may require treatment.

C. **Low grade lesions: CIN 1**
   1. Aggressive intervention in these patients is usually not indicated because a significant number of these lesions spontaneously regress and infrequently progress.
   2. LSIL regresses to normal in 47%; progression to a high grade lesion occurs in 21%, and to cancer in 0.15%.
   3. **Management.** Since spontaneous regression is observed in most women, expectant management is generally preferred for the reliable patient with biopsy confirmed CIN 1, in whom the entire lesion and limits of the transformation zone are completely visualized (ie, satisfactory colposcopic examination). If treatment is desired, ablative or excisional modalities are appropriate. An excisional procedure is the preferred diagnostic/therapeutic approach if the transformation zone is not fully visualized by colposcopy.
   4. **Expectant management.** 80 to 85% of women referred for initial colposcopy because of LSIL or HPV DNA positive ASC-US have CIN 1 or less detected on biopsy. 9 to 16% of these women will have histologically confirmed CIN 2 or 3 within two years. Expectant management of women with biopsy confirmed CIN 1 and satisfactory colposcopy consists of repeat cytology at 6 and 12 months or HPV testing at 12 months.
      a. **Colposcopy** should be repeated if repeat cytology shows ASC or greater or HPV DNA testing is positive for a high risk type.
      b. After two negative smears or a negative HPV DNA test, annual screening may be resumed.
      c. Colposcopy and repeat cytology at 12 months is an acceptable alternative to semiannual cytology or annual HPV testing.

     5. Ablation or excision
- **a.** Some women may elect to have ablation or excision of the lesion to relieve their anxiety. Immediate therapy may also be warranted in the patient at high risk for loss to follow-up.
- **b.** Endocervical sampling is recommended before ablation, and excision is recommended for patients with recurrent disease after ablation. Ablative treatment is unacceptable if colposcopy is not satisfactory. In such cases, a diagnostic and therapeutic excisional procedure should be performed.

6. Special circumstances
- **a. Pregnant and adolescent women.** Expectant management of pregnant or adolescent women with biopsy confirmed CIN 1, even in the setting of an unsatisfactory colposcopic examination, is an acceptable alternative to ablative/excisional therapy because undetected high grade disease is uncommon in this setting.
- **b. CIN 1.** Expectant management is recommended for the reliable patient in whom the entire lesion and limits of the transformation zone are completely visualized. Repeat cytology should be done at 6 and 12 months or HPV testing at 12 months.

D. High grade lesions: CIN 2/3
1. 43 to 58% of CIN 2 lesions will regress if left untreated, while 22% progress to CIN 3 and 5% progress to invasive cancer.
2. **Management.** The entire transformation zone should be eliminated. Prior to any therapeutic intervention, an assessment needs to be made as to whether a patient qualifies for ablative therapy or if she requires a more invasive excisional procedure for further diagnostic work-up.
3. **Ablative therapy.** Prerequisites for ablative treatment are:
   - **a.** Accurate histologic diagnosis/no discrepancy between cytology/colposcopy/histology
   - **b.** No evidence of microinvasion/invasion
   - **c.** No evidence of a glandular lesion (adenocarcinoma in situ or invasive adenocarcinoma)
   - **d.** Satisfactory colposcopy (eg, the transformation zone is fully visualized)
   - **e.** The lesion is limited to the ectocervix and seen in its entirety
   - **f.** There is no evidence of endocervical involvement as determined by colposcopy/endocervical curettage
4. The most commonly used ablative treatment techniques are cryotherapy and laser ablation.
5. **Excisional therapy.** Indications for excisional therapy are:
   - **a.** Suspected microinvasion
   - **b.** Unsatisfactory colposcopy (the transformation zone is not fully visualized)
   - **c.** Lesion extending into the endocervical canal
   - **d.** Endocervical curettage revealing dysplasia
   - **e.** Lack of correlation between the cytology and colposcopy/biopsies
   - **f.** Suspected adenocarcinoma in situ
   - **g.** Colposcopist unable to rule out invasive disease
   - **h.** Recurrence after an ablative procedure
6. **Excisional treatment** can be performed by cold knife conization, laser conization, or the loop electrosurgical excision procedure (LEEP). With suspected microinvasion or ACIS, cold knife conization is recommended so that margins can be evaluated without cautery artifact.
7. **Special circumstances**
   - **a. Pregnancy.** High-grade lesions discovered during pregnancy have a high rate of regression in the postpartum period. 70% of CIN 3 regress and none progress to invasive carcinoma. Treatment of CIN 2/3 is not indicated during pregnancy. The patient

should be monitored with colposcopy (without endocervical curettage) each trimester. Colposcopy and cervical cytology should be performed 6 to 12 weeks postpartum. However, conization during pregnancy is usually required in women with suspected invasive disease.

- **b. Adolescents.** Observation with colposcopy and cytology at six-month intervals for one year is acceptable for reliable adolescents with biopsy-confirmed CIN 2, provided colposcopy is satisfactory, endocervical curettage is negative. In this population, the rate of regression is high and progression to invasive cancer is extremely small.
    - **(1)** Ablation or excision is recommended for adolescents with CIN 3.
    - **(2) CIN 2/3.** Ablative and excisional procedures have equally effective cure rates. A loop electrosurgical excisional procedure (LEEP) is recommended over an ablative or other excisional procedures (cold knife cone). LEEP is an office procedure with ease of use, providing a histologic specimen at low cost and morbidity, and high rate of success.
    - **(3) Cold knife conization** is recommended for women with suspected microinvasion, unsatisfactory colposcopy (eg, the transformation zone is not fully visualized), lesion extending into the endocervical canal, and suspected adenocarcinoma in situ.
- **E. Therapeutic procedures.** The five most common techniques for treatment of CIN are:
    1. Loop electrosurgical excision procedure (LEEP)
    2. Cryotherapy (nitrous oxide or carbon dioxide)
    3. Carbon dioxide (CO_2) laser ablation
    4. Conization (cold knife or laser)
    5. These techniques were equally effective, averaging approximately 90% cure.
- **F. Loop electrosurgical excision procedure.** The loop electrosurgical excision procedure (LEEP) has become the approach of choice for treating CIN 2 and 3 because of its ease of use, low cost, and high rate of success.
- **G. Cryotherapy** refers to the application of a super-cooled probe (nitrous oxide or carbon dioxide) directly to the cervical lesion using one or more cooling and thawing cycles. The probe must be able to cover the entire lesion and the lesion cannot extend into the endocervical canal. Anesthesia is not required.
    1. Blanching extend at least 7 to 8 mm beyond the edge of the cryoprobe to reach the full depth of the cervical crypts. Typically, the cervix is frozen for two to three minutes, followed by a thaw period lasting five minutes. After the cervix has returned to a pink color, an additional two to three minute freeze application is performed.
    2. **Conization** refers to the excision of a cone shaped portion of the cervix. The procedure is usually performed using a scalpel, but laser conization is also possible. Endocervical curettage can be performed after the conization to evaluate the remaining endocervical canal.
- **H. Prognosis and follow-up.** Overall, the rate of recurrent or persistent disease is 5 to 17% despite therapy with any of the excisional or ablative techniques.
    1. **Negative margins.** There is a high rate of cure in patients who have their entire lesion excised.
    2. **Follow-up.** Cervical cytology or a combination of cytology and colposcopy with endocervical curettage every six months is suggested for follow-up after treatment of biopsy confirmed CIN 2/3. Repeat colposcopy is indicated if ASC or greater is detected. After three results negative for SIL or malignancy have been obtained,

annual follow-up is acceptable and should be continued until at least three additional consecutive negative results have been documented.

3. **Positive margins.** In contrast, patients with positive margins after LEEP or cold knife conization are at increased risk for residual disease as determined at subsequent hysterectomy or repeat conization.

4. **Follow-up.** Women who have positive margins on the specimens excised by cold knife conization or LEEP or in the concomitant endocervical curettage specimen should receive follow-up with cytology and colposcopy/biopsy/endocervical curettage (instead of immediate retreatment) if the patient is likely to be compliant with frequent monitoring. Alternatively, a repeat excisional procedure can be offered to women with positive margins who are averse to the risk of progression. Hysterectomy is an option for women who have completed childbearing.

5. **Negative histopathology.** A completely negative LEEP/cone biopsy performed for high grade lesions is also of concern, and these patients should be followed similarly to those with positive margins, with cytology and endocervical curettage every six months for at least the first three visits.

References: See page 208.

Atypical Squamous Cells on Cervical Cytology

Atypical squamous cells are commonly caused by self-limited disease, which resolves spontaneously. The risk of invasive cancer in patients with atypical squamous cells is low, 0.1 to 0.2%. However, 5 to 17% of patients with atypical squamous cells and 24 to 94% of those with ASC-high grade will have precancerous lesions at biopsy, therefore, further evaluation is necessary to determine if high-grade dysplasia is present.

I. **Evaluation of atypical squamous cells of undetermined significance (ASC-US).**
   A. Reflex HPV testing with triage of women with high risk HPV types to colposcopy is the recommended approach. Reflex testing refers to concurrent collection of cytology and HPV samples with actual testing for HPV only if indicated by abnormal cytology results.
      1. If liquid-based cytology is used, reflex HPV testing can be performed on the same specimen. If a conventional Papanicolaou (Pap) smear is obtained, a second specimen is collected for HPV DNA testing. If high risk subtypes are found, colposcopy is performed.

Risk of cervical cancer with human papilloma virus
High-risk (oncogenic or cancer-associated) types Common types: 16, 18, 31, 33, 35, 39, 45, 51, 52, 56, 58, 59, 68, 69, 82
Low-risk (non-oncogenic) types Common types: 6, 11, 40, 42, 43, 44, 54, 61, 72, 81

Management of women with combined test screening	
Results of cytology/HPV	Recommended follow-up
Negative / Negative	Routine screening in 3 years
Negative / Positive	Repeat combined test in 6 to 12 months
ASCUS / Negative	Repeat cytology in 12 months
ASCUS / Positive	Colposcopy
Greater than ASCUS / Positive or negative	Colposcopy

- **B. Special circumstances and populations**
  1. **Pregnant women** with ASC are managed in the same way as nonpregnant women, except endocervical sampling is not performed.
  2. **Infection or reactive changes.** When an infectious organism is identified or suggested, the patient should be contacted to determine if she is symptomatic. Antibiotic therapy is indicated for symptomatic infections, as well as some asymptomatic infections. After treatment of the infection, women with high risk HPV types are referred to colposcopy.
  3. **Atrophic epithelium** (a normal finding in postmenopausal women) is often characterized by nuclear enlargement, which meets one of the pathologic criteria for ASC. Administration of estrogen (eg, 0.3 mg conjugated estrogen applied as vaginal cream nightly for four weeks [1/8th of the applicator]) causes atypical atrophic, but not dysplastic, epithelium to mature into normal squamous epithelium. Hormonal therapy given for vaginal atrophy should be followed by repeat cervical cytology one week after completing treatment. If negative, cytology should be repeated again in six months. If both tests are negative, the woman can return to routine screening intervals, but if either test is positive for ASC-US or greater colposcopy should be completed.
  4. **Immunosuppressed women**, including all women who are HIV positive, with ASC-US should be referred for immediate colposcopy instead of HPV testing or serial cytology.
  5. **Adolescents.** Initial colposcopy or reflex HPV testing may be deferred in adolescents because the risk of invasive cancer is near zero and the prevalence of transient HPV infection is very high . Instead, serial cytology should be completed at six and 12 months or HPV DNA testing at 12 months with referral to colposcopy for positive results (ASC or greater, high risk HPV DNA types).
- **C. Management after colposcopy/biopsy.** Colposcopy/biopsy of women with ASC-US will either yield a histologic abnormality (eg, CIN II or III), which should be treated as appropriate, or show no abnormal findings. If no abnormal findings are found and HPV testing was not performed or showed a low-risk type, then follow-up cytological testing in 12 months is recommended.
- **D.** Women who test positive for high risk HPV types, but have CIN I or less on colposcopy/biopsy require a repeat cervical cytology at 6 and 12 months, or perform an HPV test at 12 months, with colposcopy for ASC or higher or a positive HPV test.
- **II. Evaluation of atypical squamous cells—cannot exclude high-grade squamous intraepithelial lesion (ASC-H)**
  - **A.** Most women with ASC-H on cytological examination should be referred for colposcopy and ECC (ECC is not performed in pregnancy),

without HPV testing. Twenty-four to 94% of these women will have CIN II or higher. Biopsy proven CIN II or III is treated, as appropriate.
- **B.** If no lesion or a CIN I lesion is identified, the cytology sample, colposcopy, and any biopsy specimens should be reviewed, if possible, to address any possible cytological-histological discordancy, with further management dependent upon the results. If review of cytology confirms ASC-H, follow-up cytology in six and 12 months or HPV DNA testing in 12 months is acceptable. Colposcopy should be repeated for ASC-US or greater on cytology or a positive test for high risk HPV DNA.
- **C.** In women age 30 or older with ASC-H, an acceptable alternative is to perform HPV testing for initial triaging. If high risk HPV types are present, the patient is referred for colposcopy.

References: See page 208.

Atypical and Malignant Glandular Cells on Cervical Cytology

Cervical Pap smear cytology showing atypical glandular (AGC) or endometrial carcinoma cells indicates the presence of glandular cells that could originate from the endocervical or endometrial region. The Bethesda 2001 system classifies AGC into two subcategories:

AGC (specify endocervical, endometrial, or glandular cells not otherwise specified [NOS])

AGC, favor neoplastic (specify endocervical or NOS)

Additional categories for glandular cell abnormalities are:

Endocervical adenocarcinoma in situ (AIS)

Adenocarcinoma

I. Atypical glandular cells
- **A.** A smear with AGC is associated with a premalignant or malignant lesion of the endocervix or endometrium in 10 to 40% of cases.
- **B.** Women over age 50 with AGC are at higher risk of having uterine cancer than younger women (8 and 1%, respectively). Conversely, premenopausal women with AGC are more likely to have CIN II/III or AIS than postmenopausal women.
- **C.** **Evaluation.** Presence of AGC or AIS on cervical cytology is a significant marker for neoplasia of the endometrium, as well as the squamous and glandular epithelium of the cervix. All women with atypical glandular cells or AIS should be referred for colposcopy with directed cervical biopsies and sampling of the endocervical canal. An endometrial biopsy should be performed on all women over age 35 and on younger women with unexplained or anovulatory bleeding, morbid obesity, oligomenorrhea, or an increased risk of endometrial cancer.
- **D.** Women with only atypical endometrial cells on cytology can be initially evaluated with endometrial biopsy only, rather than colposcopy. If endometrial sampling is normal, then colposcopy and endocervical curettage should be performed.
- **E.** Positive findings, such as any grade of CIN on biopsy, should be managed as appropriate.
- **F.** **Negative colposcopy/endocervical curettage.** The management of women with AGC and a negative initial colposcopy/endocervical sampling depends upon AGC subclassification.
  - **1. AGC NOS.** Women with AGC NOS who have a normal initial colposcopic evaluation and endocervical biopsy can be followed with cervical cytology at four to six month intervals until four consecutive tests are negative for intraepithelial lesions or malignancy. They are then followed with routine surveillance. However, if any abnormality (ASC or greater) is noted on follow-up cytology smears, another colposcopy is required. Women with persistent AGC NOS

(two or more cytology results) are at especially high risk of significant glandular disease and need conization if repeat colposcopy
and endometrial biopsy are nondiagnostic.

2. In women with AGC NOS and normal colposcopic evaluation and
biopsies, HPV studies may be used for further monitoring and, if
negative, repeat cytology and endocervical sampling can be done
in one year rather than in four visits over two years.

3. AGC favor neoplasia or AIS. A cold-knife conization is the best
procedure for subsequent evaluation of AGC lesions at high risk of
associated adenocarcinoma, such as AGC favor neoplasia or AIS
or persistent AGC NOS.

4. If conization and endometrial biopsies are also negative, the patient
should be evaluated for primary or metastatic disease involving the
fallopian tube, ovary, and other pelvic and abdominal organs with
pelvic ultrasound examination, colonoscopy, and computed tomography of the abdomen.

II. Endocervical adenocarcinoma

A. Endocervical adenocarcinoma in situ (AIS) and adenocarcinoma
requires evaluation and will show invasive cancer in a proportion of
women with AIS on cytology. An intermediate category: atypical
endocervical cells, favor neoplastic suggests some features of AIS but
without criteria for a definitive diagnosis.

B. Colposcopy with directed biopsy is required. A diagnostic excisional
procedure is often needed because colposcopy/biopsy can miss small
lesions of AIS or adenocarcinoma and lesions high in the canal.

References: See page 208.

Colposcopy

The colposcope provides an illuminated, magnified view of the cervix,
vagina, and vulva. Malignant and premalignant epithelium has a characteristic contour, color, and vascular pattern. The goal of colposcopy is to identify
precancerous and cancerous lesions.

I. Indications for colposcopy

A. Abnormal cytological abnormalities:

1. Persistent atypical squamous cells of undetermined significance
(ASCUS) or ASCUS with positive high-risk HPV subtypes.
2. ASCUS suggestive of high-grade lesion (ASC-H).
3. Atypical glandular cells (AGC).
4. Low grade squamous intraepithelial lesion (LSIL).
5. High-grade squamous intraepithelial lesion (HSIL).

B. Evaluation of an abnormal appearing cervix, vagina, or vulva.

II. Contraindications. Active cervicitis should be treated before the exami-
nation. Biopsies are relatively contraindicated in patients on
anticoagulations, who have a known bleeding disorder, or who are pregnant.

III. Procedure. The medical history is obtained, including age, gravity, parity,
last menstrual period, use and type of contraception, prior cervical
cytology results, allergies, significant medical history including HIV status
and history of any immunosuppressive conditions or medications, other
medications, prior cervical procedures, and smoking history. If there is
any possibility of pregnancy, a pregnancy test is obtained.

A. **Repeat cervical cytology.** If the patient has not had cervical cytology
in the last six weeks, a repeat assessment of cervical cytology is
done.

B. **Visualization.** The cervix and vagina are examined with a bright light,
and then with the colposcope. Cotton soaked in saline is used to
cleanse the cervix. Pigmented areas and obvious lesions are noted.
The cervix is examined for areas of erosion, true leukoplakia, pigmented lesions, or areas of obvious ulceration or exophytic growth.

Three to 5% acetic acid is applied to the cervix using cotton swabs and the cervix is reexamined. A green-filter examination is performed to accentuate abnormal vasculature. Iodine solution (Lugol's or Schiller's) is used to improve visualization of abnormal areas.

C. The clinician first identifies the squamocolumnar junction or transformation zone (TZ) . The clinician should differentiate between the grey-pink appearing ectocervix and the pink-red appearing endocervix. The region where the two cell types meet, termed the squamocolumnar junction, defines the "transformation" zone. The ability to see the transformation zone dictates whether the colposcopic exam is adequate (ie, the entire squamocolumnar junction is visible circumferentially around the os) or unsatisfactory.

D. **The upper one-third of the vagina**, in particular the lateral fornices, is also inspected.

E. **Biopsies** are obtained from the most abnormal appearing areas. Biopsies should be taken from inferior to superior to avoid bleeding over the target sites.

F. **Endocervical curettage** is performed in patients with HSIL, AGUS, adenocarcinoma in situ (AIS) on the endocervical margin following cone biopsy, LSIL but no visible lesion, and those with an unsatisfactory colposcopic examination. A long straight curette is used to scrape the four quadrants of the endocervical canal and an endocervical brush is employed to remove any exfoliated tissue. Endocervical curettage in not performed in pregnant women.

References: See page 208.

Contraception

Approximately 31% of births are unintended; about 22% were "mistimed," while 9% were "unwanted."

I. **Oral contraceptives**
   A. Combined (estrogen-progestin) oral contraceptives are reliable, and they have noncontraceptive benefits, which include reduction in dysmenorrhea, iron deficiency, ovarian cancer, endometrial cancer.

Combination Oral Contraceptives		
Drug	**Progestin, mg**	**Estrogen**
Monophasic combinations		
Ortho-Novum 1 /35 21, 28	Norethindrone (1)	Ethinyl estradiol (35)
Ovcon 35 21, 28	Norethindrone (0.4)	Ethinyl estradiol (35)
Brevicon 21, 28	Norethindrone (0.5)	Ethinyl estradiol (35)
Modicon 28	Norethindrone (0.5)	Ethinyl estradiol (35)
Necon 0.5/35E 21, 28	Norethindrone (0.5)	Ethinyl estradiol (35)
Nortrel 0.5/35 28	Norethindrone (0.5)	Ethinyl estradiol (35)
Necon 1 /35 21, 28	Norethindrone (1)	Ethinyl estradiol (35)
Norinyl 1 /35 21, 28	Norethindrone (1)	Ethinyl estradiol (35)
Nortrel 1 /35 21, 28	Norethindrone (1)	Ethinyl estradiol (35)

Drug	Progestin, mg	Estrogen
Loestrin 1 /20 21, 28	Norethindrone acetate (1)	Ethinyl estradiol (20)
Microgestin 1 /20 28	Norethindrone acetate (1)	Ethinyl estradiol (20)
Loestrin 1.5/30 21, 28	Norethindrone acetate (1.5)	Ethinyl estradiol (30)
Microgestin 1.5/30 28	Norethindrone acetate (1.5)	Ethinyl estradiol (30)
Alesse 21, 28	Levonorgestrel (0.1)	Ethinyl estradiol (20)
Aviane 21, 28	Levonorgestrel (0.1)	Ethinyl estradiol (20)
Lessina 28	Levonorgestrel (0.1)	Ethinyl estradiol (20)
Levlite 28	Levonorgestrel (0.1)	Ethinyl estradiol (20)
Necon 1/50 21, 28	Norethindrone (1)	Mestranol (50)
Norinyl 1150 21, 28	Norethindrone (1)	Mestranol (50)
Ortho-Novum 1/50 28	Norethindrone (1)	Mestranol (50)
Ovcon 50 28	Norethindrone (1)	Ethinyl estradiol (50)
Cyclessa 28	Desogestrel (0.1)	Ethinyl estradiol (25)
Apri 28	Desogestrel (0.15)	Ethinyl estradiol (30)
Desogen 28	Desogestrel (0.15)	Ethinyl estradiol (30)
Ortho-Cept 21, 28	Desogestrel (0.15)	Ethinyl estradiol (30)
Yasmin 28	Drospirenone (3)	Ethinyl estradiol (30)
Demulen 1 /35 21, 28	Ethynodiol diacetate (1)	Ethinyl estradiol (35)
Zovia 1 /35 21, 28	Ethynodiol diacetate (1)	Ethinyl estradiol (35)
Demulen 1/50 21, 28	Ethynodiol diacetate (1)	Ethinyl estradiol (50)
Zovia 1 /50 21, 28	Ethynodiol diacetate (1)	Ethinyl estradiol (50)
Levlen 21, 28	Levonorgestrel (0.15)	Ethinyl estradiol (30)
Levora 21, 28	Levonorgestrel (0.15)	Ethinyl estradiol (30)
Nordette 21, 28	Levonorgestrel (0.15)	Ethinyl estradiol (30)
Ortho-Cyclen 21, 28	Norgestimate (0.25)	Ethinyl estradiol (35)
Lo/Ovral 21, 28	Norgestrel (0.3)	Ethinyl estradiol (30)
Low-Ogestrel 21, 28	Norgestrel (0.3)	Ethinyl estradiol (30)

Drug	Progestin, mg	Estrogen
Ogestrel 28	Norgestrel (0.5)	Ethinyl estradiol (50)
Ovral 21, 28	Norgestrel (0.5)	Ethinyl estradiol (50)
Seasonale	Levonorgestrel (0.15)	Ethinyl estradiol (0.03)
Multiphasic Combinations		
Kariva 28	Desogestrel (0.15)	Ethinyl estradiol (20, 0, 10)
Mircette 28	Desogestrel (0.15)	Ethinyl estradiol (20, 0, 10)
Tri-Levlen 21, 28	Levonorgestrel (0.05, 0.075, 0.125)	Ethinyl estradiol (30, 40, 30)
Triphasil 21, 28	Levonorgestrel (0.05, 0.075, 0.125)	Ethinyl estradiol (30, 40, 30)
Trivora 28	Levonorgestrel (0.05, 0.075, 0.125)	Ethinyl estradiol (30, 40, 30)
Necon 10/11 21, 28	Norethindrone (0.5, 1)	Ethinyl estradiol (35)
Ortho-Novum 10/11 28	Norethindrone (0.5, 1)	Ethinyl estradiol (35)
Ortho-Novum 7/7/7 21, 28	Norethindrone (0.5, 0.75, 1)	Ethinyl estradiol (35)
Tri-Norinyl 21, 28	Norethindrone (0.5, 1, 0.5)	Ethinyl estradiol (35)
Estrostep 28	Norethindrone acetate (1)	Ethinyl estradiol (20, 30, 35)
Ortho Tri-Cyclen 21, 28	Norgestimate (0.18, 0.215, 0.25)	Ethinyl estradiol (35)

B. Pharmacology
   1. Ethinyl estradiol is the estrogen in virtually all OCs.
   2. Commonly used progestins include norethindrone, norethindrone acetate, and levonorgestrel. Ethynodiol diacetate is a progestin, which also has significant estrogenic activity. New progestins have been developed with less androgenic activity; however, these agents may be associated with deep vein thrombosis.

C. Mechanisms of action
   1. The most important mechanism of action is estrogen-induced inhibition of the midcycle surge of gonadotropin secretion, so that ovulation does not occur.
   2. Another potential mechanism of contraceptive action is suppression of gonadotropin secretion during the follicular phase of the cycle, thereby preventing follicular maturation.
   3. Progestin-related mechanisms also may contribute to the contraceptive effect. These include rendering the endometrium is less suitable for implantation and making the cervical mucus less permeable to penetration by sperm.

D. Contraindications

1. **Absolute contraindications to OCs:**
   a. Previous thromboembolic event or stroke
   b. History of an estrogen-dependent tumor
   c. Active liver disease
   d. Pregnancy
   e. Undiagnosed abnormal uterine bleeding
   f. Hypertriglyceridemia
   g. Women over age 35 years who smoke heavily (>15 cigarettes per day)

2. **Screening requirements.** Hormonal contraception can be safely provided after a careful medical history and blood pressure measurement. Pap smears are not required before a prescription for OCs.

E. Efficacy
When taken properly, OCs are a very effective form of contraception. The actual failure rate is 2 to 3% due primarily to missed pills or failure to resume therapy after the seven-day pill-free interval.

Noncontraceptive Benefits of Oral Contraceptive Pills	
Dysmenorrhea	Functional ovarian cysts
Mittelschmerz	Benign breast cysts
Metrorrhagia	Ectopic pregnancy
Premenstrual syndrome	Acne
Hirsutism	Endometriosis
Ovarian and endometrial cancer	

F. Drug interactions
The metabolism of OCs is accelerated by phenobarbital, phenytoin and rifampin. The contraceptive efficacy of an OC is likely to be decreased in women taking these drugs. Other antibiotics (with the exception of rifampin) do not affect the pharmacokinetics of ethinyl estradiol.

G. Preparations

1. There are two types of oral contraceptive pills: combination pills that contain both estrogen and progestin, and the progestin-only pill ("mini-pill"). Progestin-only pills, which are associated with more breakthrough bleeding than combination pills, are rarely prescribed except in lactating women. Combination pills are packaged in 21-day or 28-day cycles. The last seven pills of a 28-day pack are placebo pills.

2. Monophasic combination pills contain the same dose of estrogen and progestin in each of the 21 hormonally active pills. Current pills contain on average 30 to 35 μg. Pills containing less than 50 μg of ethinyl estradiol are "low-dose" pills.

3. **20 μg preparations.** Several preparations containing only 20 μg of ethinyl estradiol are now available (Lo-Estrin 1/20, Mircette, Alesse, Aviane). These are often used for perimenopausal women who want contraception with the lowest estrogen dose possible. These preparations provide enough estrogen to relieve vasomotor flashes. Perimenopausal women often experience hot flashes and premenstrual mood disturbances during the seven-day pill-free interval. Mircette, contains 10 μg of ethinyl estradiol on five of the seven "placebo" days, which reduces flashes and mood symptoms.

4. **Seasonale** is a 91-day oral contraceptive. Tablets containing the active hormones are taken for 12 weeks (84 days), followed by 1 week (7 days) of placebo tablets. Seasonale contains levonorgestrel (0.15 mg) and ethinyl estradiol (0.03 mg). Many women, especially in the first few cycles, have more spotting between menstrual periods. Seasonale is as effective and safe as traditional birth control pills.

smin contains 30 mcg of ethinyl estradiol and drospirenone. ospirenone has anti-mineralocorticoid activity. It can help prevent bating, weight gain, and hypertension, but it can increase serum otassium. Yasmin is contraindicated in patients at risk for yperkalemia due to renal, hepatic, or adrenal disease. Yasmin should not be combined with other drugs that can increase potassium, such as ACE inhibitors, angiotensin receptor blockers, potassium-sparing diuretics, potassium supplements, NSAIDs, or salt substitutes.

6. Third-generation progestins

    a. More selective progestins include norgestimate, desogestrel, and gestodene. They have some structural modifications that lower their androgen activity. Norgestimate (eg, Ortho-Cyclen or Tri-Cyclen) and desogestrel (eg, Desogen or Ortho-Cept) are the least androgenic compounds in this class. The new progestins are not much less androgenic than norethindrone.

    b. The newer OCs are more effective in reducing acne and hirsutism in hyperandrogenic women. They are therefore an option for women who have difficulty tolerating older OCs. There is an increased risk of deep venous thrombosis with the use of these agents, and they should not be routinely used.

H. Recommendations

    1. Monophasic OCs containing the second generation progestin, norethindrone (Ovcon 35) are recommended when starting a patient on OCs for the first time. This progestin has very low androgenicity when compared to other second generation progestins, and also compares favorably to the third generation progestins in androgenicity.

    2. The pill should be started on the first day of the period to provide the maximum contraceptive effect in the first cycle. However, most women start their pill on the first Sunday after the period starts. Some form of back-up contraception is needed for the first month if one chooses the Sunday start, because the full contraceptive effect might not be provided in the first pill pack.

Factors to Consider in Starting or Switching Oral Contraceptive Pills

Objective	Action	Products that achieve the objective
To minimize high risk of thrombosis	Select a product with a lower dosage of estrogen.	Alesse, Aviane, Loestrin 1/20, Levlite, Mircette
To minimize nausea, breast tenderness or vascular headaches	Select a product with a lower dosage of estrogen.	Alesse, Aviane, Levlite, Loestrin 1/20, Mircette
To minimize spotting or breakthrough bleeding	Select a product with a higher dosage of estrogen or a progestin with greater potency.	Lo/Ovral, Nordette, Ortho-Cept, Ortho-Cyclen, Ortho Tri-Cyclen
To minimize androgenic effects	Select a product containing a low-dose norethindrone or ethynodiol diacetate.	Ovcon 35, Brevicon, Demulen 1/35, Modicon
To avoid dyslipidemia	Select a product containing a low-dose norethindrone or ethynodiol diacetate.	Ovcon 35, Brevicon, Demulen 1/35, Modicon

Instructions on the Use of Oral Contraceptive Pills

Initiation of use (choose one):
The patient begins taking the pills on the first day of menstrual bleeding.
The patient begins taking the pills on the first Sunday after menstrual bleeding begins.
The patient begins taking the pills immediately if she is definitely not pregnant and
has not had unprotected sex since her last menstrual period.

Missed pill
If it has been less than 24 hours since the last pill was taken, the patient takes a pill
right away and then returns to normal pill-taking routine.
If it has been 24 hours since the last pill was taken, the patient takes both the missed
pill and the next scheduled pill at the same time.
If it has been more than 24 hours since the last pill was taken (ie, two or more missed
pills), the patient takes the last pill that was missed, throws out the other missed pills
and takes the next pill on time. Additional contraception is used for the remainder of
the cycle.

Additional contraceptive method
Use an additional contraceptive method for the first 7 days after initially starting oral
contraceptive pills.
Use an additional contraceptive method for 7 days if more than 12 hours late in taking
an oral contraceptive pill.
Use an additional contraceptive method while taking an interacting drug and for 7
days thereafter.

II. Hormonal contraceptive methods other than oral contraceptives

- **A. Contraceptive vaginal ring (NuvaRing)** delivers 15 μg ethinyl
  estradiol and 120 μg of etonogestrel daily.
  1. **Advantages of the ring** include rapid return to ovulation after
     discontinuation, lower doses of hormones, ease and convenience,
     and improved cycle control. Benefits, risks, and contraindications to
     use are similar to those with combined oral contraceptive pills,
     except for the convenience of monthly administration.
  2. In women who have not used hormonal contraception in the past
     month, the ring is inserted on or before day 5 of the menstrual
     cycle, even if bleeding is not complete, and an additional form of
     contraception should be used for the following 7 days. New rings
     should be inserted at approximately the same time of day the ring
     was removed the previous week.
  3. If the ring accidentally falls out, it may be rinsed with cool or warm
     water and replaced within 3 hours. If it is out of place for more than
     3 hours contraceptive effectiveness decreases, so an additional
     form of contraception should be used until the ring has been in-
     serted for 7 continuous days. If the ring remains in place more than
     3 but <4 weeks, it is removed and a new one is inserted after a 1-
     week ring-free interval; if the ring is left in place for >4 weeks,
     backup contraception is recommended until a new ring has been in
     place for 7 days.
- **B. Transdermal contraceptive patch**
  1. **Ortho Evra** is a transdermal contraceptive patch, which is as
     effective as oral contraceptives. Ortho Evra delivers 20 μg of ethinyl
     estradiol and 150 μg of norelgestromin daily for 6 to 13 months.
     Compliance is better with the patch. The patch is applied at the
     beginning of the menstrual cycle. A new patch is applied each week
     for 3 weeks; week 4 is patch-free. It is sold in packages of 3
     patches. Effectiveness is similar to oral contraceptives.
  2. Breakthrough bleeding during the first two cycles, dysmenorrhea,
     and breast discomfort are more common in women using the patch.
     A reaction at the site of application of the patch occurs in 1.9% of
     the women. Contraceptive efficacy may be slightly lower in women
     weighing more than 90 kg.

C. **Depot medroxyprogesterone acetate** (DMPA, Depo-Provera) is an injectable contraceptive. Deep intramuscular injection of 150 mg results in effective contraception for three to four months. Effectiveness is 99.7%.

D. Women who receive the first injection after the seventh day of the menstrual cycle should use a second method of contraception for seven days. The first injection should be administered within five days after the onset of menses, in which case alternative contraception is not necessary.

E. Ovulation is suppressed for at least 14 weeks after injection of a 150 mg dose of DMPA. Therefore, injections should repeated every three months. A pregnancy test must be administered to women who are more than two weeks late for an injection.

F. Return of fertility can be delayed for up to 18 months after cessation of DMPA. DMPA is not ideal for women who may wish to become pregnant soon after cessation of contraception.

G. Amenorrhea, irregular bleeding, and weight gain (typically 1 to 3 kg) are the most common adverse effects of DMPA. Adverse effects also include acne, headache, and depression. Fifty% of women report amenorrhea by one year. Persistent bleeding may be treated with 50 µg of ethinyl estradiol for 14 days.

H. **Medroxyprogesterone acetate/estradiol cypionate (MPA/E2C, Lunelle)** is a combined (25 mg MPA and 5 mg E2C), injectable contraceptive.

1. Although monthly IM injections are required, MPA/E2C has several desirable features:
   a. It has nearly 100% effectiveness in preventing pregnancy.
   b. Fertility returns within three to four months after it is discontinued.
   c. Irregular bleeding is less common than in women given MPA alone.

2. Weight gain, hypertension, headache, mastalgia, or other nonmenstrual complaints are common.

3. Lunelle should be considered for women who forget to take their birth control pills or those who want a discreet method of contraception. The initial injection should be given during the first 5 days of the menstrual cycle or within 7 days of stopping oral contraceptives. Lunelle injections should be given every 28 to 30 days; 33 days at the most.

III. **Barrier methods**

A. Barrier methods of contraception, such as the condom, diaphragm, cervical cap, and spermicides, have fewer side effects than hormonal contraception.

B. The diaphragm and cervical cap require fitting by a clinician and are only effective when used with a spermicide. They must be left in the vagina for six to eight hours after intercourse; the diaphragm needs to be removed after this period of time, while the cervical cap can be left in place for up to 24 hours. These considerations have caused them to be less desirable methods of contraception. A major advantage of barrier contraceptives is their efficacy in protecting against sexually transmitted diseases and HIV infection.

IV. **Intrauterine devices**

A. The currently available intrauterine devices (IUDs) are safe and effective methods of contraception:

1. **Copper T380 IUD** induces a foreign body reaction in the endometrium. It is effective for 8 to 10 years.

2. **Progesterone-releasing IUDs** inhibit sperm survival and implantation. They also decrease menstrual blood loss and relieve dysmenorrhea. **Paragard** is replaced every 10 years. **Progestasert** IUDs must be replaced after one year.

3. **Levonorgestrel IUD (Mirena)** provides effective contraception for five years.

B. **Infection**
  1. Women who are at low risk for sexually transmitted diseases do not have a higher incidence of pelvic inflammatory disease with use of an IUD. An IUD should not be inserted in women at high risk for sexually transmitted infections, and women should be screened for the presence of sexually transmitted diseases before insertion.
  2. **Contraindications to IUDs:**
     a. Women at high risk for bacterial endocarditis (eg, rheumatic heart disease, prosthetic valves, or a history of endocarditis).
     b. Women at high risk for infections, including those with AIDS and a history of intravenous drug use.
     c. Women with uterine leiomyomas which alter the size or shape of the uterine cavity.

V. **Lactation**
  A. Women who breast-feed have a delay in resumption of ovulation postpartum. It is probably safest to resume contraceptive use in the third postpartum month for those who breast-feed full time, and in the third postpartum week for those who do not breast-feed.
  B. A nonhormonal contraceptive or progesterone-containing hormonal contraceptive can be started at any time; an estrogen-containing oral contraceptive pill should not be started before the third week postpartum because women are still at increased risk of thromboembolism prior to this time. Oral contraceptive pills can decrease breast milk, while progesterone-containing contraceptives may increase breast milk.

VI. **Progestin-only agents**
  A. Progestin-only agents are slightly less effective than combination oral contraceptives. They have failure rates of 0.5% compared with the 0.1% rate with combination oral contraceptives.
  B. Progestin-only oral contraceptives (Micronor, Nor-QD, Ovrette) provide a useful alternative in women who cannot take estrogen. Progestin-only contraception is recommended for nursing mothers. Milk production is unaffected by use of progestin-only agents.
  C. If the usual time of ingestion is delayed for more than three hours, an alternative form of birth control should be used for the following 48 hours. Because progestin-only agents are taken continuously, without hormone-free periods, menses may be irregular, infrequent or absent.

VII. **Postcoital contraception**
  A. Emergency postcoital contraception consists of administration of drugs within 72 hours to women who have had unprotected intercourse (including sexual assault), or to those who have had a failure of another method of contraception (eg, broken condom).
  B. **Preparations**
    1. Menstrual bleeding typically occurs within three days after administration of most forms of hormonal postcoital contraception. A pregnancy test should be performed if bleeding has not occurred within four weeks.
    2. **Preven Emergency Contraceptive Kit** includes four combination tablets, each containing 50 μg of ethinyl estradiol and 0.25 mg of levonorgestrel, and a pregnancy test to rule out pregnancy before taking the tablets. Instructions are to take two of the tablets as soon as possible within 72 hours of coitus, and the other two tablets twelve hours later.
    3. An oral contraceptive such as Ovral (two tablets twelve hours apart) or Lo/Ovral (4 tablets twelve hours apart) can also be used.
    4. Nausea and vomiting are the major side effects. Meclizine 50 mg, taken one hour before the first dose, reduces nausea and vomiting but can cause some sedation.
    5. **Plan B** is a pill pack that contains two 0.75 mg tablets of levonorgestrel to be taken twelve hours apart. The cost is compa-

rable to the Preven kit ($20). This regimen may be more effective and better tolerated than an estrogen-progestin regimen.
6. **Copper T380 IUD.** A copper intrauterine device (IUD) placed within 120 hours of unprotected intercourse can also be used as a form of emergency contraception. An advantage of this method is that it provides continuing contraception after the initial event.

Emergency Contraception

1. Consider pretreatment one hour before each oral contraceptive pill dose, using one of the following orally administered antiemetic agents:
    Prochlorperazine (Compazine), 5 to 10 mg
    Promethazine (Phenergan), 12.5 to 25 mg
    Trimethobenzamide (Tigan), 250 mg
    Meclizine (Antivert) 50 mg
2. Administer the first dose of oral contraceptive pill within 72 hours of unprotected coitus, and administer the second dose 12 hours after the first dose. Brand name options for emergency contraception include the following:
    Preven Kit – two pills per dose (0.5 mg of levonorgestrel and 100 μg of ethinyl estradiol per dose)
    Plan B – one pill per dose (0.75 mg of levonorgestrel per dose)
    Ovral – two pills per dose (0.5 mg of levonorgestrel and 100 μg of ethinyl estradiol per dose)
    Nordette – four pills per dose (0.6 mg of levonorgestrel and 120 μg of ethinyl estradiol per dose)
    Triphasil – four pills per dose (0.5 mg of levonorgestrel and 120 μg of ethinyl estradiol per dose)

VIII. **Sterilization**
   A. Sterilization is the most common and effective form of contraception. While tubal ligation and vasectomy may be reversible, these procedures should be considered permanent.
   B. **Essure microinsert sterilization device** is a permanent, hysteroscopic, tubal sterilization device which is 99.9% effective. The coil-like device is inserted in the office under local anesthesia into the fallopian tubes where it is incorporated by tissue. After placement, women use alternative contraception for three months, after which hysterosalpingography is performed to assure correct placement. Postoperative discomfort is minimal.
   C. **Tubal ligation** is usually performed as a laparoscopic procedure in outpatients or in postpartum women in the hospital. The techniques used are unipolar or bipolar coagulation, silicone rubber band or spring clip application, and partial salpingectomy.
   D. **Vasectomy** (ligation of the vas deferens) can be performed in the office under local anesthesia. A semen analysis should be done three to six months after the procedure to confirm azoospermia.
References: See page 208.

Pregnancy Termination

Ninety% of abortions are performed in the first trimester of pregnancy. About 1.5 million legal abortions are performed each year in the United States. Before 16 weeks of gestation, legal abortion may be performed in an office setting. Major anomalies and mid-trimester premature rupture of membranes are recognized fetal indications for termination.

I. **Menstrual extraction**
   A. Many women seek abortion services within 1-2 weeks of the missed period. Abortion of these early pregnancies with a small-bore vacuum cannula is called menstrual extraction or minisuction. The only instru-

ments required are a speculum, a tenaculum, a Karman cannula, and a modified 50 mL syringe.

B. The extracted tissue is rinsed and examined in a clear dish of water or saline over a light source to detect chorionic villi and the gestational sac. This examination is performed to rule out ectopic pregnancy and to decrease the risk of incomplete abortion.

II. First-trimester vacuum curettage

A. Beyond 7 menstrual weeks of gestation, larger cannulas and vacuum sources are required to evacuate a pregnancy. Vacuum curettage is the most common method of abortion. Procedures performed before 13 menstrual weeks are called suction or vacuum curettage, whereas similar procedures carried out after 13 weeks are termed dilation and evacuation.

B. Technique

1. Uterine size and position should be assessed during a pelvic examination before the procedure. Ultrasonography is advised if there is a discrepancy of more than 2 weeks between the uterine size and menstrual dating.

2. Tests for gonorrhea and chlamydia should be obtained, and the cervix and vagina should be prepared with a germicide. Paracervical block is established with 20 mL of 1% lidocaine injected deep into the cervix at the 3, 5, 7, and 9 o'clock positions. The cervix should be grasped with a single-toothed tenaculum placed vertically with one branch inside the canal. Uterine depth is measured with a sound. Dilation then should be performed with a tapered dilator.

3. A vacuum cannula with a diameter in millimeters that is one less than the estimated gestational age should be used to evacuate the cavity. After the tissue is removed, there should be a quick check with a sharp curette, followed by a brief reintroduction of the vacuum cannula. The aspirated tissue should be examined as described previously.

4. Antibiotics are used prophylactically . Doxycycline is the best agent because of a broad spectrum of antimicrobial effect. D-negative patients should receive D (Rho[D]) immune globulin.

C. Complications

1. The most common postabortal complications are pain, bleeding, and low-grade fever. Most cases are caused by retained gestational tissue or a clot in the uterine cavity. These symptoms are best managed by a repeat uterine evacuation, performed under local anesthesia

2. **Cervical shock.** Vasovagal syncope produced by stimulation of the cervical canal can be seen after paracervical block. Brief tonic-clonic activity rarely may be observed and is often confused with seizure. The routine use of atropine with paracervical anesthesia or the use of conscious sedation prevents cervical shock.

3. **Perforation**

   a. The risk of perforation is less than 1 in every 1,000 first-trimester abortions. It increases with gestational age and is greater for parous women than for nulliparous women. Perforation is best evaluated by laparoscopy to determine the extent of the injury.

   b. Perforations at the junction of the cervix and lower uterine segment can lacerate the ascending branch of the uterine artery within the broad ligament, giving rise to severe pain, a broad ligament hematoma, and intraabdominal bleeding. Management requires laparotomy, ligation of the severed vessels, and repair of the uterine injury.

4. **Hemorrhage**

   a. Excessive bleeding may indicate uterine atony, a low-lying implantation, a pregnancy of more advanced gestational age than the first trimester, or perforation. Management requires rapid reassessment of gestational age by examination of the fetal parts already extracted and gentle exploration of the uterine cavity with a curette and forceps. Intravenous oxytocin should be administered, and the abortion should be completed. The uterus then should be massaged to ensure contraction.

   b. When these measures fail, the patient should be hospitalized and should receive intravenous fluids and have her blood cross-matched. Persistent postabortal bleeding strongly suggests retained tissue or clot (hematometra) or trauma, and laparoscopy and repeat vacuum curettage is indicated.

5. Hematometra. Lower abdominal pain of increasing intensity in the first 30 minutes suggests hematometra. If there is no fever or bleeding is brisk, and on examination the uterus is large, globular, and tense, hematometra is likely. The treatment is immediate reevacuation.

6. Ectopic pregnancy incomplete abortion, and failed abortion

   a. Early detection of ectopic pregnancy, incomplete abortion, or failed abortion is possible with examination of the specimen immediately after the abortion. The patient may have an ectopic pregnancy if no chorionic villi are found. To detect an incomplete abortion that might result in continued pregnancy, the actual gestational sac must be identified.

   b. Determination of the b-hCG level and frozen section of the aspirated tissue and vaginal ultrasonography may be useful. If the b-hCG level is >1,500-2,000 mIU, chorionic villi are not identified on frozen section, or retained tissue is identified by ultrasonography, immediate laparoscopy should be considered. Other patients may be followed closely with serial b-hCG assays until the problem is resolved. With later (>13 weeks) gestations, all of the fetal parts must be identified by the surgeon to prevent incomplete abortion.

   c. Heavy bleeding or fever after abortion suggests retained tissue. If the postabortal uterus is larger than 12-week size, preoperative ultrasonography should be performed to determine the amount of remaining tissue. When fever is present, high-dose intravenous antibiotic therapy with two or three agents should be initiated, and curettage should be performed shortly thereafter.

III. Mifepristone (RU-486) for medical abortion in the first trimester

   A. The FDA has approved mifepristone for termination of early pregnancy as follows: Eligible women are those whose last menstrual period began within the last 49 days. The patient takes 600 mg of mifepristone (three 200 mg tablets) by mouth on day 1, then 400 µg misoprostol orally two days later.

   B. A follow-up visit is scheduled on day 14 to confirm that the pregnancy has been terminated with measurement of b-hCG or ultrasonography.

IV. Second-trimester abortion. Most abortions are performed before 13 menstrual weeks. Later abortions are generally performed because of fetal defects, maternal illness, or maternal age.

A. Dilation and evacuation

   1. Transcervical dilation and evacuation of the uterus (D&E) is the method most commonly used for mid-trimester abortions before 21 menstrual weeks. In the one-stage technique, forcible dilation is performed slowly and carefully to sufficient diameter to allow insertion of large, strong ovum forceps for evacuation. The better approach is a two-stage procedure in which multiple Laminaria are used to achieve gradual dilatation over several hours before extraction. Uterine evacuation is accomplished with long, heavy forceps, using the vacuum cannula to rupture the fetal membranes, drain amniotic fluid, and ensure complete evacuation.

   2. Preoperative ultrasonography is necessary for all cases 14 weeks and beyond. Intraoperative real-time ultrasonography helps to locate fetal parts within the uterus.

3. Dilation and evacuation becomes progressively more difficult as gestational age advances, and instillation techniques are often used after 21 weeks. Dilation and evacuation can be offered in the late mid-trimester, but two sets of Laminaria tents for a total of 36-48 hours is recommended. After multistage Laminaria treatment, urea is injected into the amniotic sac. Extraction is then accomplished after labor begins and after fetal maceration has occurred.

References: See page 208.

Ectopic Pregnancy

Ectopic pregnancy occurs when the conceptus implants outside the endometrial cavity. Ectopic pregnancy typically occurs six to eight weeks after the last normal menstrual period. Normal pregnancy discomforts (eg, breast tenderness, frequent urination, nausea) are often present.

I. **Clinical evaluation**
   A. **History.** The classic symptoms of ectopic pregnancy are: Abdominal pain, amenorrhea, and vaginal bleeding
   B. Ectopic pregnancy should be suspected in any women of reproductive age with these symptoms. These symptoms are not diagnostic of ectopic pregnancy; threatened abortion presents with the same symptoms and is far more common.
   C. Blood leaking out of the fallopian tube may irritate the diaphragm and cause shoulder pain, whereas blood pooling in the cul-de-sac may cause an urge to defecate. Lightheadedness or shock suggests tubal rupture and severe intraabdominal hemorrhage.
   D. **Physical examination.** Vital signs may reveal orthostatic changes and low grade fever. Adnexal tenderness, cervical motion tenderness, abdominal tenderness, an adnexal mass, and mild uterine enlargement may also be present.

Risk Factors for Ectopic Pregnancy

Greatest Risk
Previous ectopic pregnancy
Previous tubal surgery or sterilization
Diethylstilbestrol exposure in utero
Documented tubal pathology (scarring)
Use of intrauterine contraceptive device

Greater Risk
Previous genital infections (eg, PID)
Infertility (In vitro fertilization)
Multiple sexual partners

Lesser Risk
Previous pelvic or abdominal surgery
Cigarette smoking
Vaginal douching
Age of 1st intercourse <18 years

Presenting Signs and Symptoms of Ectopic Pregnancy	
Symptom	**Percentage**
Abdominal pain	80-100%
Amenorrhea	75-95%
Vaginal bleeding	50-80%
Dizziness, fainting	20-35%
Urge to defecate	5-15%
Pregnancy symptoms	10-25%
Passage of tissue	5-10%
Adnexal tenderness	75-90%
Abdominal tenderness	80-95%
Adnexal mass	50%
Uterine enlargement	20-30%
Orthostatic changes	10-15%
Fever	5-10%

II. Diagnosis

A. **Differential diagnosis of abdominal pain in women:** Urinary tract infection, kidney stones, diverticulitis, appendicitis, ovarian neoplasms, endometriosis, endometritis, leiomyomas, pelvic inflammatory disease, and pregnancy-related conditions.

B. **Pregnancy testing** is important in premenopausal women who present with abdominal pain or vaginal bleeding.

C. Amenorrhea and abdominal pain, with or without vaginal bleeding, are common symptoms of threatened abortion, ruptured or torsed corpus luteum cyst, and degenerating uterine leiomyoma.

D. **Diagnostic tests.** Transvaginal ultrasound examination (TVS) is the most useful test for determining the location of a pregnancy. Transvaginal ultrasound is used to detect the presence (or absence) of a gestational sac within or outside of the uterus.

E. **Diagnosis of intrauterine pregnancy.** Ultrasound is most useful for identifying an intrauterine gestation. The earliest sonographic sign of an intrauterine pregnancy is the presence of a true gestational sac, which has double echogenic rings surrounding the sac. TVS will show the gestational sac at 4.5 to 5 weeks of gestation, the yolk sac appears at 5 to 6 weeks and remains until 10 weeks, and an embryo with cardiac activity is first detected at 5.5 to 6 weeks.

   1. Concomitant intrauterine and extrauterine gestation is very rare (ie, heterotopic pregnancy occurs in 1/30,000 spontaneous conceptions). Therefore, the identification of an intrauterine pregnancy effectively excludes the possibility of an ectopic pregnancy.

F. **Diagnosis of extrauterine pregnancy.** Visualization of an extrauterine gestational sac containing a yolk sac or embryo is diagnostic of ectopic pregnancy, but is detected in only a small proportion of cases.

   1. A complex adnexal mass in the presence of a positive pregnancy test and empty uterus is highly suggestive of an extrauterine gestation and is the most common sonographic abnormality.

   2. Other nonspecific findings consistent with ectopic pregnancy include a fluid filled adnexal mass surrounded by an echogenic ring (bagel sign) and free fluid in the peritoneal cavity/cul-de-sac.

G. **Human chorionic gonadotropin (hCG)** can be detected in serum and urine as early as eight days after the LH surge, if pregnancy has occurred. The hCG concentration in a normal intrauterine pregnancy rises in a curvilinear fashion until about 41 days of gestation, after which it rises more slowly to 10 weeks, and then declines until reaching a plateau in the second and third trimesters. There is a wide range in the normal hCG level.

H. **Discriminatory zone** is based upon the correlation between visibility of the gestational sac and the hCG concentration. It is defined as the serum hCG level above which a gestational sac should be visualized by ultrasound if an intrauterine pregnancy is present. In most institutions, this serum hCG level is 1500 or 2000 IU/L with transvaginal ultrasound.

1. The absence of an intrauterine gestational sac at hCG concentrations above the discriminatory zone strongly suggests an ectopic or nonviable intrauterine pregnancy, but is nondiagnostic with hCG values below the discriminatory zone. A negative ultrasound examination at hCG levels below the discriminatory zone is consistent with an early viable intrauterine pregnancy or an ectopic pregnancy or nonviable intrauterine pregnancy. Such cases are termed "pregnancy of unknown location" and 8 to 40% are ultimately diagnosed as ectopic pregnancies.

I. **Diagnostic evaluation.** The evaluation of a pregnant woman with suspected ectopic gestation begins with TVS and quantitative hCG level. TVS alone is diagnostic if a yolk sac, embryo, or embryonic cardiac activity is demonstrable.

1. **HCG above the discriminatory zone.** Visualization of an intrauterine pregnancy almost always excludes the presence of an ectopic pregnancy.

2. **If TVS does not reveal an intrauterine pregnancy and shows a complex adnexal mass,** an extrauterine pregnancy is almost certain. Embryonic cardiac activity or a gestational sac with a definite yolk sac or embryo at an extrauterine location is diagnostic of an ectopic gestation. Treatment of ectopic pregnancy should be initiated.

3. **If no complex adnexal mass can be visualized,** the diagnosis of ectopic pregnancy is less certain. Furthermore, a serum hCG >1500 IU/L without visualization of intrauterine or extrauterine pathology may represent a multiple gestation. The next step in this setting is to repeat the TVS examination and hCG concentration two days later. If an intrauterine pregnancy is still not observed on TVS, then the pregnancy is abnormal.

   a. An ectopic pregnancy can be diagnosed if the serum hCG concentration is increasing or plateaued. Treatment can be instituted.

   b. **Falling hCG concentration** is most consistent with a failed pregnancy, such as arrested pregnancy, blighted ovum, tubal abortion or spontaneously resolving ectopic pregnancy. Weekly hCG concentrations should be monitored until the result is negative for pregnancy.

   c. **HCG below the discriminatory zone.** TVS is not sensitive for determining the location of the pregnancy when the hCG level is below the discriminatory zone. A serum hCG concentration less than 1500 IU/L should be followed by repetition of hCG in three days to follow the rate of rise. HCG concentrations usually double every 1.4 to two days until six to seven weeks of gestation in viable intrauterine pregnancies (and in some ectopic gestations).

4. A normally rising hCG concentration should be evaluated with TVS when the hCG reaches the discriminatory zone. At that time, an intrauterine pregnancy or an ectopic pregnancy can be diagnosed.

5. If the hCG concentration does not double over 72 hours, then the pregnancy is abnormal (an ectopic gestation or intrauterine pregnancy that is destined to abort). A normal intrauterine pregnancy is not present.
6. If an adnexal mass is visualized on TVS, then medical or surgical treatment is administered for a presumed ectopic pregnancy. If an adnexal mass is not visualized, methotrexate may be given or a curettage may be done to determine the type of nonviable pregnancy.
7. A falling hCG concentration is most consistent with a failed pregnancy (eg, arrested pregnancy, blighted ovum, tubal abortion, spontaneously resolving ectopic pregnancy). Weekly hCG concentrations should be monitored until the result is negative for pregnancy.

III. **Management of ectopic pregnancy**
   A. Specific indications for surgery: (1) ruptured ectopic pregnancy, especially in a hemodynamically unstable woman, (2) contraindications to medical therapy, (3) lack of timely access to a medical institution for management of tubal rupture, and (4) failed medical therapy.
   B. Medical and surgical therapy are equally successful in women who are hemodynamically stable and have an hCG concentration less than 5000 mIU/mL, a small tubal diameter, and no fetal cardiac activity. There is a reduction in the efficacy of medical therapy in the setting of a high serum hCG concentration, large tubal size, and fetal cardiac activity.
   C. **Relative contraindications to methotrexate**
      1. High hCG concentration. Women with a high baseline hCG >5000 mIU/mL are more likely to require multiple courses of medical therapy or experience treatment failure; conservative laparoscopic surgery is recommended for these patients.
      2. Large ectopic size >3.5 cm.
      3. Fetal cardiac activity is a relative contraindication to medical treatment.
   D. **Contraindications.** Women who are hemodynamically unstable, not likely to be compliant with post-therapeutic monitoring (or unwilling to accept a blood transfusion), and who do not have timely access to a medical institution should be treated surgically.
      1. Specific contraindications to methotrexate include breastfeeding women, immunodeficiency, active pulmonary disease, peptic ulcer disease, hypersensitivity to the drug, and significant hepatic, renal, or hematologic disease.

Criteria for Receiving Methotrexate

Absolute indications
Hemodynamically stable without active bleeding or signs of hemoperitoneum
Nonlaparoscopic diagnosis
Patient desires future fertility
General anesthesia poses a significant risk
Patient is able to return for follow-up care
Patient has no contraindications to methotrexate

Relative indications
Unruptured mass <3.5 cm at its greatest dimension
No fetal cardiac motion detected
Patients whose bet-hCG level does not exceed 5,000 mIU/mL

Contraindications to Methotrexate Therapy

Absolute contraindications
Breast feeding
Overt or laboratory evidence of immunodeficiency
Alcoholism, alcoholic liver disease, or other chronic liver disease
Preexisting blood dyscrasias, such as bone marrow hypoplasia, leukopenia, thrombocytopenia, or significant anemia
Known sensitivity to methotrexate
Active pulmonary disease
Peptic ulcer disease
Hepatic, renal, or hematologic dysfunction
Relative contraindications
Gestational sac >3.5 cm
Embryonic cardiac motion

- E. **Methotrexate administration**
    1. The overall rate of resolution of ectopic pregnancy is about 90%.
    2. Single dose protocol. The most practical approach to therapy is administration of a single intramuscular dose of methotrexate (50 mg per square meter of body surface area).
    3. Rh(D) immune globulin should be administered if the woman is Rh(D)-negative and the blood group of her male partner is Rh(D)-positive or unknown.
    4. Measurement of serum beta-hCG concentration and ultrasound examination are performed weekly. A second dose of methotrexate is given if the serum beta-hCG concentration on Day 7 has not declined by at least 25% from the Day 0 level. A second dose of MTX is required in 15 to 20% of women.
    5. The beta-hCG concentration usually declines to less than 15 mIU/mL by 35 days post-injection, but may take as long as 109 days. Weekly assays should be obtained until a level less than 10 to 15 mIU/mL is reached.
- F. Side effects, monitoring, and complications. Adverse reactions to methotrexate are usually mild and self-limiting. The most common are stomatitis and conjunctivitis. Rare side effects include gastritis, enteritis, dermatitis, pneumonitis, alopecia, elevated liver enzymes, and bone marrow suppression.
- G. It is common to observe an increase in beta-hCG levels in the three days following therapy because of continued hCG production by syncytiotrophoblast.
- IV. **Operative management** can be accomplished by either laparoscopy or laparotomy. Linear salpingostomy or segmental resection is the procedure of choice if the fallopian tube is to be retained. Salpingectomy is the procedure of choice if the tube requires removal.

References: See page 208.

Acute Pelvic Pain

- I. **Clinical evaluation**
    - A. Assessment of acute pelvic pain should determine the patient's age, obstetrical history, menstrual history, characteristics of pain onset, duration, and palliative or aggravating factors.
    - B. **Associated symptoms** may include urinary or gastrointestinal symptoms, fever, abnormal bleeding, or vaginal discharge.
    - C. **Past medical history.** Contraceptive history, surgical history, gynecologic history, history of pelvic inflammatory disease, ectopic pregnancy, sexually transmitted diseases should be determined. Current sexual activity and practices should be assessed.

D. **Method of contraception**
1. Sexual abstinence in the months preceding the onset of pain lessons the likelihood of pregnancy-related etiologies.
2. The risk of acute PID is reduced by 50% in patients taking oral contraceptives or using a barrier method of contraception. Patients taking oral contraceptives are at decreased risk for an ectopic pregnancy or ovarian cysts.

E. **Risk factors for acute pelvic inflammatory disease.** Age between 15-25 years, sexual partner with symptoms of urethritis, prior history of PID.

II. **Physical examination**
A. Fever, abdominal or pelvic tenderness, and peritoneal signs should be sought.
B. Vaginal discharge, cervical erythema and discharge, cervical and uterine motion tenderness, or adnexal masses or tenderness should be noted.

III. **Laboratory tests**
A. **Pregnancy testing** will identify pregnancy-related causes of pelvic pain. Serum beta-HCG becomes positive 7 days after conception. A negative test virtually excludes ectopic pregnancy.
B. **Complete blood count.** Leukocytosis suggest an inflammatory process; however, a normal white blood count occurs in 56% of patients with PID and 37% of patients with appendicitis.
C. **Urinalysis.** The finding of pyuria suggests urinary tract infection. Pyuria can also occur with an inflamed appendix or from contamination of the urine by vaginal discharge.
D. **Testing for Neisseria gonorrhoeae and Chlamydia trachomatis** are necessary if PID is a possibility.
E. **Pelvic ultrasonography** is of value in excluding the diagnosis of an ectopic pregnancy by demonstrating an intrauterine gestation. Sonography may reveal acute PID, torsion of the adnexa, or acute appendicitis.
F. **Diagnostic laparoscopy** is indicated when acute pelvic pain has an unclear diagnosis despite comprehensive evaluation.

III. **Differential diagnosis of acute pelvic pain**
A. **Pregnancy-related causes.** Ectopic pregnancy, spontaneous, threatened or incomplete abortion, intrauterine pregnancy with corpus luteum bleeding.
B. **Gynecologic disorders.** PID, endometriosis, ovarian cyst hemorrhage or rupture, adnexal torsion, Mittelschmerz, uterine leiomyoma torsion, primary dysmenorrhea, tumor.
C. **Nonreproductive tract causes**
1. **Gastrointestinal.** Appendicitis, inflammatory bowel disease, mesenteric adenitis, irritable bowel syndrome, diverticulitis.
2. **Urinary tract.** Urinary tract infection, renal calculus.

IV. **Approach to acute pelvic pain with a positive pregnancy test**
A. In a female patient of reproductive age, presenting with acute pelvic pain, the first distinction is whether the pain is pregnancy-related or non-pregnancy-related on the basis of a serum pregnancy test.
B. In the patient with acute pelvic pain associated with pregnancy, the next step is localization of the tissue responsible for the hCG production. Transvaginal ultrasound should be performed to identify an intrauterine gestation. Ectopic pregnancy is characterized by a noncystic adnexal mass and fluid in the cul-de-sac.

V. **Approach to acute pelvic pain in non-pregnant patients with a negative HCG**
A. **Acute PID** is the leading diagnostic consideration in patients with acute pelvic pain unrelated to pregnancy. The pain is usually bilateral, but may be unilateral in 10%. Cervical motion tenderness, fever, and cervical discharge are common findings.
B. **Acute appendicitis** should be considered in all patients presenting with acute pelvic pain and a negative pregnancy test. Appendicitis is charac-

terized by leukocytosis and a history of a few hours of periumbilical pain followed by migration of the pain to the right lower quadrant. Neutrophilia occurs in 75%. A slight fever exceeding 37.3°C, nausea, vomiting, anorexia, and rebound tenderness may be present.

C. **Torsion of the adnexa** usually causes unilateral pain, but pain can be bilateral in 25%. Intense, progressive pain combined with a tense, tender adnexal mass is characteristic. There is often a history of repetitive, transitory pain. Pelvic sonography often confirms the diagnosis. Laparoscopic diagnosis and surgical intervention are indicated.

D. **Ruptured or hemorrhagic corpus luteal cyst** usually causes bilateral pain, but it can cause unilateral tenderness in 35%. Ultrasound aids in diagnosis.

E. **Endometriosis** usually causes chronic or recurrent pain, but it can occasionally cause acute pelvic pain. There usually is a history of dysmenorrhea and deep dyspareunia. Pelvic exam reveals fixed uterine retrodisplacement and tender uterosacral and cul-de-sac nodularity. Laparoscopy confirms the diagnosis.

References: See page 208.

Chronic Pelvic Pain

Chronic pelvic pain (CPP) is menstrual or nonmenstrual pain of at least six months' duration, located below the umbilicus and severe enough to cause functional disability or require treatment. Gynecologic conditions account for 90% of cases of CPP. Gastrointestinal diseases, such as irritable bowel syndrome, are the next most common category.

I. **Differential diagnosis**

A. **Endometriosis** is the most common etiology of CPP in populations with a low prevalence of sexually transmitted infections. Endometriosis is found in up to 70% of patients with CPP.

B. **Chronic pelvic inflammatory disease (PID)** is one of the most common gynecologic conditions causing CPP in practices with a high prevalence of sexually transmitted diseases.

C. **Mental-health issues.** Somalization disorder, drug seeking behavior and narcotic dependency, physical and sexual abuse, and depression are commonly diagnosed in women with CPP.

D. **Fibromyalgia.** Women with fibromyalgia sometimes present with CPP. Two criteria must be present for diagnosing fibromyalgia. The patient reports pain in all four quadrants of the body, and detection of at least 11 separate areas (eg, knees, shoulders, elbows, neck) that are tender to physical pressure.

E. **Irritable bowel syndrome (IBS)** is a gastrointestinal syndrome characterized by chronic abdominal pain and altered bowel habits in the absence of any organic cause.

F. **Interstitial cystitis** is characterized by urinary urgency, bladder discomfort, and a sense of inadequate emptying of the bladder. Dyspareunia is often present. Cystoscopy is diagnostic.

Some Causes of Chronic Pelvic Pain by System	
Gynecologic	**Systemic diseases**
Endometriosis Adenomyosis Leiomyomata Adhesions Ovarian cyst/mass Pelvic inflammatory disease Endosalpingiosis Cervical stenosis Pelvic relaxation	Fibromyalgia Depression Somatization Substance abuse
Urologic	**Gastrointestinal**
Interstitial cystitis Urethral disorders	Irritable bowel Diverticulitis Inflammatory bowel disease Constipation Hernia

II. History

A. **Characteristics** of the pain should be noted, including location, intensity quality, duration, temporal pattern, precipitating factors (eg, exertion, sexual activity, menses, pregnancy), relationship to urination and defecation, and radiation.

B. **Hormonal versus nonhormonal**

1. Pelvic pain associated with severe dysmenorrhea and/or pain at the time of ovulation is likely due to endometriosis or adenomyosis. Women with endometriosis report premenstrual spotting, dyspareunia, dyschezia, poor relief of symptoms with nonsteroidal anti-inflammatory drugs, progressively worsening symptoms, inability to attend work or school during menses, and the presence of pelvic pain unrelated to menses more often than women with primary dysmenorrhea.

2. Nonhormonally responsive diseases should be considered for pain that is not related to menses, including chronic pelvic inflammatory disease, adhesions/inflammation from previous pelvic surgery, irritable bowel syndrome, diverticulitis, fibromyalgia, and interstitial cystitis.

III. Physical examination

A. Surgical scars, hernias, and masses should be sought. Pelvic examination should include an evaluation for physical findings consistent with endometriosis, adenomyosis, or leiomyomata. Tender areas should be identified.

B. **Physical findings characteristic of endometriosis** are uterosacral ligament abnormalities (eg, nodularity or thickening, focal tenderness), lateral displacement of the cervix caused by endometriosis, and cervical stenosis.

C. **Adnexal enlargement** may be palpable if an endometrioma is present.

D. Nongynecologic physical findings that are observed more frequently among women with endometriosis are red hair color, scoliosis, and dysplastic nevi.

E. **Adenomyosis and leiomyomata.** Women with adenomyosis can have a slightly enlarged, globular, tender uterus. Uterine myomas are characterized by enlarged, mobile uterus with an irregular contour.

F. **Chronic pelvic inflammatory disease** is characterized by uterine tenderness or cervical motion tenderness. Adhesions resulting from a surgical procedure can cause pain, especially with movement of viscera. An adnexal mass suggests an ovarian neoplasm. Adnexa tenderness suggests an inflammatory process. In women with uterine prolapse, the cervix/uterus may be observed protruding from the vagina.

Physical Examination in Women with Chronic Pelvic Pain
Pelvic Examination
Tenderness present? Nodularity present? Pelvic mass?
Abdominal examination
Abdominal distension? Tenderness present?
Straight leg raising test
Does leg rasing induce pain in the right or left lower quadrant?

IV. **Laboratory and imaging tests for women with CPP include:**
   A. Complete blood count with differential and erythrocyte sedimentation rate
   B. Pregnancy test.
   C. Urinalysis.
   D. Pelvic ultrasound.
   E. Additional evaluations include testing for chlamydia and gonorrhea infection and CA-125 (if ascites present).
   F. Pelvic ultrasound is highly sensitive for detecting pelvic masses, including both ovarian cysts and uterine leiomyomas.
V. **Pharmacologic treatment**
   A. **High probability of endometriosis**
      1. Nonsteroldal anti-inflammatory medications should be prescribed at doses in the upper end of the dose range (eg, ibuprofen 800 mg orally every six hours). If the first NSAID tried is not effective, another should be given.
      2. Oral contraceptive pills (OCPs) prescribed as monthly cycles.
      3. OCPs prescribed as "long cycles," with three to four months of continuous dosing of the active pill followed by one week off the pill are effective in women who fail cyclic therapy.
      4. OCPs and NSAIDS can be prescribed individually or in combination.

Summary of Recommendations for Treatment of Chronic Pelvic Pain American College of Obstetricians and Gynecologists	
Intervention	**Indication**
Combined oral contraceptive pills	Primary dysmenorrhea
GnRH agonists	Endometriosis, irritable bowel syndrome (may be given empirically in women with symptoms consistent with endometriosis)
Nonsteroidal anti-inflammatory drugs	Dysmenorrhea, moderate pain

Intervention	Indication
Progestins (daily, high dose)	Endometriosis, pelvic congestion syndrome
Laparoscopic ablation/resection of endometriosis	Stage I-III endometriosis
Presacral neurectomy	Centrally located dysmenorrhea
Uterine nerve ablation	Centrally located dysmenorrhea
Adjunctive psychotherapy	CPP

- **B. Second-line agents consist of one of the following:**
  1. Continuous progestin treatment. Medroxyprogesterone acetate (50 mg orally daily), norethindrone acetate (eg, Aygestin 5 mg orally daily), norgestrel (eg, Ovrette 0.075 mg orally daily), or norethindrone (eg, Micronor, Nor-QD 0.35 mg orally daily) for a two-month trial.
  2. Danazol 200 to 400 mg/day in two divided doses initially, may be increased to 800 mg/day in two divided doses to achieve amenorrhea. Therapy may be continued up to nine months.
  3. Empiric use of a gonadotropin-releasing hormone (GnRH) agonist analogue (eg, leuprolide [3.75 mg intramuscularly every four weeks] or nafarelin [200 µg intranasally twice daily]) for 2 months. An add-back regimen should be considered.
  4. Surgical intervention, such as laparoscopy or cystoscopy, can be considered if medical interventions are not successful or as an initial procedure to exclude neoplasia or an endometrioma.
- **C. Low probability of endometriosis.** Women in whom a particular disease process is suspected, such as adenomyosis, uterine leiomyomata, irritable bowel syndrome, interstitial cystitis, diverticulitis, or fibromyalgia should undergo further diagnostic testing and disease-specific treatment.
  1. Women with suspected pelvic inflammatory disease infection can be treated with doxycycline 100 mg orally twice daily for 14 days.
  2. NSAIDs can be prescribed at doses in the upper end of the dose range (eg, ibuprofen 800 mg orally every six hours).
  3. Antidepressants, opioids, anticonvulsants, and psychotherapy are used for treatment of chronic pain.
- **VI. Surgical approach**
  - **A.** Many causes of CPP, such as endometriosis, chronic pelvic inflammatory disease, and of a pelvic mass, require a surgical procedure to determine a definitive diagnosis. In addition to providing a diagnosis of endometriosis, surgical excision of the endometriosis implants can be performed during the laparoscopy.
  - **B. Hysterectomy** is effective in relieving chronic pelvic pain in some women, who have completed child bearing.
  - **C. Presacral neurectomy** refers to interruption of the sympathetic innervation of the uterus. The procedure can be performed via laparoscopy or laparotomy. PSN is most effective for relieving midline pelvic pain.

References: See page 208.

Endometriosis

Endometriosis is characterized by the presence of endometrial tissue on the ovaries, fallopian tubes or other abnormal sites, causing pain or infertility. Women are usually 25 to 29 years old at the time of diagnosis. Approximately 24% of women who complain of pelvic pain are subsequently found to have endometriosis. The overall prevalence of endometriosis is estimated to be 5 to 10%.

I. Clinical evaluation

A. Endometriosis should be considered in any woman of reproductive age who has pelvic pain. The most common symptoms are dysmenorrhea, dyspareunia, and low back pain that worsens during menses. Rectal pain and painful defecation may also occur. Other causes of secondary dysmenorrhea and chronic pelvic pain (eg, upper genital tract infections, adenomyosis, adhesions) may produce similar symptoms.

Differential Diagnosis of Endometriosis

Generalized pelvic pain
Pelvic inflammatory disease
Endometritis
Pelvic adhesions
Neoplasms, benign or malignant
Ovarian torsion
Sexual or physical abuse
Nongynecologic causes

Dysmenorrhea
Primary
Secondary (adenomyosis, myomas, infection, cervical stenosis)

Dyspareunia
Musculoskeletal causes (pelvic relaxation, levator spasm)
Gastrointestinal tract (constipation, irritable bowel syndrome)
Urinary tract (urethral syndrome, interstitial cystitis)
Infection
Pelvic vascular congestion
Diminished lubrication or vaginal expansion because of insufficient arousal

Infertility
Male factor
Tubal disease (infection)
Anovulation
Cervical factors (mucus, sperm antibodies, stenosis)
Luteal phase deficiency

B. Infertility may be the presenting complaint for endometriosis. Infertile patients often have no painful symptoms.

C. **Physical examination.** The physician should palpate for a fixed, retroverted uterus, adnexal and uterine tenderness, pelvic masses or nodularity along the uterosacral ligaments. A rectovaginal examination should identify uterosacral, cul-de-sac or septal nodules. Most women with endometriosis have normal pelvic findings.

II. Treatment

A. Confirmatory laparoscopy is usually required before treatment is instituted. In women with few symptoms, an empiric trial of oral contraceptives or progestins may be warranted to assess pain relief.

B. **Medical treatment**

1. Initial therapy also should include a nonsteroidal anti-inflammatory drug.

   a. Naproxen (Naprosyn) 500 mg followed by 250 mg PO tid-qid prn [250, 375,500 mg].

   b. Naproxen sodium (Aleve) 200 mg PO tid prn.

   c. Naproxen sodium (Anaprox) 550 mg, followed by 275 mg PO tid-qid prn.

   d. Ibuprofen (Motrin) 800 mg, then 400 mg PO q4-6h prn.

   e. Mefenamic acid (Ponstel) 500 mg PO followed by 250 mg q6h prn.

2. **Progestational agents.** Progestins are similar to combination OCPs in their effects on FSH, LH and endometrial tissue. They may be associated with more bothersome adverse effects than OCPs. Progestins are effective in reducing the symptoms of endometriosis. Oral progestin regimens may include once-daily administration of medroxyprogesterone at the lowest effective dosage (5 to 20 mg). Depot medroxyprogesterone may be given intramuscularly every

two weeks for two months at 100 mg per dose and then once a month for four months at 200 mg per dose.

3. **Oral contraceptive pills (OCPs)** suppress LH and FSH and prevent ovulation. Combination OCPs alleviate symptoms in about three quarters of patients. Oral contraceptives can be taken continuously (with no placebos) or cyclically, with a week of placebo pills between cycles. The OCPs can be discontinued after six months or continued indefinitely.

4. **Danazol (Danocrine)** has been highly effective in relieving the symptoms of endometriosis, but adverse effects may preclude its use. Adverse effects include headache, flushing, sweating and atrophic vaginitis. Androgenic side effects include acne, edema, hirsutism, deepening of the voice and weight gain. The initial dosage should be 800 mg per day, given in two divided oral doses. The overall response rate is 84 to 92%.

Medical Treatment of Endometriosis

Drug	Dosage	Adverse effects
Danazol (Danocrine)	800 mg per day in 2 divided doses	Estrogen deficiency, androgenic side effects
Oral contraceptives	1 pill per day (continuous or cyclic)	Headache, nausea, hypertension
Medroxyprogesterone (Provera)	5 to 20 mg orally per day	Same as with other oral progestins
Medroxyprogesterone suspension (Depo-Provera)	100 mg IM every 2 weeks for 2 months; then 200 mg IM every month for 4 months or 150 mg IM every 3 months	Weight gain, depression, irregular menses or amenorrhea
Norethindrone (Aygestin)	5 mg per day orally for 2 weeks; then increase by 2.5 mg per day every 2 weeks up to 15 mg per day	Same as with other oral progestins
Leuprolide (Lupron)	3.75 mg IM every month for 6 months	Decrease in bone density, estrogen deficiency
Goserelin (Zoladex)	3.6 mg SC (in upper abdominal wall) every 28 days	Estrogen deficiency
Nafarelin (Synarel)	400 mg per day: 1 spray in 1 nostril in a.m.; 1 spray in other nostril in p.m.; start treatment on day 2 to 4 of menstrual cycle	Estrogen deficiency, bone density changes, nasal irritation

C. **GnRH agonists.** These agents (eg, leuprolide [Lupron], goserelin [Zoladex]) inhibit the secretion of gonadotropin. GnRH agonists are contraindicated in pregnancy and have hypoestrogenic side effects. They produce a mild degree of bone loss. Because of concerns about osteopenia, "add-back" therapy with low-dose estrogen has been recommended. The dosage of leuprolide is a single monthly 3.75-mg depot injection given intramuscularly. Goserelin, in a dosage of 3.6 mg, is administered subcutaneously every 28 days. A nasal spray (nafarelin [Synarel]) may be used twice daily. The response rate is similar to that with danazol; about 90% of patients experience pain relief.

D. Surgical treatment
   1. Surgical treatment is the preferred approach to infertile patients with advanced endometriosis. Laparoscopic ablation of endometriosis lesions may result in a 13% increase in the probability of pregnancy.
   2. Definitive surgery, which includes hysterectomy and oophorectomy, is reserved for women with intractable pain who no longer desire pregnancy.

References: See page 208.

Primary Amenorrhea

Amenorrhea (absence of menses) results from dysfunction of the hypothalamus, pituitary, ovaries, uterus, or vagina. It is often classified as either primary (absence of menarche by age 16) or secondary (absence of menses for more than three cycle intervals or six months in women who were previously menstruating).

I. Etiology
   A. Primary amenorrhea is usually the result of a genetic or anatomic abnormality. Common etiologies of primary amenorrhea:
   1. Chromosomal abnormalities causing gonadal dysgenesis: 45%
   2. Physiologic delay of puberty: 20%
   3. Müllerian agenesis: 15%
   4. Transverse vaginal septum or imperforate hymen: 5%
   5. Absent production of gonadotropin-releasing hormone (GnRH) by the hypothalamus: 5%
   6. Anorexia nervosa: 2%
   7. Hypopituitarism: 2%

Causes of Primary and Secondary Amenorrhea	
Abnormality	**Causes**
Pregnancy	
Anatomic abnormalities	
Congenital abnormality in Mullerian development	Isolated defect Testicular feminization syndrome 5-Alpha-reductase deficiency Vanishing testes syndrome Defect in testis determining factor
Congenital defect of urogenital sinus development	Agenesis of lower vagina Imperforate hymen
Acquired ablation or scarring of the endometrium	Asherman's syndrome Tuberculosis
Disorders of hypothalamic-pituitary ovarian axis Hypothalamic dysfunction Pituitary dysfunction Ovarian dysfunction	

Causes of Amenorrhea due to Abnormalities in the Hypothalamic-Pituitary-Ovarian Axis	
Abnormality	**Causes**

Hypothalamic dysfunction	Functional hypothalamic amenorrhea
	    Weight loss, eating disorders
	    Exercise
	    Stress
	    Severe or prolonged illness
	Congenital gonadotropin-releasing hormone deficiency
	Inflammatory or infiltrative diseases
	Brain tumors - eg, craniopharyngioma
	Pituitary stalk dissection or compression
	Cranial irradiation
	Brain injury - trauma, hemorrhage, hydrocephalus
	Other syndromes - Prader-Willi, Laurence-Moon-Biedl

Pituitary dysfunction	Hyperprolactinemia Other pituitary tumors- acromegaly, corticotroph adenomas (Cushing's disease) Other tumors - meningioma, germinoma, glioma Empty sella syndrome Pituitary infarct or apoplexy

Ovarian dysfunction	Ovarian failure (menopause)
	    Spontaneous
	    Premature (before age 40 years)
	    Surgical

Other	Hyperthyroidism Hypothyroidism Diabetes mellitus Exogenous androgen use

II. Diagnostic evaluation of primary amenorrhea

A. Step I: Evaluate clinical history:

1. Signs of puberty may include a growth spurt, absence of axillary and pubic hair, or apocrine sweat glands, or absence of breast development. Lack of pubertal development suggests ovarian or pituitary failure or a chromosomal abnormality.
2. Family history of delayed or absent puberty suggests a familial disorder.
3. Short stature may indicate Turner syndrome or hypothalamic-pituitary disease.
4. Poor health may be a manifestation of hypothalamic-pituitary disease. Symptoms of other hypothalamic-pituitary disease include headaches, visual field defects, fatigue, or polyuria and polydipsia.
5. Virilization suggests polycystic ovary syndrome, an androgen-secreting ovarian or adrenal tumor, or the presence of Y chromosome material.
6. Recent stress, change in weight, diet, or exercise habits; or illness may suggest hypothalamic amenorrhea.
7. Heroin and methadone can alter hypothalamic gonadotropin secretion.
8. Galactorrhea is suggestive of excess prolactin. Some drugs cause amenorrhea by increasing serum prolactin concentrations, including metoclopramide and antipsychotic drugs.

B. **Step II: Physical examination**
1. An evaluation of pubertal development should include current height, weight, and arm span (normal arm span for adults is within 5 cm of height) and an evaluation of the growth chart.
2. Breast development should be assessed by Tanner staging.
3. The genital examination should evaluate clitoral size, pubertal hair development, intactness of the hymen, depth of the vagina, and presence of a cervix, uterus, and ovaries. If the vagina can not be penetrated with a finger, rectal examination may allow evaluation of the internal organs. Pelvic ultrasound is also useful to determine the presence or absence of müllerian structures.
4. The skin should be examined for hirsutism, acne, striae, increased pigmentation, and vitiligo.
5. Classic physical features of Turner syndrome include low hair line, web neck, shield chest, and widely spaced nipples.

C. **Step III: Basic laboratory testing**
1. **If a normal vagina or uterus are not obviously present** on physical examination, pelvic ultrasonography should be performed to confirm the presence or absence of ovaries, uterus, and cervix. Ultrasonography can be useful to exclude vaginal or cervical outlet obstruction in patients with cyclic pain.

   a. **Uterus absent**
      (1) If the uterus is absent, evaluation should include a karyotype and serum testosterone. These tests should distinguish abnormal müllerian development (46, XX karyotype with normal female serum testosterone concentrations) from androgen insensitivity syndrome (46, XY karyotype and normal male serum testosterone concentrations).
      (2) Patients with 5-alpha reductase deficiency also have a 46, XY karyotype and normal male serum testosterone concentrations but, in contrast to the androgen insensitivity syndrome which is associated with a female phenotype, these patients undergo striking virilization at the time of puberty (secondary sexual hair, muscle mass, and deepening of the voice).

2. **Uterus present**. For patients with a normal vagina and uterus and no evidence of an imperforate hymen, vaginal septum, or congenital absence of the vagina. Measurement of serum beta human chorionic gonadotropin to exclude pregnancy and of serum FSH, prolactin, and TSH.

   a. A high serum FSH concentration is indicative of primary ovarian failure. A karyotype is then required and may demonstrate complete or partial deletion of the X chromosome (Turner syndrome) or the presence of Y chromatin. The presence of a Y chromosome is associated with a higher risk of gonadal tumors and makes gonadectomy mandatory.
   b. A low or normal serum FSH concentration suggests functional hypothalamic amenorrhea, congenital GnRH deficiency, or other disorders of the hypothalamic-pituitary axis. Cranial MR imaging is indicated in most cases of hypogonadotropic hypogonadism to evaluate hypothalamic or pituitary disease. Cranial MRI is recommended for all women with primary hypogonadotropic hypogonadism, visual field defects, or headaches.
   c. Serum prolactin and thyrotropin (TSH) should be measured, especially if galactorrhea is present.
   d. If there are signs or symptoms of hirsutism, serum testosterone and dehydroepiandrosterone sulfate (DHEA-S) should be measured to assess for an androgen-secreting tumor.
   e. If hypertension is present, blood tests should be drawn for evaluate for CYP17 deficiency. The characteristic findings are elevations in serum progesterone (>3 ng/mL) and deoxy-

corticosterone and low values for serum 17-alpha-hydroxy-progesterone (<0.2 ng/mL).

III. Treatment

A. Treatment of primary amenorrhea is directed at correcting the underlying pathology; helping the woman to achieve fertility, if desired; and prevention of complications of the disease.

B. **Congenital anatomic lesions or Y chromosome material** usually requires surgery. Surgical correction of a vaginal outlet obstruction is necessary before menarche, or as soon as the diagnosis is made after menarche. Creation of a neovagina for patients with müllerian failure is usually delayed until the women is emotionally mature. If Y chromosome material is found, gonadectomy should be performed to prevent gonadal neoplasia. However, gonadectomy should be delayed until after puberty in patients with androgen insensitivity syndrome. These patients have a normal pubertal growth spurt and feminize at the time of expected puberty.

C. **Ovarian failure** requires counseling about the benefits and risks of hormone replacement therapy.

D. **Polycystic ovary syndrome** is managed with measures to reduce hirsutism, resume menses, and fertility and prevent of endometrial hyperplasia, obesity, and metabolic defects.

E. **Functional hypothalamic amenorrhea** can usually be reversed by weight gain, reduction in the intensity of exercise, or resolution of illness or emotional stress. For women who want to continue to exercise, estrogen-progestin replacement therapy should be given to those not seeking fertility to prevent osteoporosis. Women who want to become pregnant can be treated with gonadotropins or pulsatile GnRH.

F. **Hypothalamic or pituitary dysfunction** that is not reversible (eg, congenital GnRH deficiency) is treated with either exogenous gonadotropins or pulsatile GnRH if the woman wants to become pregnant.

References: See page 208.

Secondary Amenorrhea

Amenorrhea (absence of menses) can be a transient, intermittent, or permanent condition resulting from dysfunction of the hypothalamus, pituitary, ovaries, uterus, or vagina. Amenorrhea is classified as either primary (absence of menarche by age 16 years) or secondary (absence of menses for more than three cycles or six months in women who previously had menses). Pregnancy is the most common cause of secondary amenorrhea.

I. Diagnosis of secondary amenorrhea

A. **Step 1: Rule out pregnancy**. A pregnancy test is the first step in evaluating secondary amenorrhea. Measurement of serum beta subunit of hCG is the most sensitive test.

B. **Step 2: Assess the history**
1. Recent stress; change in weight, diet or exercise habits; or illnesses that might result in hypothalamic amenorrhea should be sought.
2. Drugs associated with amenorrhea, systemic illnesses that can cause hypothalamic amenorrhea, recent initiation or discontinuation of an oral contraceptive, androgenic drugs (danazol) or high-dose progestin, and antipsychotic drugs should be evaluated.
3. Headaches, visual field defects, fatigue, or polyuria and polydipsia may suggest hypothalamic-pituitary disease.
4. Symptoms of estrogen deficiency include hot flashes, vaginal dryness, poor sleep, or decreased libido.
5. Galactorrhea is suggestive of hyperprolactinemia. Hirsutism, acne, and a history of irregular menses are suggestive of hyperandrogenism.

6. A history of obstetrical catastrophe, severe bleeding, dilatation and curettage, or endometritis or other infection that might have caused scarring of the endometrial lining suggests Asherman's syndrome.

C. **Step 3: Physical examination.** Measurements of height and weight, signs of other illnesses, and evidence of cachexia should be assessed. The skin, breasts, and genital tissues should be evaluated for estrogen deficiency. The breasts should be palpated, including an attempt to express galactorrhea. The skin should be examined for hirsutism, acne, striae, acanthosis nigricans, vitiligo, thickness or thinness, and easy bruisability.

D. **Step 4: Basic laboratory testing.** In addition to measurement of serum hCG to rule out pregnancy, minimal laboratory testing should include measurements of serum prolactin, thyrotropin, and FSH to rule out hyperprolactinemia, thyroid disease, and ovarian failure (high serum FSH). If there is hirsutism, acne or irregular menses, serum dehydroepiandrosterone sulfate (DHEA-S) and testosterone should be measured.

E. **Step 5: Follow-up laboratory evaluation**
   1. **High serum prolactin concentration.** Prolactin secretion can be transiently increased by stress or eating. Therefore, serum prolactin should be measured at least twice before cranial imaging is obtained, particularly in those women with small elevations (<50 ng/mL). These women should be screened for thyroid disease with a TSH and free T4 because hypothyroidism can cause hyperprolactinemia.
   2. Women with verified high serum prolactin values should have a cranial MRI unless a very clear explanation is found for the elevation (eg, antipsychotics). Imaging should rule out a hypothalamic or pituitary tumor.
   3. **High serum FSH concentration.** A high serum FSH concentration indicates the presence of ovarian failure. This test should be repeated monthly on three occasions to confirm. A karyotype should be considered in most women with secondary amenorrhea age 30 years or younger.

Causes of Primary and Secondary Amenorrhea	
Abnormality	**Causes**
Pregnancy	
Anatomic abnormalities	
Congenital abnormality in Müllerian development	Isolated defect Testicular feminization syndrome 5-Alpha-reductase deficiency Vanishing testes syndrome Defect in testis determining factor
Congenital defect of urogenital sinus development	Agenesis of lower vagina Imperforate hymen
Acquired ablation or scarring of the endometrium	Asherman's syndrome Tuberculosis

Disorders of hypothalamic-pituitary ovarian axis
   Hypothalamic dysfunction
   Pituitary dysfunction
   Ovarian dysfunction	

Causes of Amenorrhea due to Abnormalities in the Hypothalamic-Pituitary-Ovarian Axis	
Abnormality	**Causes**

Hypothalamic dysfunction	Functional hypothalamic amenorrhea
	    Weight loss, eating disorders
	    Exercise
	    Stress
	    Severe or prolonged illness
	Congenital gonadotropin-releasing hormone deficiency
	Inflammatory or infiltrative diseases
	Brain tumors - eg, craniopharyngioma
	Pituitary stalk dissection or compression
	Cranial irradiation
	Brain injury - trauma, hemorrhage, hydrocephalus
	Other syndromes - Prader-Willi, Laurence-Moon-Biedl

Pituitary dysfunction	Hyperprolactinemia Other pituitary tumors- acromegaly, corticotroph adenomas (Cushing's disease) Other tumors - meningioma, germinoma, glioma Empty sella syndrome Pituitary infarct or apoplexy

Ovarian dysfunction	Ovarian failure (menopause)
	    Spontaneous
	    Premature (before age 40 years)
	    Surgical

Other	Hyperthyroidism Hypothyroidism Diabetes mellitus Exogenous androgen use

Drugs Associated with Amenorrhea	
Drugs that Increase Prolactin	Antipsychotics Tricyclic antidepressants Calcium channel blockers
Drugs with Estrogenic Activity	Digoxin, marijuana, oral contraceptives
Drugs with Ovarian Toxicity	Chemotherapeutic agents

4. **High serum androgen concentrations**. A high serum androgen value may suggest the diagnosis of polycystic ovary syndrome or may suggest an androgen-secreting tumor of the ovary or adrenal gland. Further testing for a tumor might include a 24-hour urine collection for cortisol and 17-ketosteroids, determination of serum 17-hydroxyprogesterone after intravenous injection of corticotropin (ACTH), and a dexamethasone suppression test. Elevation of 17-ketosteroids, DHEA-S, or 17-hydroxyprogesterone is more consistent with an adrenal, rather than ovarian, source of excess androgen.

5. **Normal or low serum gonadotropin concentrations and all other tests normal**
   a. This result is one of the most common outcomes of laboratory testing in women with amenorrhea. Women with hypothalamic amenorrhea (caused by excessive exercise or weight loss) have normal to low serum FSH values. Cranial MRI is indicated in all women without an clear explanation for hypogonadotropic hypogonadism and in most women who have visual field defects or headaches. No further testing is required if the onset of amenorrhea is recent or is easily explained (eg, weight loss, excessive exercise) and there are no symptoms suggestive of other disease.
   b. High serum transferrin saturation may indicate hemochromatosis, high serum angiotensin-converting enzyme values suggest sarcoidosis, and high fasting blood glucose or hemoglobin A1c values indicate diabetes mellitus.

6. **Normal serum prolactin and FSH concentrations with history of uterine instrumentation preceding amenorrhea**
   a. Evaluation for Asherman's syndrome should be completed. A progestin challenge should be performed (medroxyprogesterone acetate 10 mg for 10 days). If withdrawal bleeding occurs, an outflow tract disorder has been ruled out. If bleeding does not occur, estrogen and progestin should be administered.
   b. Oral conjugated estrogens (0.625 to 2.5 mg daily for 35 days) with medroxyprogesterone added (10 mg daily for days 26 to 35); failure to bleed upon cessation of this therapy strongly suggests endometrial scarring. In this situation, a hysterosalpingogram or hysteroscopy can confirm the diagnosis of Asherman syndrome.

II. **Treatment**
   A. **Athletic women** should be counseled on the need for increased caloric intake or reduced exercise. Resumption of menses usually occurs.
   B. **Nonathletic women who are underweight** should receive nutritional counseling and treatment of eating disorders.
   C. **Hyperprolactinemia** is treated with a dopamine agonist. Cabergoline (Dostinex) or bromocriptine (Parlodel) are used for most adenomas. Ovulation, regular menstrual cycles, and pregnancy may usually result.
   D. **Ovarian failure** should be treated with hormone replacement therapy.
   E. **Hyperandrogenism** is treated with measures to reduce hirsutism, resume menses, and fertility and preventing endometrial hyperplasia, obesity, and metabolic defects.
   F. **Asherman's syndrome** is treated with hysteroscopic lysis of adhesions followed by long-term estrogen administration to stimulate regrowth of endometrial tissue.

References: See page 208.

Menopause

Menopause is defined as the cessation of menstrual periods, menopause occurs at a mean age of 51.4 years in normal women.

I. **Definitions**
   A. **Menopausal transition** begins with variation in menstrual cycle length and an elevated FSH concentration and ends with the final menstrual period (12 months of amenorrhea). Stage -2 (early) is characterized by variable cycle length (>7 days different from normal menstrual cycle length, which is 21 to 35 days). Stage -1 (late) is characterized by ≥ 2 skipped cycles and an interval of amenorrhea ≥ 60 days; women at this stage often have hot flashes as well.
   B. **Perimenopause** begins in stage -2 of the menopausal transition and ends 12 months after the last menstrual period.

    C. Menopause is defined by 12 months of amenorrhea after the final menstrual period. It results from complete, or near complete, ovarian follicular depletion and absence of ovarian estrogen secretion.

    D. Postmenopause. Stage +1 (early) is defined as the first five years after the final menstrual period. It is characterized by further and complete decline in ovarian function and accelerated bone loss; many women in this stage continue to have hot flashes. Stage +2 (late) begins five years after the final menstrual period and ends with death.

II. Epidemiology

    A. The average age at menopause is 51 years; however, for 5% of women it occurs after age 55 (late menopause), and for another 5%, between ages 40 to 45 years (early menopause). Menopause that occurs before age 40 years is premature ovarian failure.

    B. The age of menopause is reduced by about two years in women who smoke. Women who have never had children and who have had regular cycles tend to have an earlier age of menopause.

III. Clinical manifestations

    A. Bleeding patterns. Chronic anovulation and progesterone deficiency in this transition period may cause long periods of unopposed estrogen exposure and result in anovulatory bleeding and endometrial hyperplasia.

    B. Oligomenorrhea (irregular cycles) for six or more months, or an episode of heavy dysfunctional bleeding is an indication for endometrial surveillance. Endometrial biopsy is the standard to rule out the occurrence of endometrial hyperplasia.

    C. Irregular or heavy bleeding during the menopausal transition may be treated with low-dose oral contraceptives or intermittent progestin therapy.

    D. Hot flashes

        1. The most common symptom during menopause is the hot flash, occurring in up to 75%. Hot flashes are self-limited, usually resolving without treatment within one to five years, although some women will continue to have hot flashes until after age 70.

        2. Hot flashes begin as the sudden sensation of heat in the upper chest and face that rapidly becomes generalized. The sensation of heat lasts from two to four minutes, is often associated with perspiration and occasionally palpitations, and is often followed by chills and shivering, and sometimes anxiety. Hot flashes usually occur several times per day and are common at night.

    E. Genitourinary symptoms

        1. Vaginal dryness. The vagina and urethra are very sensitive to estrogen, and estrogen deficiency leads to thinning of the vaginal epithelium. This results in vaginal atrophy (atrophic vaginitis), causing symptoms of vaginal dryness, itching and often, dyspareunia.

        2. The vagina typically appears pale, with lack of the normal rugae and often has visible blood vessels or petechial hemorrhages.

        3. Sexual dysfunction. Estrogen deficiency causes a decrease in blood flow to the vagina and vulva, decreased vaginal lubrication, and sexual dysfunction.

        4. Atrophic urethritis results from low estrogen production after the menopause, predisposing to stress and urge urinary incontinence. The prevalence of incontinence increases with age.

IV. Diagnosis

    A. Menopause is defined as 12 months of amenorrhea in a woman over age 45 in the absence of other causes. Further evaluation is not necessary for women in this group.

    B. The best approach to diagnosing the menopausal transition is an assessment of menstrual cycle history and menopausal symptoms (vasomotor flushes, mood changes, sleep disturbances). Measuring serum FSH, estradiol, or inhibin levels is usually not necessary. Serum FSH concentrations increase across the menopausal transition, but at times may be suppressed into the normal premenopausal range (after a recent ovulation).

C. **Differential diagnosis.** Hyperthyroidism should be considered in the differential diagnosis because irregular menses, sweats (although different from typical hot flashes), and mood changes are all potential clinical manifestations of hyperthyroidism. Other etiologies for menstrual cycle changes that should be considered include pregnancy, hyperprolactinemia, and thyroid disease. Atypical hot flashes and night sweats may be caused by medications, carcinoid, pheochromocytoma, or underlying malignancy.

V. **Treatment of menopausal symptoms in women not taking systemic estrogen**

A. Many women cannot or choose not to take estrogen to treat symptoms of estrogen deficiency at menopause because of an increased risk of breast cancer and cardiovascular disease.

B. Therapy prevents bone loss and fracture, but does not confir a protective effect on the heart. Continuous combined therapy with conjugated estrogen (0.625 mg/day) and medroxyprogesterone acetate (2.5 mg/day) is ineffective for either primary or secondary prevention of CHD, and slightly increases risk. Other risks included an increased risk of stroke, venous thromboembolism, and breast cancer.

C. **Patient selection.** Estrogen is a reasonable short-term option for most symptomatic postmenopausal women, with the exception of those with a history of breast cancer, coronary heart disease, a previous venous thromboembolic event or stroke, or those at high risk for these complications. Short-term therapy is six months to five years.

D. **Vasomotor instability.** Hot flashes can result in sleep disturbances, headache, and irritability. Although estrogen is the gold standard for relief of hot flashes, a number of other drugs have been shown to be somewhat better than placebo. Venlafaxine (Effexor, 75 mg daily) reduces hot flashes by 61%. Mouth dryness, anorexia, nausea, and constipation are common. Gabapentin (Neurontin) has been used for hot flashes at a dose of 200mg orally once daily to 400mg orally four times daily.

E. **Urogenital atrophy**

1. Both systemic and vaginal estrogen are effective for genitourinary atrophy; however, vaginal estrogen has lesser systemic levels than estrogen tablets.

2. **Moisturizers and lubricants.** The long-acting vaginal moisturizer, Replens, produces a moist film over the vaginal tissue. A water soluble lubricant, such as Astroglide and K-Y Personal Lubricant, should be used at the time of intercourse.

3. **Low-dose vaginal estrogen**

   a. **Estrogen Cream (Premarin)** 0.5 g of cream, or one-eighth of an applicatorful daily into the vagina for three weeks followed by twice weekly administration thereafter. Estrace, which is crystalline estradiol, can also by given by vaginal applicator at a dose of one-eighth of an applicator or 0.5 g (which contains 50 microgram of estradiol).

   b. **Vaginal ring** is a silastic ring impregnated with estradiol (Estring, Phadia) involves insertion of a silastic ring that delivers 6 to 9 mcg of estradiol to the vagina daily for a period of three months.

   c. With low-dose vaginal estrogen, a progestin is not necessary.

F. **Osteoporosis.** Estrogen is no longer a primary therapy for osteoporosis. Exercise, and daily intake of calcium (1500 mg/day) and vitamin D (400 to 800 IU/day) are recommended for prevention of bone loss in perimenopausal and postmenopausal women.

VI. **Treatment of menopausal symptoms with hormone therapy**

A. Estrogen prevents bone loss and fracture, but is not cardioprotective, and slightly increases risk. Other risks seen with combined therapy included an increased risk of stroke, venous thromboembolism, and breast cancer.

B. Menopausal symptoms
1. **Hot flashes**. Estrogen therapy remains the gold standard for relief of menopausal symptoms, in particular, hot flashes, and therefore is a reasonable option for most postmenopausal women, with the exception of those with a history of breast cancer, CHD, a previous venous thromboembolic event or stroke, or those at high risk for these complications. In otherwise healthy women, the absolute risk of an adverse event is extremely low.
2. Short-term therapy (with a goal of symptom management) is less than five years.
3. **Adding a progestin.** Endometrial hyperplasia and cancer can occur after as little as six months of unopposed estrogen therapy; as a result, a progestin should be added in women who have not had a hysterectomy. Women who have undergone hysterectomy should not receive a progestin.
4. Hormone preparations: Combined, continuous conjugated estrogens (0.625 mg) and medroxyprogesterone acetate (MPA 2.5 mg) is commonly used. However, low dose estrogen is a better option (eg, 0.3 mg conjugated estrogens or 0.5 mg estradiol).
5. **A low-estrogen oral contraceptive** (20 mcg of ethinyl estradiol) remains an appropriate treatment for perimenopausal women who seek relief of menopausal symptoms, and who also desire contraception, and in some instances need bleeding control (in cases of dysfunctional uterine bleeding). Most of these women are between the ages of 40 and 50 years and are still candidates for oral contraception.
6. When women taking a low-dose oral contraceptive during menopause reach age 50 or 51 years, options include stopping the pill altogether, or changing to an estrogen replacement regimen if necessary for symptoms. Tapering the oral contraceptive by one pill per week is recommended.

References: See page 208.

Premenstrual Syndrome and Premenstrual Dysphoric Disorder

Premenstrual syndrome (PMS) is characterized by physical and behavioral symptoms that occur repetitively in the second half of the menstrual cycle and interfere with some aspects of the woman's life. Premenstrual dysphoric disorder (PMDD) is the most severe form of PMS, with the prominence anger, irritability, and internal tension. PMS affects up to 75% of women with regular menstrual cycles, while PMDD affects only 3 to 8% of women.

I. Symptoms
A. The most common physical manifestation of PMS is abdominal bloating, which occurs in 90% of women with this disorder; breast tenderness and headaches are also common, occurring in more than 50% of cases.
B. The most common behavioral symptom of PMS is an extreme sense of fatigue which is seen in more than 90%. Other frequent behavioral complaints include irritability, tension, depressed mood, labile mood (80%), increased appetite (70%), and forgetfulness and difficulty concentrating (50%).

Symptom Clusters Commonly Noted in Patients with PMS	
Affective Symptoms Depression or sadness Irritability Tension Anxiety Tearfulness or crying easily Restlessness or jitteriness Anger Loneliness Appetite change Food cravings Changes in sexual interest Pain Headache or migraine Back pain Breast pain Abdominal cramps General or muscular pain	**Cognitive or performance** Mood instability or mood swings Difficulty in concentrating Decreased efficiency Confusion Forgetfulness Accident-prone Social avoidance Temper outbursts Energetic **Fluid retention** Breast tenderness or swelling Weight gain Abdominal bloating or swelling Swelling of extremities **General somatic** Fatigue or tiredness Dizziness or vertigo Nausea Insomnia

C. Other common findings include acne, oversensitivity to environmental stimuli, anger, easy crying, and gastrointestinal upset. Hot flashes, heart palpitations, and dizziness occur in 15 to 20% of patients. Symptoms should occur in the luteal phase only.

UCSD Criteria for Premenstrual Syndrome

At least one of the following affective and somatic symptoms during the five days before menses in each of the three previous cycles:
Affective symptoms: depression, angry outbursts, irritability, anxiety, confusion, social withdrawal
Somatic symptoms: breast tenderness, abdominal bloating, headache, swelling of extremities Symptoms relieved from days 4 through 13 of the menstrual cycle

DSM-IV Criteria for Premenstrual Dysphoric Disorder

* Five or more symptoms
* At least one of the following four symptoms:
  Markedly depressed mood, feelings of hopelessness, or self deprecating thoughts
  Marked anxiety, tension, feeling of being "keyed up" or "on edge"
  Marked affective lability
  Persistent and marked anger or irritability or increase in interpersonal conflicts
* Additional symptoms that may be used to fulfill the criteria:
  Decreased interest in usual activities
  Subjective sense of difficulty in concentrating
  Lethargy, easy fatigability, or marked lack of energy
  Marked change in appetite, overeating, or specific food cravings
  Hypersomnia or insomnia
  Subjective sense of being overwhelmed or out of control
* Other physical symptoms such as breast tenderness or swelling, headaches, joint or muscle pain, a sensation of bloating, or weight gain
* Symptoms occurring during last week of luteal phase
* Symptoms are absent postmenstrually
* Disturbances that interfere with work or school or with usual social activities and relationships
* Disturbances that are not an exacerbation of symptoms of another disorder

Differential Diagnosis of Premenstrual Syndrome	
Affective disorder (eg, depression, anxiety, dysthymia, panic) Anemia Anorexia or bulimia Chronic medical conditions (eg, diabetes mellitus) Dysmenorrhea	Endometriosis Hypothyroidism Oral contraceptive pill use Perimenopause Personality disorder Substance abuse disorders

D. Differential diagnosis

1. PMDD should be differentiated from premenstrual exacerbation of an underlying major psychiatric disorder, as well as medical conditions such as hyper- or hypothyroidism.
2. About 13% of women with PMS are found to have a psychiatric disorder alone with no evidence of PMS, while 38% had premenstrual exacerbation of underlying depressive and anxiety disorders.
3. 39% of women with PMDD meet criteria for mood or anxiety disorders.
4. The assessment of patients with possible PMS or PMDD should begin with the history, physical examination, chemistry profile, complete blood count, and serum TSH. The history should focus in particular on the regularity of menstrual cycles. Appropriate gynecologic endocrine evaluation should be performed if the cycles are irregular (lengths less than 25 or >36 days).
5. The patient should be asked to record symptoms prospectively for two months. If the patient fails to demonstrate a symptom free interval in the follicular phase, she should be evaluated for a mood or anxiety disorder.

II. Nonpharmacologic therapy

A. Relaxation therapy and cognitive behavioral therapy have shown some benefit. Behavioral measures include keeping a symptom diary, getting adequate rest and exercise, and making dietary changes.

B. Sleep disturbances, ranging from insomnia to excessive sleep, are common. A structured sleep schedule with consistent sleep and wake times is recommended. Sodium restriction may minimize bloating, fluid retention, and breast swelling and tenderness. Caffeine restriction and aerobic exercise often reduce symptoms.

III. Dietary Supplementation

A. Vitamin E supplementation is a treatment for mastalgia. The administration of 400 IU per day of vitamin E during the luteal phase improves affective and somatic symptoms.

B. Calcium carbonate in a dosage of 1200 mg per day for three menstrual cycles results in symptom improvement in 48% of women with PMS.

IV. Pharmacologic Therapy

A. Fluoxetine (Sarafem) and sertraline (Zoloft) have been approved for the treatment of PMDD. SSRIs are recommended as initial drug therapy in women with PMS and PMDD. Common side effects of SSRIs include insomnia, drowsiness, fatigue, nausea, nervousness, headache, mild tremor, and sexual dysfunction.

B. Fluoxetine (Sarafem) 20 mg or sertraline (Zoloft) 50 mg, taken in the morning, is best tolerated and sufficient to improve symptoms. Fluoxetine or sertraline can be given during the 14 days before the menstrual period.

C. Benefit has also been demonstrated for citalopram (Celexa) during the 14 days before the menstrual period.

D. **Diuretics.** Spironolactone (Aldactone) is the only diuretic that has been shown to effectively relieve breast tenderness and fluid retention. Spironolactone is administered only during the luteal phase.

E. Prostaglandin Inhibitors. Nonsteroidal anti-inflammatory
(NSAIDs) are traditional therapy for primary dysmenorrhea a
menorrhagia. These agents include mefenamic acid (Ponstel) and
naproxen sodium (Anaprox, Aleve).

References: See page 208.

Prescription Medications Commonly Used in the Treatment of Premenstrual Syndrome (PMS)

Drug class and representative agents	Dosage	Recommendations	Side effects
SSRIs			
Fluoxetine (Sarafem)	10 to 20 mg per day	First-choice agents for the treatment of PMDD. Effective in alleviating behavioral and physical symptoms of PMS and PMDD. Administer during luteal phase (14 days before menses).	Insomnia, drowsiness, fatigue, nausea, nervousness, headache, mild tremor, sexual dysfunction
Sertraline (Zoloft)	50 to 150 mg per day		
Paroxetine (Paxil)	10 to 30 mg per day		
Fluvoxamine (Luvox)	25 to 50 mg per day		
Citalopram (Celexa)	20 to 40 mg per day		
Diuretics			
Spironolactone (Aldactone)	25 to 100 mg per day luteal phase	Effective in alleviating breast tenderness and bloating.	Antiestrogenic effects, hyperkalemia
NSAIDs			
Naproxen sodium (Anaprox)	275 to 550 mg twice daily	Effective in alleviating various physical symptoms of PMS. Any NSAID should be effective.	Nausea, gastric ulceration, renal dysfunction. Use with caution in women with pre-existing gastrointestinal or renal disease.
Mefenamic acid (Ponstel)	250 mg tid with meals		
Androgens			
Danazol (Danocrine)	100 to 400 mg twice daily	Somewhat effective in alleviating mastalgia when taken during luteal phase.	Weight gain, decreased breast size, deepening of voice. Monitor lipid profile and liver function.

	Dosage	Recommendations	Side effects
	3.75 mg IM every month or 11.25 mg IM every three months	Somewhat effective in alleviating physical and behavioral symptoms of PMS. Side effect profile and cost limit use.	Hot flashes, cardiovascular effects, and osteoporosis
Goserelin (Zoladex)	3.6 mg SC every month or 10.8 mg SC every three months		
Nafarelin (Synarel)	200 to 400 mcg intranasally twice daily		

Abnormal Vaginal Bleeding

Menorrhagia (excessive bleeding) is most commonly caused by anovulatory menstrual cycles. Occasionally it is caused by thyroid dysfunction, infections or cancer.

I. Pathophysiology of normal menstruation
   A. In response to gonadotropin-releasing hormone from the hypothalamus, the pituitary gland synthesizes follicle-stimulating hormone (FSH) and luteinizing hormone (LH), which induce the ovaries to produce estrogen and progesterone.
   B. During the follicular phase, estrogen stimulation causes an increase in endometrial thickness. After ovulation, progesterone causes endometrial maturation. Menstruation is caused by estrogen and progesterone withdrawal.
   C. **Abnormal bleeding** is defined as bleeding that occurs at intervals of less than 21 days, more than 36 days, lasting longer than 7 days, or blood loss >80 mL.

II. Clinical evaluation of abnormal vaginal bleeding
   A. A menstrual and reproductive history should include last menstrual period, regularity, duration, frequency; the number of pads used per day, and intermenstrual bleeding.
   B. Stress, exercise, weight changes and systemic diseases, particularly thyroid, renal or hepatic diseases or coagulopathies, should be sought. The method of birth control should be determined.
   C. Pregnancy complications, such as spontaneous abortion, ectopic pregnancy, placenta previa and abruptio placentae, can cause heavy bleeding. Pregnancy should always be considered as a possible cause of abnormal vaginal bleeding.

III. Puberty and adolescence – menarche to age 16
   A. Irregularity is normal during the first few months of menstruation; however, soaking more than 25 pads or 30 tampons during a menstrual period is abnormal.
   B. Absence of premenstrual symptoms (breast tenderness, bloating, cramping) is associated with anovulatory cycles.
   C. Fever, particularly in association with pelvic or abdominal pain may, indicate pelvic inflammatory disease. A history of easy bruising sug-

gests a coagulation defect. Headaches and visual changes suggest a pituitary tumor.

D. Physical findings
1. Pallor not associated with tachycardia or signs of hypovolemia suggests chronic excessive blood loss secondary to anovulatory bleeding, adenomyosis, uterine myomas, or blood dyscrasia.
2. Fever, leukocytosis, and pelvic tenderness suggests PID.
3. Signs of impending shock indicate that the blood loss is related to pregnancy (including ectopic), trauma, sepsis, or neoplasia.
4. Pelvic masses may represent pregnancy, uterine or ovarian neoplasia, or a pelvic abscess or hematoma.
5. Fine, thinning hair, and hypoactive reflexes suggest hypothyroidism.
6. Ecchymoses or multiple bruises may indicate trauma, coagulation defects, medication use, or dietary extremes.

E. Laboratory tests
1. CBC and platelet count and a urine or serum pregnancy test should be obtained.
2. Screening for sexually transmitted diseases, thyroid function, and coagulation disorders (partial thromboplastin time, INR, bleeding time) should be completed.
3. **Endometrial sampling** is rarely necessary for those under age 20.

F. Treatment of infrequent bleeding
1. Therapy should be directed at the underlying cause when possible. If the CBC and other initial laboratory tests are normal and the history and physical examination are normal, reassurance is usually all that is necessary.
2. Ferrous gluconate, 325 mg bid-tid, should be prescribed.

G. Treatment of frequent or heavy bleeding
1. Treatment with nonsteroidal anti-inflammatory drugs (NSAIDs) improves platelet aggregation and increases uterine vasoconstriction. NSAIDs are the first choice in the treatment of menorrhagia because they are well tolerated and do not have the hormonal effects of oral contraceptives.
   a. **Mefenamic acid (Ponstel)** 500 mg tid during the menstrual period.
   b. **Naproxen (Anaprox, Naprosyn)** 500 mg loading dose, then 250 mg tid during the menstrual period.
   c. **Ibuprofen (Motrin, Nuprin)** 400 mg tid during the menstrual period.
   d. Gastrointestinal distress is common. NSAIDs are contraindicated in renal failure and peptic ulcer disease.
2. Iron should also be added as ferrous gluconate 325 mg tid

H. Patients with hypovolemia or a hemoglobin level below 7 g/dL should be hospitalized for hormonal therapy and iron replacement.
1. Hormonal therapy consists of estrogen (Premarin) 25 mg IV q6h until bleeding stops. Thereafter, oral contraceptive pills should be administered q6h x 7 days, then taper slowly to one pill qd.
2. If bleeding continues, IV vasopressin (DDAVP) should be administered. Hysteroscopy may be necessary, and dilation and curettage is a last resort. Transfusion may be indicated in severe hemorrhage.
3. Iron should also be added as ferrous gluconate 325 mg tid.

IV. Primary childbearing years – ages 16 to early 40s
A. Contraceptive complications and pregnancy are the most common causes of abnormal bleeding in this age group. Anovulation accounts for 20% of cases.
B. Adenomyosis, endometriosis, and fibroids increase in frequency as a woman ages, as do endometrial hyperplasia and endometrial polyps. Pelvic inflammatory disease and endocrine dysfunction may also occur.
C. **Laboratory tests**
1. CBC and platelet count, Pap smear, and pregnancy test.

2. Screening for sexually transmitted diseases, thyroid-stimulating hormone, and coagulation disorders (partial thromboplastin time, INR, bleeding time).
3. If a non-pregnant woman has a pelvic mass, ultrasonography or hysterosonography (with uterine saline infusion) is required.

D. Endometrial sampling

1. Long-term unopposed estrogen stimulation in anovulatory patients can result in endometrial hyperplasia, which can progress to adeno-carcinoma; therefore, in perimenopausal patients who have been anovulatory for an extended interval, the endometrium should be biopsied.
2. Biopsy is also recommended before initiation of hormonal therapy for women over age 30 and for those over age 20 who have had prolonged bleeding.
3. Hysteroscopy and endometrial biopsy with a Pipelle aspirator should be done on the first day of menstruation (to avoid an unexpected pregnancy) or anytime if bleeding is continuous.

E. Treatment

1. Medical protocols for anovulatory bleeding (dysfunctional uterine bleeding) are similar to those described above for adolescents.
2. **Hormonal therapy**
   a. In women who do not desire immediate fertility, hormonal therapy may be used to treat menorrhagia.
   b. A 21-day package of oral contraceptives is used. The patient should take one pill three times a day for 7 days. During the 7 days of therapy, bleeding should subside, and, following treatment, heavy flow will occur. After 7 days off the hormones, another 21-day package is initiated, taking one pill each day for 21 days, then no pills for 7 days.
   c. Alternatively, medroxyprogesterone (Provera), 10-20 mg per day for days 16 through 25 of each month, will result in a reduction of menstrual blood loss. Pregnancy will not be prevented.
   d. Patients with severe bleeding may have hypotension and tachycardia. These patients require hospitalization, and estrogen (Premarin) should be administered IV as 25 mg q4-6h until bleeding slows (up to a maximum of four doses). Oral contraceptives should be initiated concurrently as described above.
3. Iron should also be added as ferrous gluconate 325 mg tid.
4. Surgical treatment can be considered if childbearing is completed and medical management fails to provide relief.

V. Premenopausal, perimenopausal, and postmenopausal years--age 40 and over

A. Anovulatory bleeding accounts for about 90% of abnormal vaginal bleeding in this age group. However, bleeding should be considered to be from cancer until proven otherwise.

B. History, physical examination and laboratory testing are indicated as described above. Menopausal symptoms, personal or family history of malignancy and use of estrogen should be sought. A pelvic mass requires an evaluation with ultrasonography.

C. Endometrial carcinoma

1. In a perimenopausal or postmenopausal woman, amenorrhea preceding abnormal bleeding suggests endometrial cancer. Endometrial evaluation is necessary before treatment of abnormal vaginal bleeding.
2. Before endometrial sampling, determination of endometrial thickness by transvaginal ultrasonography is useful because biopsy is often not required when the endometrium is less than 5 mm thick.

D. Treatment

1. Cystic hyperplasia or endometrial hyperplasia without cytologic atypia is treated with depo-medroxyprogesterone, 200 mg IM, then 100 to 200 mg IM every 3 to 4 weeks for 6 to 12 months.

Endometrial hyperplasia requires repeat endometrial biopsy every 3 to 6 months.
2. Atypical hyperplasia requires fractional dilation and curettage, followed by progestin therapy or hysterectomy.
3. If the patient's endometrium is normal (or atrophic) and contraception is a concern, a low-dose oral contraceptive may be used. If contraception is not needed, estrogen and progesterone therapy should be prescribed.
4. **Surgical management**
   a. **Vaginal or abdominal hysterectomy** is the most absolute curative treatment.
   b. **Dilatation and curettage** can be used as a temporizing measure to stop bleeding.
   c. **Endometrial ablation and resection** by laser, electrodiathermy "rollerball," or excisional resection are alternatives to hysterectomy.

References: See page 208.

Endometrial Hyperplasia

Endometrial hyperplasia is an endmetrial abnormality characterized by abnormal proliferation of endometrial glands, resulting in an increased gland-to-stroma ratio. The proliferating glands vary in size and shape and may show cytological atypia, which may progress to endometrial cancer. Endometrial hyperplasia is caused by chronic estrogen stimulation unopposed by the counterbalancing effects of progesterone.

I. **Classification**
   A. The World Health Organization classification of endometrial hyperplasia is based upon two factors:
      1. Simple or complex glandular/stromal architectural pattern
      2. The presence or absence of nuclear atypia
   B. **Simple versus complex.** Simple hyperplasia is characterized by glands that are cystically dilated with only occasional outpouching; mitoses of the glandular cells may be present.
   C. **Complex hyperplasia** consists of endometrial glands that are back-to-back with luminal outpouching and minimal intervening stroma. The gland-to-stroma ratio is higher in complex compared to simple hyperplasia.
   D. **Atypia.** Simple atypical hyperplasia is characterized by atypical cells lining glands that are separated by significant amounts of normal stroma. Complex atypical hyperplasia consists of back-to-back crowding of glands lined by atypical cells.
   E. Women with simple hyperplasia without atypia are least likely to develop endometrial carcinoma, whereas women with complex hyperplasia with atypia are most likely to develop carcinoma.
   F. Endometrial carcinoma is more than 10-fold more likely in atypical hyperplasia (simple or complex). Cancer occurs after a diagnosis of simple, complex, simple atypical, and complex atypical hyperplasia in 1, 3, 8, and 29% of cases, respectively.
II. **Risk factors** for endometrial hyperplasia are the same as those for endometrial cancer. The risk for both disorders is increased 10-fold in women who use unopposed estrogen replacement therapy.

Risk factors for Endometrial Cancer	
Risk factor	**Relative risk (RR)**
Increasing age	NA
Unopposed estrogen therapy	2-10
Late menopause (after age 55)	2
Nulliparity	2
Polycystic ovary syndrome (chronic anovulation)	3
Obesity	2-4
Diabetes	3
Hereditary nonpolyposis colorectal cancer	22-50% lifetime risk
Tamoxifen	2/1000
Early menarche	NA
Estrogen secreting tumor	NA
Family history of endometrial, ovarian, breast, or colon cancer	NA

III. **Etiology.** Exposure of the endometrium to continuous estrogen unopposed by progesterone can lead to endometrial hyperplasia.
   A. **Endogenous estrogen.** The most common cause of endogenous unopposed estrogen is chronic anovulation. Chronic anovulation is associated with the polycystic ovary syndrome (PCOS) and the perimenopausal period. Excessive estradiol from an ovarian tumor (eg, granulosa cell tumor) may also cause endometrial hyperplasia.
   B. **Obese women** have high levels of endogenous estrogen resulting from conversion of androstenedione to estrone and of androgens to estradiol.
   C. **Exogenous estrogen.** Continuous exposure to unopposed estrogen (0.625 mg of conjugated estrogens orally daily) results in an increased incidence of endometrial hyperplasia. 62% of women who receive only estrogen develop endometrial hyperplasia.
IV. **Clinical manifestations.** Endometrial hyperplasia should be suspected in women with heavy, prolonged, frequent (ie, less than 21 days), or irregular uterine bleeding. Abnormal uterine bleeding in perimenopausal or postmenopausal women is the most common clinical symptom of endometrial neoplasia, although such bleeding is usually (80%) due to a benign condition. Postmenopausal bleeding requires evaluation.
V. **Diagnostic evaluation**
   A. **Indications for endometrial biopsy**
      1. **Abnormal uterine bleeding.** An endometrial biopsy should be performed in all women with abnormal uterine bleeding in whom endometrial hyperplasia or carcinoma is a possibility.
      2. **Atypical glandular cells** detected by cervical cytology should be investigated with an endometrial biopsy to determine whether endometrial hyperplasia or carcinoma is the cause.
      3. **Endometrial cells.** Asymptomatic women with benign appearing endometrial cells noted on cervical cytology should undergo endometrial biopsy if they are at increased risk of endometrial cancer (eg, postmenopausal; family or personal history of ovarian, breast, colon, or endometrial cancer; tamoxifen use; chronic anovulation; obesity; estrogen therapy; prior endometrial hyperplasia; diabetes).

Women Who Should Undergo Evaluation for Endometrial Hyperplasia or Endometrial Cancer

Over age 40 years with abnormal uterine bleeding
Under age 40 years with abnormal uterine bleeding and risk factors (eg, chronic anovulation, obesity, tamoxifen)
Failure to respond to medical treatment of abnormal uterine bleeding
Postmenopausal women with uterus receiving unopposed estrogen replacement therapy
Presence of atypical glandular cells on Papanicolaou smear
Presence of endometrial cells on Papanicolaou smear in a woman >40 year of age
Women with hereditary nonpolyposis colorectal cancer

- B. **Indications for additional diagnostic evaluation**
  1. **Endometrial hyperplasia with atypia.** If endometrial hyperplasia with atypia is diagnosed by office biopsy, further evaluation is needed to exclude a coexistent endometrial adenocarcinoma, which is present in 25%. Dilation and curettage (D&C) can be performed to rule out endometrial cancer. Given a risk of endometrial cancer of 35 to 43% in these women, hysterectomy should be considered, especially in postmenopausal women or those no longer considering future fertility.
  2. **Nondiagnostic office biopsy.** Endometrial hyperplasia/cancer needs to be excluded in women with a nondiagnostic office biopsy. Dilatation and curettage or hysteroscopy with directed biopsy is required.
  3. **Persistent bleeding.** Endometrial hyperplasia/cancer needs to be excluded if abnormal uterine bleeding persists after a benign endometrial biopsy or treatment of endometrial pathology. Transvaginal sonography with or without hysteroscopy/directed biopsy should be performed to determine the cause of bleeding.
  4. **Postmenopausal women.** Further diagnostic evaluation of simple or complex endometrial hyperplasia without atypia is unnecessary in pre- or peri-menopausal women. Obesity can be considered the probable etiology of endometrial hyperplasia in menopausal women.
- VI. **Treatment.** Simple or complex endometrial hyperplasia without atypia is treated in order to control abnormal uterine bleeding and to prevent progression to cancer, although this risk is very low (<1 to 3%). Atypical endometrial hyperplasia is treated for the same reasons, except the risk of a subsequent diagnosis of endometrial cancer is much higher (17 to 53%).
  - A. **Premenopausal women**
    1. **No atypia.** Treatment consists of treatment with progestins with follow-up sampling to document regression. Medroxyprogesterone acetate (MPA) 10 mg daily should be prescribed for 12 to 14 days each month for three to six months. Regression occurs in 80% with hyperplasia without atypia treated with MPA. Micronized progesterone (100 to 200 mg) in a vaginal cream is an alternative to MPA.
       - a. Ovulation induction is another option for younger women with endometrial hyperplasia without atypia who desire pregnancy.
       - b. Insertion of a levonorgestrel containing intrauterine contraception (IUC) is also effective.
       - c. After treatment, preventative treatment should be initiated if the patient has not resumed normal cyclic menstrual function. A rebiopsy is required if abnormal uterine bleeding recurs.
    2. **With atypia.** Endometrial hyperplasia with atypia on initial endometrial biopsy is further evaluated by D&C. If the diagnosis is confirmed and there is no coexistent adenocarcinoma, treatment

with continuous oral megestrol acetate 40 mg twice per day every day is initiated in women who wish to preserve childbearing potential. Medroxyprogesterone acetate 10 mg/day is an alternative.

- **a.** A repeat endometrial biopsy should be performed in three months. Hysterectomy is recommended if atypical hyperplasia persists.
- **b.** Once endometrial sampling has demonstrated regression with no evidence of hyperplasia, the patient should pursue fertility options. If childbearing is delayed, progestin therapy should be continued. Options include megestrol acetate, MPA, oral contraceptive pills, depot medroxyprogesterone acetate, or a progestin releasing intrauterine contraception. Repeating an endometrial biopsy every 6 to 12 months should be considered initially.
- **c.** Hysterectomy is the treatment of choice for women who are not planning future pregnancy or who are unable to comply with medical therapy and follow-up endometrial sampling.

B. Postmenopausal women

1. **No atypia.** If ovarian/adrenal tumors and use of exogenous hormone therapy have been excluded, treatment with continuous medroxyprogesterone acetate (MPA) 10 mg daily for three months should be started. An endometrial biopsy should be performed immediately after cessation of therapy. This regimen results in regression of simple and/or complex endometrial hyperplasia to normal endometrium after three months of therapy in 86%.
2. **If follow-up endometrial biopsy shows persistent endometrial hyperplasia** without atypia and the patient continues to have bleeding, then a hysterectomy should be offered or she can continue treatment with follow up biopsies every 6 to 12 months. If endometrial hyperplasia has regressed, then treatment is discontinued.
3. If the woman is taking hormone replacement therapy at diagnosis of endometrial hyperplasia, the hormones should be discontinued and MPA initiated as described above. If MPA treatment is successful, and resumption of hormone replacement therapy is desired, then concurrent progestin treatment at higher doses and for longer intervals is advised with a repeat endometrial biopsy in three to six months.
4. **Postmenopausal women** with endometrial hyperplasia unrelated to exogenous estrogen or an ovarian neoplasm are often obese. These patients should lose weight and be treated with MPA as described above.
5. **With atypia.** Endometrial hyperplasia with atypia is considered a premalignant condition, preferably treated with hysterectomy. If hysterectomy is not an option, continuous oral megestrol acetate at doses of 40 mg two to four times per day (or MPA 10 mg/day) can be administered after coexistent endometrial cancer has been excluded by hysteroscopy with directed biopsies. An endometrial biopsy should be performed after three months of therapy.

Options for Progestin Treatment for Prevention of Endometrial Hyperplasia

Oral contraceptive pills
Levonorgestrel-releasing intrauterine device
Depot medroxyprogesterone acetate (150 mg IM) every three months
Intermittent progestin therapy taken daily for 12-14 days per month:
    medroxyprogesterone acetate (5-10 mg)
    norethindrone acetate (5-15 mg)
    micronized progesterone in a vaginal cream (100-200 mg)
Continuous combined estrogen replacement therapy

Progestin Treatment of Endometrial Hyperplasia Without Atypia

Medroxyprogesterone acetate (MPA) 10 mg daily for 12-14 days each month for 3-6 months
Micronized progesterone 100-200 mg daily in a vaginal cream for 12-14 days each month for 3-6 months
Insertion of a levonorgestrel containing intrauterine device

References: See page 208.

Breast Cancer Screening and Diagnosis

Breast cancer is the second most commonly diagnosed cancer among women, after skin cancer. Approximately 182,800 new cases of invasive breast cancer are diagnosed in the United States per year. The incidence of breast cancer increases with age. White women are more likely to develop breast cancer than black women. The incidence of breast cancer in white women is about 113 cases per 100,000 women and in black women, 100 cases per 100,000.

I. Risk factors

Risk Factors for Breast Cancer	
Age >50 years	Age >30 at first birth
Prior history of breast cancer	Obesity
Family history	High socioeconomic status
Early menarche, before age 12	Atypical hyperplasia on biopsy
Late menopause, after age 50	Ionizing radiation exposure
Nulliparity	

A. Family history is highly significant in a first-degree relative (ie, mother, sister, daughter), especially if the cancer has been diagnosed premenopausally. Women who have premenopausal first-degree relatives with breast cancer have a three- to fourfold increased risk of breast cancer. Having several second-degree relatives with breast cancer may further increase the risk of breast cancer. Most women with breast cancer have no identifiable risk factors.

B. Approximately 8% of all cases of breast cancer are hereditary. About one-half of these cases are attributed to mutations in the BRCA1 and BRCA2 genes. Hereditary breast cancer commonly occurs in premenopausal women. Screening tests are available that detect BRCA mutations.

II. Diagnosis and evaluation

A. **Clinical evaluation of a breast mass** should assess duration of the lesion, associated pain, relationship to the menstrual cycle or exogenous hormone use, and change in size since discovery. The presence of nipple discharge and its character (bloody or tea-colored, unilateral or bilateral, spontaneous or expressed) should be assessed.

B. **Menstrual history.** The date of last menstrual period, age of menarche, age of menopause or surgical removal of the ovaries, previous pregnancies should be determined.

C. **History of previous breast biopsies**, cyst aspiration, dates and results of previous mammograms should be determined.

D. **Family history** should document breast cancer in relatives and the age at which family members were diagnosed.

III. Physical examination

A. The breasts should be inspected for asymmetry, deformity, skin retraction, erythema, peau d'orange (breast edema), and nipple retraction, discoloration, or inversion.

B. **Palpation**
   1. The breasts should be palpated while the patient is sitting and then supine with the ipsilateral arm extended. The entire breast should be palpated systematically. The mass should be evaluated for size, shape, texture, tenderness, fixation to skin or chest wall.
   2. mass that is suspicious for breast cancer is usually solitary, discrete and hard. In some instances, it is fixed to the skin or the muscle. A suspicious mass is usually unilateral and nontender. Sometimes, an area of thickening may represent cancer. Breast cancer is rarely bilateral. The nipples should be expressed for discharge.

3. The axillae should be palpated for adenopathy, with an assessment of size of the lymph nodes, number, and fixation.

C. Mammography. Screening mammograms are recommended every year for asymptomatic women 40 years and older. Unfortunately, only 60% of cancers are diagnosed at a local stage.

Screening for Breast Cancer in Women	
Age	American Cancer Society guidelines
20 to 39 years	Clinical breast examination every three years Monthly self-examination of breasts
Age 40 years and older	Annual mammogram Annual clinical breast examination Monthly self-examination of breasts

IV. Methods of breast biopsy

A. Palpable masses. Fine-needle aspiration biopsy (FNAB) has a sensitivity ranging from 90-98%. Nondiagnostic aspirates require surgical biopsy.

1. The skin is prepped with alcohol and the lesion is immobilized with the nonoperating hand. A 10 mL syringe, with a 14 gauge needle, is introduced in to the central portion of the mass at a 90° angle. When the needle enters the mass, suction is applied by retracting the plunger, and the needle is advanced. The needle is directed into different areas of the mass while maintaining suction on the syringe.

2. Suction is slowly released before the needle is withdrawn from the mass. The contents of the needle are placed onto glass slides for pathologic examination. Excisional biopsy is done when needle biopsies are negative but the mass is clinically suspected of malignancy.

B. Stereotactic core needle biopsy. Using a computer-driven stereotactic unit, the lesion is localized in three dimensions, and an automated biopsy needle obtains samples. The sensitivity and specificity of this technique are 95-100% and 94-98%, respectively.

C. Nonpalpable lesions

1. Needle localized biopsy

a. Under mammographic guidance, a needle and hookwire are placed into the breast parenchyma adjacent to the lesion. The patient is taken to the operating room along with mammograms for an excisional breast biopsy.

b. The skin and underlying tissues are infiltrated with 1% lidocaine with epinephrine. For lesions located within 5 cm of the nipple, a periareolar incision may be used or use a curved incision located over the mass and parallel to the areola. Incise the skin and subcutaneous fat, then palpate the lesion and excise the mass.

c. After removal of the specimen, a specimen x-ray is performed to confirm that the lesion has been removed. The specimen can then be sent fresh for pathologic analysis.

d. Close the subcutaneous tissues with a 4-0 chromic catgut suture, and close the skin with 4-0 subcuticular suture.

2. Ultrasonography. Screening is useful to differentiate between solid and cystic breast masses when a palpable mass is not well seen on a mammogram. Ultrasonography is especially helpful in young women with dense breast tissue when a palpable mass is not visualized on a mammogram. Ultrasonography is not used for

routine screening because microcalcifications are not visualized and the yield of carcinomas is negligible.
References: See page 208.

Evaluation of Breast Lumps in Primary Care

About 16% of women ages 40 to 69 will have breast complaints; the complaint is for a breast lump or lumpiness in 40%. Breast cancer is found in 11% of women complaining of a lump. Breast cancer is found in 8% of abnormal screening mammograms and 2% of abnormal screening clinical breast examinations. The vast majority of breast lumps are caused by benign breast disease.

I. Diagnostic evaluation
A. History in women with a breast lump:
1. Its precise location
2. How it was first noted (accidentally, by breast self-examination, clinical breast examination, or mammogram)
3. How long it has been present
4. Presence of nipple discharge
5. Any change in size
6. Whether the lump waxes and wanes at times in the menstrual cycle. Benign cysts may be more prominent premenstrually and regress in size during the follicular phase.
7. Assessment should evaluate past history of breast cancer or breast biopsy, and risk factors for breast cancer (eg, age, family history of breast cancer, age of menarche, age at first pregnancy, age at menopause, alcohol use, and hormonal replacement therapy).
8. Older age, previous history of breast cancer, and family history in a first degree relative increase the chance that a palpable breast lump is cancerous on biopsy.

B. Breast tissue in healthy women is often lumpy, and sometimes general lumpiness, rather than a distinct lump, is felt. The physical examination should determine whether a dominant mass is present.

C. If the initial physical examination does not confirm the presence of a dominant mass, either the patient should be asked to return for a follow-up examination in 2 to 3 months. Women who have not had a mammogram in the preceding year and are eligible for regular screening should have a mammogram.

D. Classic characteristics of cancerous lesions:
1. Single lesion
2. Hard
3. Immovable
4. Irregular borders
5. Size >2 cm

E. Clinical evaluation of breast lumps:
1. **Lump contour.** Smooth, well-demarcated lumps are usually benign.
2. **Breast pain.** Although usually painless, breast cancer can be accompanied by pain.
3. **Nipple discharge.** Discharge is uncommon in cancer and, if present, is unilateral.
4. **Lymph node examination.** Careful examination of the axillae and supraclavicular area.

F. Clinical follow-up. In women under the age of 35 years who present with a breast lump with no suspicious physical findings, it is sometimes advised that the patient return three to ten days after the onset of the next menstruation.

Risk Factors for Developing Breast Cancer			
Risk factors	**Low risk**	**High risk**	**Relative risk**
Deleterious BRCA1/BRCA2 genes	Negative	Positive	3-7
Mother or sister with breast cancer	No	Yes	2.6
Age	30 to 34	70 to 74	18.0
Age at menarche	>14	<12	1.5
Age at first birth	<20	>30	1.9-3.5
Age at menopause	<45	>55	2.0
Use of contraceptive pills	Never	Past/current use	1.2
Hormone replacement therapy	Never	Current	1.4
Alcohol	None	2 to 5 drinks/day	1.4
Breast density on mammography (%)	0	≥ 75	1.8-6
Bone density	Lowest quartile	Highest quartile	2.7-3.5
History of a benign breast biopsy	No	Yes	1.7
History of atypical hyperplasia on biopsy	No	Yes	3.7

1. **Diagnostic mammography** is part of the evaluation of woman age 35 or older who has a breast mass to search for other lesions and to evaluate the mass. Certain mammographic features suggest malignancy:
   a. Increased density
   b. Irregular margins
   c. Spiculation
   d. Clustered irregular microcalcifications
2. Mammography usually cannot determine whether a lump is benign. The sensitivity and specificity of diagnostic mammography in women not reporting a breast lump is 82.3 and 91.2% respectively; in women with a self-reported breast lump, the sensitivity and specificity is 87.3 and 84.5%, respectively.
3. Mammography misses 10 to 20% of clinically palpable breast cancers. Thus, a negative mammogram should not stop further investigation if a suspicious lump is felt.
4. Diagnostic mammography is not ordered routinely in women under age 35. The breast tissue in younger women is often too dense to evaluate the lump.

G. **Ultrasonography** can determine whether a breast mass is a simple or complex cyst or a solid tumor. It is most useful in the following:
   1. Women under age 35
   2. Evaluation of a non-palpable mass detected on screening mammography
   3. Patient declining aspiration of a mass
   4. Mass that is too small or deep for aspiration

H. The risk of cancer is low if the lesion is a simple cyst on ultrasound.

I. The negative predictive value of ultrasound in the patient with a palpable breast mass and a non-suspicious mammogram is over 97%.

J. **Fine needle aspiration biopsy (FNAB)** can be useful in determining if a palpable lump is a simple cyst. The mass is stabilized between the fingers of one hand, and a 22 to 24-gauge needle is inserted. Local anesthesia may be used, but is not always required.

1. FNAB is especially valuable in evaluating cystic breast lesions and can be therapeutic if all of the fluid is removed. There are three possible sample findings with FNAB:

   a. **Non-bloody fluid.** Fluid that is obtained and is not bloody does not need to be sent for analysis. The mass should disappear with the removal of fluid and the patient can be reassured and checked in four to six weeks to ensure that the cyst has not reappeared; recurrence suggests the need for surgical referral.

   b. **Bloody fluid** from patients with otherwise benign examinations should be sent for pathological analysis; cancer is found in 7% of such cases The patient should be checked in four to six weeks to ensure that the cyst has not reappeared. If cytologic examination is suspicious, or if there is a residual mass after aspiration, the patient should be referred to a breast surgeon.

   c. **No fluid**. When no fluid is obtained and the mass turns out to be solid, cells can be obtained for cytologic analysis with FNAB by aspirating cells from the solid mass.

2. **Core needle biopsy**. Core needle biopsy uses a larger needle (14 to 18 gauge, compared with 22 to 24 gauge), and thereby provides histologic material. Core needle biopsies are often performed using stereotactic mammographic equipment or ultrasound guidance.

K. **Triple diagnosis** refers to the use of physical examination, mammography, and FNAB for diagnosing palpable breast lumps. Very few breast cancers are missed using triple diagnosis. Recommendations for follow-up with the triple diagnosis approach are:

1. Women in whom all three tests suggest benign disease are followed with physical examination every three to six months for one year to make sure the mass is stable or regresses.

2. Women in whom all three tests suggest malignancy are referred for definitive therapy.

3. Women with any one of the tests suggesting malignancy undergo excisional biopsy.

II. Guidelines for breast lump evaluation

A. Women age 35 and older

1. If the initial physical examination does not confirm the presence of a dominant mass, a follow-up examination in 2 to 3 months should be completed. Women who have not had a mammogram in the preceding year and are eligible for regular screening, should have a mammogram.

2. Women with a dominant mass should undergo either ultrasonography or a fine needle aspiration biopsy (FNAB). Diagnostic mammography should be obtained if ultrasound or FNAB results suggest the lesion is not a simple cyst.

3. Ultrasound should be obtained for palpable lumps that do not feel cystic. If ultrasound demonstrates a solid mass, the patient should undergo definitive diagnosis with FNAB, core needle biopsy, or excisional biopsy.

4. Ultrasound or FNAB should be performed for lumps that feel cystic.

5. If ultrasound demonstrates a simple cyst, no invasive evaluation is indicated. If a complex cyst or solid mass is present on ultrasound, the patient should undergo definitive diagnosis with FNAB, core needle biopsy, or excisional biopsy.

6. If FNAB is performed first and yields clear fluid and the mass disappears, the patient can be reassured and followed in four to six weeks to check for recurrence or reaccumulation. Recurrence requires surgical referral. Bloody fluid should be sent for cytology.

7. If fluid is not obtained, cellular material should be sent for cytology. If the sample does not contain adequate material, the patient should be sent for surgical evaluation.

      8. If cellular material is obtained that is atypical or suspicious for
cancer, the patient should be referred for a core-needle biopsy or
excisional biopsy.

  B. Women younger than age 35
    1. Evaluation of a breast mass in a young woman should follow the
procedure recommended for women age 35 and older, with the
following exceptions:
      a. If a dominant mass is found but is not suspicious for cancer, the
patient may be asked to return three to ten days after the next
menstruation for reevaluation. Further investigation is indicated if
the lump remains palpable.
      b. Diagnostic mammography should not be performed in the initial
evaluation of women under age 35.

Benign Breast Disease

Benign breast disease includes breast pain, breast lumps, or nipple discharge. The most common cause of breast nodularity and tenderness is
fibrocystic change, which occurs in 60% of premenopausal women.

I. Benign breast lesions, which are discovered by breast palpation or
mammography, have been subdivided into those that are associated with
an increased risk of breast cancer and those that are not.
  A. No increased risk of breast cancer
    1. Fibrocystic changes consist of an increased number of cysts or
fibrous tissue in an otherwise normal breast. Fibrocystic changes
do not constitute a disease state.
    2. Fibrocystic disease is diagnosed when fibrocystic changes occur
in conjunction with pain, nipple discharge, or a degree of lumpiness
sufficient to cause suspicion of cancer.
    3. Duct ectasia is characterized by distention of subareolar ducts.
    4. Solitary papillomas consist of papillary cells that grow from the
wall of a cyst into its lumen.
    5. Simple fibroadenomas are benign solid tumors, usually presenting
as a well-defined, mobile mass.
  B. Increased risk of breast cancer
    1. Ductal hyperplasia without atypia is the most common lesion
associated with increased risk of breast cancer.
    2. Sclerosing adenosis consists of lobular tissue that has undergone
hyperplastic change.
    3. Diffuse papillomatosis refers to the formation of multiple
papillomas.
    4. Complex fibroadenomas are tumors that contain cysts >3 mm in
diameter, sclerosing adenosis, epithelial calcification, or papillary
apocrine changes.
    5. Atypical hyperplasia is associated with a four to sixfold increased
risk of breast cancer.
    6. Radial scars are benign breast lesions of uncertain pathogenesis
that are occasionally detected by mammography. Thus, histologic
confirmation is required to exclude spiculated carcinoma.

II. Symptoms and signs of benign breast disease
  A. Women with fibrocystic changes can have breast tenderness during
the luteal phase of the menstrual cycle. Fibrocystic disease is characterized by more severe or prolonged pain.
  B. Women in their 30s sometimes present with multiple breast nodules 2
to 10 mm in size as a result of proliferation of glandular cells.
  C. Women in their 30s and 40s present with solitary or multiple cysts.
Acute enlargement of cysts may cause severe, localized pain of
sudden onset. Nipple discharge is common, varying from pale green
to brown.

III. **Differential diagnosis**
  A. **Breast pain**
    1. Women with mastitis usually complain of the sudden onset of pain, fever, erythema, tenderness, and induration.
    2. Large pendulous breasts may cause pain due to stretching of Cooper's ligaments.
    3. Hidradenitis suppurativa can present as breast nodules and pain.
    4. Chest wall pain induced by trauma or trauma-induced fat necrosis, intercostal neuralgia, costochondritis, underlying pleuritic lesions, or arthritis of the thoracic spine can mimic benign breast disease.
  B. **Nipple discharge** is uncommon in cancer and, if present, is unilateral. Approximately 3% of cases of unilateral nipple discharge are due to breast cancer; a mass is usually also present.
    1. Nonspontaneous, nonbloody, or bilateral nipple discharge is unlikely to be due to cancer.
      a. Purulent discharge is often caused by mastitis or a breast abscess.
      b. Milky discharge commonly occurs after childbearing and can last several years; it also may be associated with oral contraceptives or tricyclic antidepressants. Serum prolactin should be measured if the discharge is sustained, particularly if it is associated with menstrual abnormalities.
      c. A green, yellow, white, grey, or brown discharge can be caused by duct ectasia.
    2. Evaluation of nipple discharge for suspected cancer may include cytology and galactography. Occult blood can be detected with a guaiac test.

IV. **Clinical evaluation**
  A. **History**
    1. The relationship of symptoms to the menstrual cycles, the timing of onset of breast lumps and their subsequent course, the color and location of nipple discharge, and hormone use should be assessed.
    2. Risk factors for breast cancer should be determined, including menarche before age 12 years, first live birth at age $\geq$30 years, and menopause at age $\geq$55 years; the number of previous breast biopsies, the presence of atypical ductal hyperplasia on biopsy, obesity, nulliparity, increased age, the amount of alcohol consumed, and the number and ages of first-degree family members with breast cancer with two such relatives with breast cancer at any early age should be determined.
  B. **Physical examination.** The examination is performed when the breasts are least stimulated, seven to nine days after the onset of menses. The four breast quadrants, subareolar areas, and the axillae should be systematically examined with the woman both lying and sitting with her hands on her hips.
    1. **The specific goals of the examination are to:**
      a. Delineate and document breast masses
      b. Elicit discharge from a nipple
      c. Identify localized areas of tenderness
      d. Detect enlarged axillary or supraclavicular lymph nodes
      e. Detect skin changes, noting the symmetry and contour of the breasts, position of the nipples, scars, dimpling, edema or erythema, ulceration or crusting of the nipple
    2. **"Classic" characteristics of breast cancers:**
      a. Single lesion
      b. Hard
      c. Immovable
      d. Irregular border
      e. Size $\geq$2 cm
  C. **Mammography**
    1. Although 90% or more of palpable breast masses in women in their 20s to early 50s are benign, excluding breast cancer is a crucial

step in the evaluation. Mammography is recommended for any woman age 35 years or older who has a breast mass.

2. Mammography usually is not ordered routinely in women under age 35 years. The breast tissue in younger women is often too dense to evaluate the lump. Ultrasonography is useful in these women to evaluate lumps and to assess for cysts.

3. Round dense lesions on mammography often represent cystic fluid. Solid and cystic lesions can often be distinguished by ultrasonography and mammography, and needle aspiration under ultrasound guidance further documents the cystic nature of the lesion.

D. **Breast pain.** Women who present with breast pain as their only symptom often undergo mammography. Only 0.4% of women with breast pain have breast cancer. The vast majority of women have normal findings (87%); benign abnormalities are noted in 9%.

E. **Ductal lavage.** The cytologic detection of cellular atypia can identify women with a higher risk of developing breast cancer.

V. **Treatment**

A. **Fibrocystic disease.** The major aim of therapy in fibrocystic disease is to relieve breast pain or discomfort. Symptomatic relief also may be achieved with a soft brassiere with good support, acetaminophen or a nonsteroidal anti-inflammatory drug, or both.

1. Breast pain or discomfort may be relieved with a thiazide diuretic.

2. **Avoidance of caffeine** may provide some patients with relief of pain.

3. **Vitamin E,** 400 IU twice daily reduces breast pain.

4. **Evening primrose oil** in doses of 1500-3000 mg daily, relieves breast pain in 30 to 80%.

5. **Danazol** in doses of 100 to 200 mg daily reduces breast pain. Common side effects include weight gain, acne, hirsutism, bloating, and amenorrhea.

6. **Tamoxifen** reduces breast pain in about 70% of women. It is safe and well-tolerated as 10 mg twice daily, or bromocriptine 1.25 to 5 mg daily can be tried.

7. **Oral contraceptives.** The frequency of fibrocystic changes decreases with prolonged oral contraceptive therapy. Oral contraceptives containing 19-norprogestins, such as norlutate, have androgenic properties that are beneficial.

References: See page 208.

Sexual Assault

Sexual assault is defined as any sexual act performed by one person on another without the person's consent. Sexual assault includes genital, anal, or oral penetration by a part of the accused's body or by an object. It may result from force, the threat of force, or the victim's inability to give consent. The annual incidence of sexual assault is 200 per 100,000 persons.

I. **Psychological effects**

A. A woman who is sexually assaulted loses control over her life during the period of the assault. Her integrity and her life are threatened. She may experience intense anxiety, anger, or fear. After the assault, a "rape-trauma" syndrome often occurs. The immediate response may last for hours or days and is characterized by generalized pain, headache, chronic pelvic pain, eating and sleep disturbances, vaginal symptoms, depression, anxiety, and mood swings.

B. The delayed phase is characterized by flashbacks, nightmares, and phobias.

II. Medical evaluation

A. Informed consent must be obtained before the examination. Acute injuries should be stabilized. About 1% of injuries require hospitalization and major operative repair, and 0.1% of injuries are fatal.

B. A history and physical examination should be performed. A chaperon should be present during the history and physical examination to reassure the victim and provide support. The patient should be asked to state in her own words what happened, identify her attacker if possible, and provide details of the act(s) performed if possible.

Clinical Care of the Sexual Assault Victim

Medical
- Obtain informed consent from the patient
- Obtain a gynecologic history
- Assess and treat physical injuries
- Obtain appropriate cultures and treat any existing infections
- Provide prophylactic antibiotic therapy and offer immunizations
- Provide therapy to prevent unwanted conception
- Offer baseline serologic tests for hepatitis B virus, human immunodeficiency virus (HIV), and syphilis
- Provide counseling
- Arrange for follow-up medical care and counseling

Legal
- Provide accurate recording of events
- Document injuries
- Collect samples (pubic hair, fingernail scrapings, vaginal secretions, saliva, blood-stained clothing)
- Report to authorities as required
- Assure chain of evidence

C. Previous obstetric and gynecologic conditions should be sought, particularly infections, pregnancy, use of contraception, and date of the last menstrual period. Preexisting pregnancy, risk for pregnancy, and the possibility of preexisting infections should be assessed.

D. **Physical examination** of the entire body and photographs or drawings of the injured areas should be completed. Bruises, abrasions, and lacerations should be sought. Superficial or extensive lacerations of the hymen and vagina, injury to the urethra, and occasionally rupture of the vaginal vault into the abdominal cavity may be noted. Bite marks are common.

   1. **Pelvic examination** should assess the status of the reproductive organs, collect samples from the cervix and vagina, and test for Neisseria gonorrhoeae and Chlamydia trachomatis.

   2. **A Wood light** should be used to find semen on the patient's body: dried semen will fluoresce. Sperm and other Y-chromosome-bearing cells may be identified from materials collected from victims.

E. **A serum sample** should be obtained for baseline serology for syphilis, herpes simplex virus, hepatitis B virus, and HIV.

F. **Trichomonas** is the most frequently acquired STD. The risk of acquiring human immunodeficiency virus (HIV) <1% during a single act of heterosexual intercourse, but the risk depends on the population involved and the sexual acts performed. The risk of acquiring gonorrhea is 6-12%, and the risk of acquiring syphilis is 3%.

G. **Hepatitis B virus** is 20 times more infectious than HIV during sexual intercourse. Hepatitis B immune globulin (0.06 mL of hepatitis B immune globulin per kilogram) should be administered intramuscularly as soon as possible within 14 days of exposure. It is followed by the standard three-dose immunization series with hepatitis B vaccine (0, 1, and 6 months), beginning at the time of hepatitis B immune globulin administration.

H. Emergency contraception. If the patient is found to be at risk for pregnancy as a result of the assault, emergency contraception should be offered. The risk of pregnancy after sexual assault is 2-4% in victims not already using contraception. One dose of combination oral contraceptive tablets is given at the time the victim is seen and an additional dose is given in 12 hours. Emergency contraception can be effective up to 120 hours after unprotected coitus. Metoclopramide (Reglan), 20 mg with each dose of hormone, is prescribed for nausea. A pregnancy test should be performed at the 2-week return visit if conception is suspected.

Emergency Contraception

1. Consider pretreatment one hour before each oral contraceptive pill dose, using one of the following orally administered antiemetic agents:
   Prochlorperazine (Compazine), 5 to 10 mg
   Promethazine (Phenergan), 12.5 to 25 mg
   Trimethobenzamide (Tigan), 250 mg
2. Administer the first dose of oral contraceptive pill within 72 hours of intercourse, and administer the second dose 12 hours after the first dose. Brand name options for emergency contraception include the following:
   Preven Kit--two pills per dose (0.5 mg of levonorgestrel and 100 µg of ethinyl estradiol per dose)
   Ovral--two pills per dose (0.5 mg of levonorgestrel and 100 µg of ethinyl estradiol per dose)
   Plan B--one pill per dose (0.75 mg of levonorgestrel per dose)
   Nordette--four pills per dose (0.6 mg of levonorgestrel and 120 µg of ethinyl estradiol per dose)
   Triphasil--four pills per dose (0.5 mg of levonorgestrel and 120 µg of ethinyl estradiol per dose)

Screening and Treatment of Sexually Transmissible Infections Following Sexual Assault

Initial Examination

Infection
- Testing for and gonorrhea and chlamydia from specimens from any sites of penetration or attempted penetration
- Wet mount and culture or a vaginal swab specimen for Trichomonas
- Serum sample for syphilis, herpes simplex virus, hepatitis B virus, and HIV

Pregnancy Prevention
Prophylaxis
- Hepatitis B virus vaccination and hepatitis B immune globulin.
- Empiric recommended antimicrobial therapy for chlamydial, gonococcal, and trichomonal infections and for bacterial vaginosis:
  Ceftriaxone, 125 mg intramuscularly in a single dose, plus
  Metronidazole, 2 g orally in a single dose, plus
  Doxycycline 100 mg orally two times a day for 7 days
  Azithromycin (Zithromax) is used if the patient is unlikely to comply with the 7 day course of doxycycline; single dose of four 250 mg caps.
  If the patient is penicillin-allergic, ciprofloxacin 500 mg PO or ofloxacin 400 mg PO is substituted for ceftriaxone. If the patient is pregnant, erythromycin 500 mg PO qid for 7 days is substituted for doxycycline.
  HIV prophylaxis consists of zidovudine (AZT) 200 mg PO tid, plus lamivudine (3TC) 150 mg PO bid for 4 weeks.

Follow-Up Examination (2 weeks)
• Cultures for N gonorrhoeae and C trachomatis (not needed if prophylactic treatment has been provided) • Wet mount and culture for T vaginalis • Collection of serum sample for subsequent serologic analysis if test results are positive

Follow-Up Examination (12 weeks)

Serologic tests for infectious agents:
   T pallidum
   HIV (repeat test at 6 months)
   Hepatitis B virus (not needed if hepatitis B virus vaccine was given)

III. Emotional care
   A. The physician should discuss the injuries and the probability of infection or pregnancy with the victim, and she should be allowed to express her anxieties.
   B. Anxiolytic medication may be useful; lorazepam (Ativan) 1-5 mg PO tid prn anxiety.
   C. The patient should be referred to personnel trained to handle rape-trauma victims within 1 week.

IV. Follow-up care
   A. The patient is seen for medical follow-up in 2 weeks for documentation of healing of injuries.
   B. Repeat testing includes syphilis, hepatitis B, and gonorrhea and chlamydia cultures. HIV serology should be repeated in 3 months and 6 months.
   C. A pregnancy test should be performed if conception is suspected.

References: See page 208.

Osteoporosis

Over 1.3 million osteoporotic fractures occur each year in the United States. The risk of all fractures increases with age; among persons who survive until age 90, 33% of women will have a hip fracture. The lifetime risk of hip fracture for white women at age 50 is 16%. Osteoporosis is characterized by low bone mass, microarchitectural disruption, and increased skeletal fragility.

Risk Factors for Osteoporotic Fractures	
Personal history of fracture as an adult History of fracture in a first-degree relative Current cigarette smoking Low body weight (less than 58 kg [127 lb]) Female sex Estrogen deficiency (menopause before age 45 years or bilateral ovariectomy, prolonged premenopausal amenorrhea [>one year])	White race Advanced age Lifelong low calcium intake Alcoholism Inadequate physical activity Recurrent falls Dementia Impaired eyesight despite adequate correction Poor health/frailty

I. Screening for osteoporosis and osteopenia
   A. Normal bone density is defined as a bone mineral density (BMD) value within one standard deviation of the mean value in young adults of the same sex and race.
   B. Osteopenia is defined as a BMD between 1 and 2.5 standard deviations below the mean.

C. **Osteoporosis** is defined as a value more than 2.5 standard deviations below the mean; this level is the fracture threshold. These values are referred to as T-scores (number of standard deviations above or below the mean value).

D. **Dual x-ray absorptiometry**. In dual x-ray absorptiometry (DXA), two photons are emitted from an x-ray tube. DXA is the most commonly used method for measuring bone density because it gives very precise measurements with minimal radiation. DXA measurements of the spine and hip are recommended.

II. **Recommendations for screening for osteoporosis of the National Osteoporosis Foundation**

A. All women should be counseled about the risk factors for osteoporosis, especially smoking cessation and limiting alcohol. All women should be encouraged to participate in regular weight-bearing and exercise.

B. Measurement of BMD is recommended for all women 65 years and older regardless of risk factors. BMD should also be measured in all women under the age of 65 years who have one or more risk factors for osteoporosis (in addition to menopause). The hip is the recommended site of measurement.

C. All adults should be advised to consume at least 1,200 mg of calcium per day and 400 to 800 IU of vitamin D per day. A daily multivitamin (which provides 400 IU) is recommended. In patients with documented vitamin D deficiency, osteoporosis, or previous fracture, two multivitamins may be reasonable, particularly if dietary intake is inadequate and access to sunlight is poor.

D. Treatment is recommended for women without risk factors who have a BMD that is 2 SD below the mean for young women, and in women with risk factors who have a BMD that is 1.5 SD below the mean.

III. **Nonpharmacologic therapy of osteoporosis in women**

A. **Diet.** An optimal diet for treatment (or prevention) of osteoporosis includes an adequate intake of calories (to avoid malnutrition), calcium, and vitamin D.

B. **Calcium.** Postmenopausal women should be advised to take 1000 to 1500 mg/day of elemental calcium, in divided doses, with meals.

C. **Vitamin D** total of 800 IU daily should be taken.

D. **Exercise.** Women should exercise for at least 30 minutes three times per week. Any weight-bearing exercise regimen, including walking, is acceptable.

E. **Cessation of smoking** is recommended for all women because smoking cigarettes accelerates bone loss.

IV. **Drug therapy of osteoporosis in women**

A. Selected postmenopausal women with osteoporosis or at high risk for the disease should be considered for drug therapy. Particular attention should be paid to treating women with a recent fragility fracture, including hip fracture, because they are at high risk for a second fracture.

B. Candidates for drug therapy are women who already have postmenopausal osteoporosis (less than -2.5) and women with osteopenia (T score -1 to -2.5) soon after menopause.

C. **Bisphosphonates**

1. **Alendronate (Fosamax)** (10 mg/day or 70 mg once weekly) or **risedronate (Actonel)** (5 mg/day or 35 mg once weekly) are good choices for the treatment of osteoporosis. Bisphosphonate therapy increases bone mass and reduces the incidence of vertebral and nonvertebral fractures.

2. Alendronate (5 mg/day or 35 mg once weekly) and risedronate (5 mg/day of 35 mg once weekly) have been approved for prevention of osteoporosis.

3. Alendronate or risedronate should be taken with a full glass of water 30 minutes before the first meal or beverage of the day. Patients should not lie down for at least 30 minutes after taking the dose to avoid the unusual complication of pill-induced esophagitis.

4. Alendronate is well tolerated and effective for at least seven years.

5. The bisphosphonates (alendronate or risedronate) and raloxifene are first-line treatments for *prevention* of osteoporosis. The bisphosphonates are first-line therapy for *treatment* of osteoporosis. Bisphosphonates are preferred for prevention and treatment of osteoporosis because they increase bone mineral density more than raloxifene.

D. Selective estrogen receptor modulators

1. **Raloxifene (Evista)** (5 mg daily or a once-a-week preparation) is a selective estrogen receptor modulator (SERM) for prevention and treatment of osteoporosis. It increases bone mineral density and reduces serum total and low-density-lipoprotein (LDL) cholesterol. It also appears to reduce the incidence of vertebral fractures and is one of the first-line drugs for prevention of osteoporosis.
2. Raloxifene is somewhat less effective than the bisphosphonates for the prevention and treatment of osteoporosis. Venous thromboembolism is a risk.

Treatment Guidelines for Osteoporosis

Calcium supplements with or without vitamin D supplements or calcium-rich diet
Weight-bearing exercise
Avoidance of alcohol tobacco products
Alendronate (Fosamax)
Risedronate (Actonel)
Raloxifene (Evista)

Agents for Treating Osteoporosis

Medication	Dosage	Route
Calcium	1,000 to 1,500 mg per day	Oral
Vitamin D	400 IU per day (800 IU per day in winter in northern latitudes)	Oral
Alendronate (Fosamax)	**Prevention:** 5 mg per day or 35 mg once-a-week **Treatment:** 10 mg per day or 70 mg once-a-week	Oral
Risedronate (Actonel)	5 mg daily or 35 mg once weekly	Oral
Raloxifene (Evista)	60 mg per day	Oral

E. Monitoring the response to therapy

1. Bone mineral density and a marker of bone turnover should be measured at baseline, followed by a repeat measurement of the marker in three months.
2. If the marker falls appropriately, the drug is having the desired effect, and therapy should be continued for two years, at which time bone mineral density can be measured again. The anticipated three-month decline in markers is 50% with alendronate.

F. Estrogen/progestin therapy

1. Estrogen-progestin therapy is no longer a first-line approach for the treatment of osteoporosis in postmenopausal women because of increases in the risk of breast cancer, stroke, venous thromboembolism, and coronary disease.
2. Indications for estrogen-progestin in postmenopausal women include persistent menopausal symptoms and patients with an

indication for antiresorptive therapy who cannot tolerate the other drugs.

References: See page 208.

Infertility

Infertility is defined as failure of a couple of reproductive age to conceive after 12 months or more of regular coitus without using contraception. Infertility is considered primary when it occurs in a woman who has never established a pregnancy and secondary when it occurs in a woman who has a history of one or more previous pregnancies. Fecundability is defined as the probability of achieving a pregnancy within one menstrual cycle. It is estimated that 10% to 20% of couples are infertile.

I. Diagnostic evaluation
A. History
1. The history should include the couple's ages, the duration of infertility, previous infertility in other relationships, frequency of coitus, and use of lubricants (which can be spermicidal). Mumps orchitis, renal disease, radiation therapy, sexually transmitted diseases, chronic disease such as tuberculosis, major stress and fatigue, or a recent history of acute viral or febrile illness should be sought. Exposure to radiation, chemicals, excessive heat from saunas or hot tubs should be investigated.
2. Pelvic inflammatory disease, previous pregnancies, douching practices, work exposures, alcohol and drug use, exercise, and history of any eating disorders should be evaluated.
3. Menstrual cycle length and regularity and indirect indicators of ovulation, such as Mittelschmerz, mid-cycle cervical mucus change and premenstrual molimina, should be assessed.

B. Physical examination for the woman
1. Vital signs, height, and weight should be noted. Hypertension hair distribution, acne, hirsutism, thyromegaly, enlarged lymph nodes, abdominal masses or scars, galactorrhea, or acanthosis nigricans (suggestive of diabetes) should be sought.
2. Pelvic examination should include a Papanicolaou smear and bimanual examination to assess uterine size and any ovarian masses.
3. Testing for Chlamydia trachomatis, Mycoplasma hominis, and Ureaplasma urealyticum are recommended.

C. Physical examination for the man
1. Height, weight, and hair distribution, gynecomastia, palpable lymph nodes or thyromegaly should be sought.
2. The consistency, size, and position of both testicles and the presence of varicocele or abnormal location of the urethral meatus on the penis should be noted. Testing for Chlamydia, Ureaplasma, and Mycoplasma should be completed.

D.
The cornerstone of any infertility evaluation relies on the assessment of six basic elements: (1) semen analysis, (2) sperm-cervical mucus interaction, (3) ovulation, (4) tubal patency, and (5) uterine and (6) peritoneal abnormalities. Couples of reproductive age who have intercourse regularly without contraception have approximately a 25-30% chance of conceiving in a given menstrual cycle and an 85% chance of conceiving within 1 year.

E. Semen analysis.
The specimen is routinely obtained by masturbation and collected in a clean glass or plastic container. It is customary to have the man abstain from ejaculation for at least 2 days before producing the specimen. Criteria for a normal semen analysis include a sperm count >20 million sperm/mL with at least 50% motility and 30% normal morphology.

Semen Analysis Interpretation		
Semen Parameter	**Normal Values**	**Poor Prognosis**
Sperm concentration	>20 x 106/mL	<5 million/ mL
Sperm motility	>50% progressive motility	<10% motility
Sperm morphology	>50% normal	<4% normal
Ejaculate volume	>2 cc	<2 cc

F. The postcoital test (PCT) is used to assess sperm-cervical mucus interaction after intercourse. The PCT provides information regarding cervical mucus quality and survivability of sperm after intercourse. The PCT should be performed 8 hours after intercourse and 1 to 2 days before the predicted time of ovulation, when there is maximum estrogen secretion unopposed by progesterone.

G. Ovulation assessment

1. Commonly used methods used to assess ovulation include measuring a rise in basal body temperature (BBT), identifying an elevation in the midluteal phase serum progesterone concentration, luteal phase endometrial biopsy, and detection of luteinizing hormone (LH) in the urine. The BBT chart is used to acquire information regarding ovulation and the duration of the luteal phase. Female patients are instructed to take their temperature upon awaking each morning before any physical activity. A temperature rise of 0.4°F (0.22°C) for 2 consecutive days is indicative of ovulation. The initial rise in serum progesterone level occurs between 48 hours before ovulation and 24 hours after ovulation. For this reason, a rise in temperature is useful in establishing that ovulation has occurred, but it should not be used to predict the onset of ovulation in a given cycle.

2. Another test used to assess ovulation is a midluteal phase serum progesterone concentration. A blood sample is usually obtained for progesterone 7 days after the estimated day of ovulation. A concentration >3.0 ng/mL is consistent with ovulation, while a concentration >10 ng/mL signifies adequate luteal phase support.

3. Alternatively, urine LH kits can be used to assess ovulation. Unlike the rise in BBT and serum progesterone concentrations, which are useful for retrospectively documenting ovulation, urinary LH kits can be used to predict ovulation. Ovulation usually occurs 24 to 36 hours after detecting the LH surge.

H. Tubal patency can be evaluated by hysterosalpingography (HSG) and/or by chromopertubation during laparoscopy.

Timing of the Infertility Evaluation	
Test	**Day**
Hysterosalpingogram	day 7-10
Postcoital Test	day 12-14
Serum Progesterone	day 21-23
Endometrial Biopsy	day 25-28

II. Differential diagnosis and treatment

A. The differential diagnosis of infertility includes ovarian (20%), pelvic (25%), cervical (10%), and male (35%) factors. In approximately 10% of cases no explanation is found. Optimal frequency of coitus is every other day around the time of ovulation; however, comparable pregnancy rates are achieved by 3-4 times weekly intercourse throughout the cycle.

B. Ovarian factor infertility

1. An ovarian factor is suggested by irregular cycles, abnormal BBT charts, midluteal phase serum progesterone levels less than 3 ng/mL, or luteal phase defect documented by endometrial biopsy. Ovulatory dysfunction may be intrinsic to the ovaries or caused by thyroid, adrenal, prolactin, or central nervous system disorders. Emotional stress, changes in weight, or excessive exercise should be sought because these disorders can result in ovulatory dysfunction. Luteal phase deficiency is most often the result of inadequate ovarian progesterone secretion.

2. **Clomiphene citrate (Clomid, CC)** is the most cost-effective treatment for the treatment of infertility related to anovulation or oligo ovulation. The usual starting dose of CC is 50 mg/day for 5 days, beginning on the second to sixth day after induced or spontaneous bleeding. Ovulation is expected between 7 and 10 days after the last dose of CC.

3. Ovulation on a specified dosage of CC should be confirmed with a midluteal phase serum progesterone assay, BBT rise, pelvic ultrasonography, or urinary ovulation-predictor kits. In the event ovulation does not occur with a specified dose of CC, the dose can be increased by 50 mg/day in a subsequent cycle. The maximum dose of CC should not exceed 250 mg/day. The addition of dexamethasone is advocated for women with elevated dehydroepiandrosterone sulfate levels who remain anovulatory despite high doses of CC. The incidence of multiple gestations with CC is 5% to 10%. Approximately 33% of patients will become pregnant within five cycles of treatment. Treatment with CC for more than six ovulatory cycles is not recommended because of low success rates.

4. **Human menopausal gonadotropins (hMG, Pergonal, Metrodin)** ovulation induction with is another option for the treatment of ovulatory dysfunction. Because of its expense and associated risk of multiple gestations, gonadotropin therapy should be reserved for patients who remain refractory to CC therapy. The pregnancy rate with gonadotropin therapy is 25% per cycle. This is most likely the result of recruitment of more follicles with gonadotropin therapy. The incidence of multiple gestations with gonadotropin therapy is 25% to 30%.

5. **Luteal phase deficiency** is treated with progesterone, usually prescribed as an intravaginal suppository at a dose of 25 mg twice a day until 8 to 10 weeks of gestation.

6. **Women with ovulatory dysfunction** secondary to ovarian failure or poor ovarian reserve should consider obtaining oocytes from a donor source.

C. Pelvic factor infertility

1. Pelvic factor infertility is caused by conditions that affect the fallopian tubes, peritoneum, or uterus. Tubal factor infertility is a common sequela of salpingitis. Appendicitis, ectopic pregnancy, endometriosis, and previous pelvic or abdominal surgery can also damage the fallopian tubes and cause adhesion formation.

2. Endometriosis is another condition involving the peritoneal cavity that is commonly associated with infertility. Uterine abnormalities are responsible for infertility in about 2% of cases. Examples of uterine abnormalities associated with infertility are congenital deformities of

the uterus, leiomyomas, and intrauterine scarification or adhesions (Asherman's syndrome).
3. The mainstay of treatment of pelvic factor infertility relies on laparoscopy and hysteroscopy. In many instances, tubal reconstructive surgery, lysis of adhesions, and ablation and resection of endometriosis can be accomplished laparoscopically.

D. **Cervical factor infertility**
1. Cervical factor infertility is suggested when well-timed PCTs are consistently abnormal in the presence of a normal semen analysis. Cervical factor infertility results from inadequate mucus production by the cervical epithelium, poor mucus quality, or the presence of antisperm antibodies.
2. Patients with an abnormal PCT should be screened for an infectious etiology. The presence of immotile sperm or sperm shaking in place and not demonstrating forward motion is suggestive of immunologically related infertility. Sperm-cervical mucus and antisperm antibody testing are indicated when PCTs are repeatedly abnormal, despite normal-appearing cervical mucus and normal semen analysis.

E. **Male factor infertility** includes conditions that affect sperm production, sperm maturation, and sperm delivery. Intrauterine insemination is frequently used to treat men with impaired semen parameters.

F. **Unexplained Infertility**
1. The term unexplained infertility should be used only after a thorough infertility investigation has failed to reveal an identifiable source and the duration of infertility is 24 months or more. History, physical examination, documentation of ovulation, endometrial biopsy, semen analyses, PCT, hysterosalpingogram, and laparoscopy should have been completed.
2. Because couples with unexplained infertility lack an identifiable causative factor of their infertility, empirical treatment with clomiphene therapy increases the spontaneous pregnancy rate to 6.8% per cycle compared with 2.8% in placebo-control cycles. For optimal results, gonadotropins should be used for ovulation induction. Intrauterine insemination, in vitro fertilization and gamete intrafallopian transfer (GIFT) are additional options.

References: See page 208.

Sexual Dysfunction

Almost two-thirds of the women may have had sexual difficulties at some time. Fifteen% of women experience pain with intercourse, 18-48% experience difficulty becoming aroused, 46% note difficulty reaching orgasm, and 15-24% are not orgasmic.

I. **Clinical evaluation of sexual dysfunction.** Sexual difficulty can be caused by a lack of communication, insufficient stimulation, a lack of understanding of sexual response, lack of nurturing, physical discomfort, or fear of infection.

II. **Treatment of sexual dysfunction**
A. **Lack of arousal**
1. Difficulty becoming sexually aroused may occur if there is insufficient foreplay or if either partner is emotionally distracted. Arousal phase dysfunction may be manifest by insufficient vasocongestion.
2. Treatment consists of Sensate Focus exercises. In these exercises, the woman and her partner take turns caressing each other's body, except for the genital area. When caressing becomes pleasurable for both partners, they move on to manual genital stimulation, and then to further sexual activity.

B. **Lack of orgasm**
   1. Lack of orgasm should be considered a problem if the patient or her partner perceives it as one. Ninety% of women are able to experience orgasm.
   2. **At-home methods of overcoming dysfunction**
      a. The patient should increase self-awareness by examining her body and genitals at home. The patient should identify sensitive areas that produce pleasurable feelings. The intensity and duration of psychologic stimulation may be increased by sexual fantasy.
      b. If, after completing the above steps, an orgasm has not been reached, the patient may find that the use of a vibrator on or around the clitoris is effective.
      c. Once masturbation has resulted in orgasm, the patient should masturbate with her partner present and demonstrate pleasurable stimulation techniques.
      d. Once high levels of arousal have been achieved, the couple may engage in intercourse. Manual stimulation of the clitoris during intercourse may be beneficial.

C. **Dyspareunia**
   1. Dyspareunia consists of pain during intercourse. Organic disorders that may contribute to dyspareunia include hypoestrogenism, endometriosis, ovaries located in the cul-de-sac, fibroids, and pelvic infection.
   2. Evaluation for dyspareunia should include careful assessment of the genital tract and an attempt to reproduce symptoms during bimanual examination.

D. **Vaginismus**
   1. Vaginismus consists of spasm of the levator ani muscle, making penetration into the vagina painful. Some women may be unable to undergo pelvic examination.
   2. **Treatment of vaginismus**
      a. **Vaginal dilators**. Plastic syringe covers or vaginal dilators are available in sets of 4 graduated sizes. The smallest dilator (the size of the fifth finger) is placed in the vagina by the woman. As each dilator is replaced with the next larger size without pain, muscle relaxation occurs.
      b. **Muscle awareness exercises**
         (1) The examiner places one finger inside the vaginal introitus, and the woman is instructed to contract the muscle that she uses to stop urine flow. The woman then inserts her own finger into the vagina and contracts. The process is continued at home.
         (2) Once a woman can identify the appropriate muscles, vaginal contractions can be done without placing a finger in the vagina.

F **Medications that interfere with sexual function**. The most common of medications that interfere with sexual function are antihypertensive agents, anti-psychotics, and antidepressants.

Medications Associated With Sexual Dysfunction in Women		
Medication	**Decreased Libido**	**Delayed or No Orgasm**
Amphetamines and anorexic drugs		X
Cimetidine	X	

Medication	Decreased Libido	Delayed or No Orgasm
Diazepam		X
Fluoxetine		X
Imipramine		X
Propranolol	X	

References: See page 208.

Urinary Incontinence

I. **Terminology**
   A. **Urinary incontinence** is involuntary leakage of urine.
   B. **Urgency** is the complaint of a sudden and compelling desire to pass urine, that is difficult to defer.
   C. **Urge incontinence** is the complaint of involuntary leakage accompanied by urgency. Common precipitants include running water, hand washing, and exposure to cold.
   D. **Stress incontinence** is involuntary leakage with effort, exertion, sneezing, or coughing.
   E. Mixed incontinence is the complaint of involuntary leakage associated with urgency and also with exertion, effort, sneezing, or coughing.
   F. **Overactive bladder** is a symptom syndrome consisting of urgency, frequency, and nocturia, with or without urge incontinence.
   G. **Hesitancy** describes difficulty in initiating voiding.
   H. **Straining to void** is the muscular effort used either to initiate, maintain, or improve the urinary stream.

II. **Types of urinary incontinence**
   A. **Incontinence related to reversible conditions.** Incontinence affects up to one-third of community-dwelling older persons and is often caused by medical and functional factors. Medications often precipitate or worsen urinary incontinence in older individuals.
   B. **Urge incontinence.** The etiology of the overactive bladder syndrome is uninhibited bladder contractions (called detrusor overactivity).
   C. **Most common causes of detrusor overactivity:**
      1. Age-related changes
      2. Interruption of central nervous system (CNS) inhibitory pathways (eg, by stroke, cervical stenosis)
      3. Bladder irritation caused by infection, bladder stones, inflammation, or neoplasms
      4. Detrusor overactivity in many cases may be idiopathic.
      5. Urge urinary incontinence in younger women may be due to interstitial cystitis, characterized by urgency and frequent voiding of small amounts of urine, often with dysuria or pain.
   D. **Urge urinary incontinence** in frail older persons frequently coexists with impaired detrusor contractile function, a condition termed detrusor hyperactivity with impaired contractility (DHIC). DHIC is characterized by urgency and an elevated postvoid residual in the absence of outlet obstruction.
   E. **Stress incontinence** occurs when increases in intraabdominal pressure overcome sphincter closure mechanisms. Stress urinary incontinence is the most common cause of urinary incontinence in younger women, second most common cause in older women, and may occur in older men after transurethral or radical prostatectomy.

1. **Causes of stress incontinence:**
   a. Stress urinary incontinence in women most often results from impaired urethral support from pelvic endofascia and muscles.
   b. Stress urinary incontinence is less frequently caused failure of urethral closure, called intrinsic sphincter deficiency (ISD). This usually results from operative trauma and scarring, but it can also occur with postmenopausal mucosal atrophy. Unlike the episodic, stress-maneuver-related leakage of stress urinary incontinence, ISD leakage typically is continual.

F. **Mixed incontinence** is the most common type of urinary incontinence in women, caused by detrusor overactivity and impaired urethral sphincter function.

G. **Overflow incontinence** is dribbling and/or continuous leakage associated with incomplete bladder emptying caused by impaired detrusor contractility and/or bladder outlet obstruction. The postvoid residual is elevated, and there may be a weak urinary stream, dribbling, intermittency, hesitancy, frequency, and nocturia. Stress-related leakage may occur.
   1. Outlet obstruction is the second most common cause of urinary incontinence in older men (after detrusor overactivity), resulting from benign prostatic hyperplasia, prostate cancer, or urethral stricture.

III. **Diagnostic evaluation**
   A. **History.** The onset and course of incontinence and associated lower urinary tract symptoms.
   B. Leakage frequency, volume, timing, and associated symptoms (eg, urgency, effort maneuvers, urinary frequency, nocturia, hesitancy, interrupted voiding, incomplete emptying, straining to empty, sense of warning).
   C. Precipitants: medications, caffeinated beverages, alcohol, physical activity, cough, laughing, sound of water.
   D. Bowel and sexual function (impaction can cause overflow urinary incontinence; bowel control and sexual function share sacral cord innervation with voiding).
   E. Status of other medical conditions, parity, and medications, along with their temporal relationship to urinary incontinence onset.

Key Questions in Evaluating Patients for Urinary Incontinence

Do you leak urine when you cough, laugh, lift something or sneeze? How often?
Do you ever leak urine when you have a strong urge on the way to the bathroom? How often?
How frequently do you empty your bladder during the day?
How many times do you get up to urinate after going to sleep? Is it the urge to urinate that wakes you?
Do you ever leak urine during sex?
Do you wear pads that protect you from leaking urine? How often do you have to change them?
Do you ever find urine on your pads or clothes and were unaware of when the leakage occurred?
Does it hurt when you urinate?
Do you ever feel that you are unable to completely empty your bladder?

Drugs That Can Influence Bladder Function

Drug	Side effect
Antidepressants, antipsychotics, sedatives/hypnotics	Sedation, retention (overflow)
Diuretics	Frequency, urgency (OAB)

Drug	Side effect
Caffeine	Frequency, urgency (OAB)
Anticholinergics	Retention (overflow)
Alcohol	Sedation, frequency (OAB)
Narcotics	Retention, constipation, sedation (OAB and overflow)
Alpha-adrenergic blockers	Decreased urethral tone (stress incontinence)
Alpha-adrenergic agonists	Increased urethral tone, retention (overflow)
Beta-adrenergic agonists	Inhibited detrusor function, retention (overflow)

IV. **Physical examination**
   A. **General examination** should include the level of alertness and functional status. Vital signs should include orthostatic vital signs.
   B. **Neck examination** should investigate limitations in cervical lateral rotation and lateral flexion, interosseous muscle wasting, and an abnormal Babinski reflex. These changes suggest cervical spondylosis or stenosis, with secondary interruption of inhibitory tracts to the detrusor, thus causing detrusor overactivity.
   C. **Back examination** may reveal dimpling or a hair tuft at the spinal cord base, suggestive of occult dysraphism (incomplete spina bifida). Evidence of prior laminectomy should be sought.
   D. **Cardiovascular examination** should look for evidence of volume overload (eg, rales, pedal edema).
   E. **Abdomen** should be palpated for masses, tenderness, and bladder distention.
   F. **Extremities** should be examined for joint mobility and function.
   G. **Genital examination** in women should include inspection of the vaginal mucosa for atrophy (thinning, pallor, loss of rugae), narrowing of the introitus by posterior synechia, vault stenosis, and inflammation (erythema, petechiae, telangiectasia, friability). A bimanual examination should be done to evaluate for masses or tenderness.
      1. The adequacy of pelvic support may be assessed by a split-speculum exam, removing the top blade of the speculum and holding the bottom blade firmly against the posterior vaginal wall. While the woman to coughs, assess whether the urethra remains firmly fixed or swings quickly forward (urethral hypermobility) and for bulging of the anterior vaginal wall (cystocoele).
      2. Check for rectocele by turning the single blade of the speculum to support the anterior vaginal wall and having the patient cough again.
      3. Uncircumcised men should be checked for phimosis, paraphimosis, and balanitis.
   H. **Rectal examination** should check for masses and fecal impaction, and for prostate consistency and symmetry in men (estimation of prostate size by digital examination is unreliable).
   I. **Neurologic examination** assess sacral root integrity, including perineal sensation, resting and volitional tone of the anal sphincter, anal wink (anal contraction in response to a light scratch of the perineal skin lateral to the anus), and the bulbocavernosus reflex (anal contraction in response to a light squeeze of the clitoris or glans

penis). Cognitive status and affect should be assessed, as well as motor strength and tone (especially with regard to mobility), and vibration and peripheral sensation for peripheral neuropathy.

J. **Clinical testing**
  1. **Stress test** is best done when the patient has not recently voided and is in a standing position with a relaxed perineum. The patient should give a single vigorous cough. A pad is held underneath the perineum, and the physician or nurse observes directly whether there is leakage from the urethra.
     a. **Leakage instantaneous with cough** suggests impaired sphincter function, while a several-second delay before leakage suggests an effort-induced uninhibited detrusor contraction.
  2. **Postvoid residual volume (PVR)** by catheterization or ultrasound. Elevated PVR is found most commonly in:
     a. Frail elderly men with symptoms of bladder outlet obstruction
     b. Patients with symptoms of decreased bladder emptying or abdominal distention
     c. Women with previous anti-incontinence surgery
     d. Persons with suprasacral and sacral spinal cord injury
     e. Patients who have failed empiric antimuscarinic drug therapy
     f. A PVR of less than 50 mL is considered adequate emptying, and a PVR >200 mL is suggestive of either detrusor weakness or obstruction.
K. **Laboratory tests.** Renal function tests, glucose, calcium, and, in older people, a vitamin B12 level should be obtained. A urinalysis should be performed. Urine cytology and cystoscopy are indicated only if there is hematuria or pelvic pain.
L. **Urodynamic testing** is not usually necessary in the evaluation of urinary incontinence.

V. **Treatment of urinary incontinence**
  A. **Lifestyle.** Adequate fluid intake (up to two liters per day); avoidance of caffeinated beverages and alcohol; minimizing evening intake; management of constipation, smoking cessation; and treatment of pulmonary disease if cough is exacerbating incontinence.
  B. **Behavioral therapy**
     1. **Cognitively intact patients**
        a. **Bladder training** involves timed voiding every two hours while awake. Bladder relaxation techniques involve having the patients sit down when an urge occurs and concentrate on making the urge decrease and pass by taking a deep breath, contracting their pelvic muscles. Once in control of the urge, they walk to a bathroom and void.
        b. **Supplemental biofeedback** may be helpful for some patients in addition to bladder training.
     2. **Cognitively impaired patients.** Prompted voiding involves regular monitoring of continence: prompting to toilet on a scheduled basis, and praise when individuals are continent and attempt to toilet.
  C. **Pelvic muscle (Kegel) exercises** (PME) strengthen the urethral closure mechanism with small numbers of isometric repetitions at maximal exertion. The basic recommended regimen is three sets of 8 to 12 slow velocity contractions sustained for six to eight seconds each, performed three or four times a week and continued for at least 15 to 20 weeks.

VI. **Pharmacological therapy.** Medications are not useful in the treatment of with stress incontinence.
  A. **Antimuscarinics.** Anticholinergics with antimuscarinic effects are frequently prescribed for urge incontinence. These agents result in a 40% higher rate of cure or improvement; dry mouth is common.
     1. **Oxybutynin (Ditropan)** has direct antispasmodic effects and inhibits the action of acetylcholine on smooth muscle. Oxybutynin is available in both immediate release (IR), extended release (ER), and transdermal formulations. Efficacy is similar.

    a. The initial dosage for IR is 2.5 mg two to three times daily, followed by titration as needed up to 20 mg/day in divided doses. The ER formulation is started at 5 mg once daily and titrated up to 20 to 30 mg once daily. The transdermal patch is available at 3.8 mg and should be changed twice a week.

    b. Anticholinergic side effects, especially dry mouth, can limit therapy; dry mouth is less frequent with extended release and transdermal preparations. The postvoid residual should be monitored in older patients. Worsening of urinary incontinence can result from subclinical retention.

  2. Tolterodine (Detrol LA, 1 to 2 mg twice a day immediate release, 2 to 4 mg per day extended release) has similar efficacy to oxybutynin. It causes dry mouth less frequently than oxybutynin IR 5 mg three times daily, but has similar side effects to ER oxybutynin 10 mg/day. Tolterodine is more expensive than generic oxybutynin IR. Oxybutynin and tolterodine have similar clinical efficacy, but tolterodine causes less dry mouth.

  3. Trospium (Sanctura, 20 mg twice daily) is approved for the treatment of overactive bladder. Dose should be reduced to 20 mg once a day in the elderly and renal impairment. Trospium must be taken on an empty stomach. Dry mouth occurs in 22% and constipation in 10%.

  4. Solifenacin (Vesicare, 5 to 10 mg daily) and **darifenacin (Enablex,** 7.5 to 15 mg daily) are approved for overactive bladder. Solifenacin and darifenacin are more selective for the M-3 muscarinic receptor in the bladder. Incontinence episodes decrease with solifenacin, similar to tolterodine (58%). The rate of dry mouth is 14% and the rate of constipation is 7%.

  5. Duloxetine (Cymbalta) is a serotonin and norepinephrine reuptake inhibitor that is only approved for major depression and neuropathic pain. It stimulates pudendal motor neuron alpha adrenergic and 5-hydroxytryptamine-2 receptors. 40 mg twice daily results in significant decreases in the frequency of incontinence compared with placebo (50 to 54%). Nausea is common. Duloxetine is contraindicated in chronic liver disease.

B. Stress incontinence may be treated with topical estrogen. Up to 2 g of vaginal cream daily, intravaginal estrogen rings, or dissolving tablets (Vagifem) are effective for urinary incontinence. Topical estrogen is applied as 0.3 mg of conjugated estrogens or 0.5 mg of estradiol daily for three weeks, and then twice a week thereafter.

Medications Used to Treat Urinary Incontinence	
Drug	**Dosage**
Stress Incontinence	
Estrogen dissolving tablets (Vagifem)	One tablet inserted vaginally once daily for the first two weeks. Then one tablet twice weekly
Vaginal estrogen ring (Estring)	Insert into vagina every three months
Vaginal estrogen cream	0.5 g, apply in vagina every night

Drug	Dosage
Overactive bladder	
Oxybutynin transdermal (Oxytrol)	39 cm^2 patch 2 times/week
Oxybutynin ER (Ditropan XL)	5 to 15 mg, every morning
Tolterodine LA (Detrol LA)	2-4 mg qd
Generic oxybutynin	2.5 to 10 mg, two to four times daily
Tolterodine (Detrol)	1 to 2 mg, two times daily
Trospium (Sanctura)	20 mg twice daily
Solifenacin (Vesicare)	5 to 10 mg daily
Darifenacin (Enablex)	7.5 to 15 mg daily
Duloxetine (Cymbalta)	20 mg twice daily, and increasing to 40 mg twice daily after two weeks

VII. **Surgery**
  A. **Urge incontinence.** Potential surgical treatments for severe cases of intractable urge urinary incontinence are sacral nerve modulation and augmentation cystoplasty; however, these are not first-line treatments.
  B. **Stress incontinence.** Surgery offers the highest cure rates for stress urinary incontinence. However, it is invasive and potentially morbid.
    1. **Bladder neck suspension procedures** such as the transvaginal Burch colposuspension are used to treat urethral hypermobility and stress urinary incontinence.
    2. **Sling procedures** (using material to support the urethra or bladder neck) including tension-free vaginal tape (TVT) are increasingly being used for stress incontinence in women.
    3. **Periurethral bulking injections** with collagen are preferable for intrinsic sphincter deficiency.
VIII. **Continence pessaries** may benefit women with stress urinary incontinence related to pelvic floor prolapse or laxity. The use of these devices may be very appealing to women, who wish to avoid surgery.
References: See page 208.

Acute Cystitis

Cystitis is an infection of the bladder. Acute cystitis in the healthy nonpregnant adult woman is considered to be uncomplicated. A complicated infection is associated with a condition that increases the risk of failing therapy. About 7.8% of girls and 1.6% of boys have had a symptomatic UTI. Approximately 50 to 60% of adult women have had a UTI at some time during their life. Young sexually active women have 0.5 episodes of acute cystitis per year.

I. **Microbiology Clinical features**
  A. Escherichia coli is the causative pathogen in 80 to 85% of episodes of acute uncomplicated cystitis. Staphylococcus saprophyticus is responsible for most other episodes, while Proteus mirabilis, Klebsiella species, enterococci or other uropathogens are isolated from a small proportion of patients.

    B. Acute uncomplicated cystitis is characterized by dysuria, usually in combination with frequency, urgency, suprapubic pain, and/or hematuria. Fever (>38ºC), flank pain, costovertebral angle tenderness, and nausea or vomiting suggest pyelonephritis

    C. Vaginitis should be considered if there is vaginal discharge or odor, pruritus, dyspareunia, external dysuria, and the absence of frequency or urgency.

II. Diagnosis

    A. **Physical examination** should include temperature, abdominal examination, and assessment for costovertebral angle tenderness. A pelvic examination is indicated if symptoms of urethritis or vaginitis are present.

    B. **Urinalysis.** Pyuria is usually present with acute cystitis; its absence strongly suggests a noninfectious cause for the symptoms. An unspun voided midstream urine specimen should be examined with a hemocytometer; 10 or more leukocytes per mm^3 is considered abnormal. White blood cell casts in the urine are diagnostic of upper tract infection. Hematuria is common with UTI but not in urethritis or vaginitis. Microscopic evaluation of the urine for bacteriuria is generally not recommended for acute uncomplicated cystitis because pathogens in low quantities ($\leq$10^4 CFU/mL) are difficult to find on the wet mount or Gram stain.

    C. **Indications for voided midstream urine cultures**
        1. Suspected complicated infection.
        2. The symptoms are not characteristic of UTI.
        3. The patient has persistent symptoms of UTI following treatment.
        4. UTI symptoms recur less than one month after treatment of a previous UTI.

    D. **Acute urethral syndrome.** A CFU count $\geq$10^2/mL should be considered positive on a midstream urine specimen in women with acute symptoms and pyuria. Some women with acute dysuria have neither bacteriuria nor pyuria. The symptoms usually resolve after antimicrobial therapy.

    E. **Urine dipsticks**
        1. Dipsticks detect the presence of leukocyte esterase and nitrite; the former detect pyuria and the latter Enterobacteriaceae which convert urinary nitrate to nitrite. The leukocyte esterase test is a practical screening test with a sensitivity of 75 to 96% and specificity of 94 to 98%. A microscopic evaluation for pyuria or a culture is indicated with a negative leukocyte esterase test with urinary symptoms.
        2. The nitrite test is fairly sensitive and specific for detecting $\geq$10^5 Enterobacteriaceae CFU per mL of urine. However, it lacks adequate sensitivity for detection of "low count" UTIs, or, in some cases, infections caused by common uropathogenic species.

III. Treatment

    A. **E. coli Resistance**
        1. One-third or more of isolates demonstrate resistance to ampicillin and sulfonamides; these agents should not be used for empiric therapy. An increasing proportion of uropathogens demonstrate resistance to trimethoprim and/or TMP-SMX.
        2. The prevalence of resistance to nitrofurantoin among E. coli is less than 5%, although non-E. coli uropathogens are often resistant.
        3. Resistance to the fluoroquinolones remains well below 5%.

    B. **S. saprophyticus resistance.** Three% are resistant to TMP-SMX, 1% to cephalothin, 0% to nitrofurantoin, and 0.4% to ciprofloxacin.

    C. **Recommendation**
        1. Because of increasing fluoroquinolone resistance, TMP-SMX should be the first-line treatment for acute cystitis if the woman:
            a. Has no history of allergy to the drug.
            b. Has not been on antibiotics, especially TMP-SMX, in the past three months.

    c. Has not been hospitalized recently.
    d. If the prevalence of E. coli resistance to TMP-SMX in the area is not known to be more than 20% among women with acute uncomplicated cystitis.

  2. **A fluoroquinolone** is an appropriate choice for women who have an allergy to TMP-SMX or risk factors for TMP-SMX resistance and who have moderate to severe symptoms.

Oral Antibiotics for Acute Uncomplicated Cystitis		
Drug, dose	**Dose and interval**	**Duration**
Levofloxacin (Levaquin)	250 mg q24h	3 days
Ciprofloxacin (Cipro)	100 to 250 mg q12h **OR** 500 mg q24h	3 days 3 days
Gatifloxacin (Tequin)	400 mg single dose **OR** 200 mg q24h	3 days
Trimethoprim-sulfamethoxazole (Bactrim)	160/800 mg q12h	3 days
Trimethoprim	100 mg q12h	3 days
Cefpodoxime proxetil (Vantin)	100 mg q12h	3-7days
Nitrofurantoin macrocrystals (Macrobid)	50 mg q6h	7 days
Nitrofurantoin monohydrate macrocrystals (Macrobid)	100 mg q12h	7 days
Amoxicillin-clavulanate (Augmentin)	500 mg q12h	7 days

  3. **Nitrofurantoin (Macrodantin** [for seven days]) should be used for women with mild-to-moderate symptoms who have allergy to TMP-SMX or risk factors for TMP-SMX resistance.
  4. Urinary analgesia (phenazopyridine [Pyrimidine] 200 mg orally TID) is offered to those with severe dysuria (10%).
    Phenazopyridine is usually given for only one to two days.
  5. Routine post-treatment cultures in non-pregnant women who have become asymptomatic after an episode of cystitis are not indicated. In patients whose symptoms do not resolve, urine culture and antimicrobial susceptibility testing should be performed. Empiric therapy should include a fluoroquinolone unless such an agent was used initially.

IV. Acute complicated cystitis

A. Urinary tract infection may lead to serious complications in the person who is pregnant, very young or old, diabetic, immunocompromised, or who has an abnormal genitourinary tract.

B. **Clinical presentation.** Acute complicated cystitis generally presents with dysuria, frequency, urgency, suprapubic pain, and/or hematuria. Fever (>38°C), flank pain, costovertebral angle tenderness, and nausea or vomiting suggest the infection has extended beyond the bladder.

C. **Bacteriology.** The spectrum of uropathogens causing complicated cystitis is much broader than that causing uncomplicated cystitis. Infection with Proteus, Klebsiella, Pseudomonas, Serratia, and Providencia species, and enterococci, staphylococci and fungi is more common in complicated cystitis. These uropathogens, including E. coli, are much more likely to be resistant to common antimicrobials.

D. **Diagnosis.** Pyuria is present in almost all patients with complicated cystitis. Urine cultures with susceptibility testing should be obtained in complicated cystitis. A Gram stain may be helpful since the presence of Gram positive cocci, suggestive of enterococci, may influence the choice of empiric antibiotics.

E. **Treatment**
1. Complicated cystitis should be treated with an oral fluoroquinolone such as ciprofloxacin, levofloxacin, or gatifloxacin. The fluoroquinolones are well tolerated, provide a broad spectrum of activity covering most expected pathogens (including P. aeruginosa), and achieve high levels in the urine and urinary tract tissue. The recommended dose for ciprofloxacin (Cipro) is 500 mg PO twice daily, for levofloxacin (Levaquin) is 500 mg PO once daily, and for gatifloxacin (Tequin) is 400 mg PO once daily, each for 7 to 14 days.
2. Amoxicillin, nitrofurantoin and sulfa drugs are poor choices for empiric therapy in complicated cystitis because of the high prevalence of resistance.
3. Parenteral therapy is occasionally indicated for the treatment of complicated cystitis caused by multiply-resistant uropathogens, or for those patients who are allergic or intolerant to fluoroquinolones. Parenteral levofloxacin (500 mg) or gatifloxacin (400 mg), ceftriaxone (1 g), or an aminoglycoside (3 to 5 mg/kg of gentamicin or tobramycin) can be administered once daily. Patients initially given parenteral therapy can be switched to oral agents, usually a fluoroquinolone, after clinical improvement.
4. Gram positive cocci, suggestive of enterococci, may require the addition of ampicillin (1 g every six hours) or amoxicillin (500 mg PO every eight hours) to a treatment regimen.
5. If the patient does not show improvement within 24 to 48 hours, a repeat urine culture and ultrasound or computerized tomography should be considered to rule out urinary tract pathology.
6. The recommended duration of treatment for acute complicated cystitis is 7 to 14 days. A follow-up urine culture is not indicated in the asymptomatic patient.

V. Cystitis in young men.
A small number of 15- to 50-year-old men suffer acute uncomplicated UTIs. Risk factors include homosexuality, intercourse with an infected female partner, and lack of circumcision.

A. Dysuria, frequency, urgency, suprapubic pain, or hematuria are typical of cystitis in men. The absence of pyuria suggests a non-infectious diagnosis. A midstream urine culture is recommended.

B. **Other causes of infection.** Urethritis must be considered in sexually active men; examination for penile ulcerations and urethral discharge, evaluation of a urethral swab specimen Gram stain, and diagnostic tests for N. gonorrheae and C. trachomatis are warranted. A urethral

Gram stain demonstrating leukocytes and predominant Gram negative rods suggests E. coli urethritis.

C. **Chronic prostatitis** should also be considered, particularly in men who have had recurrent UTIs.

D. **Treatment of cystitis.** The etiologic agents causing uncomplicated urinary tract infections in men are similar to those in women. Thus, the TMP-SMX (Bactrim) is appropriate for empiric use in men, although 7-day regimens are recommended. Nitrofurantoin and beta-lactams should not be used in men with cystitis since they do not achieve reliable tissue concentrations and would be ineffective for occult prostatitis. Fluoroquinolones provide the best antimicrobial spectrum and prostatic penetration.

References: See page 208.

Acute Pyelonephritis

Urinary tract infections (UTIs) are common, especially in young children and sexually active women. UTI is defined either as a lower tract (acute cystitis) or upper tract (acute pyelonephritis) infection.

I. Clinical features

A. Acute uncomplicated pyelonephritis is suggested by flank pain, nausea/vomiting, fever (>38°C) and/or costovertebral angle tenderness. Frequency, dysuria, and suprapubic pain are found in the majority of patients whether infection is localized to the upper or lower tract.

B. Fever $\geq 37.8°C$ is strongly correlated with acute pyelonephritis. The examination should focus on temperature, abdomen, and costovertebral angle tenderness.

C. **Pelvic examination** may be indicated since pelvic inflammatory disease is a condition often mistaken for acute uncomplicated pyelonephritis. Pelvic examination does not need to be performed, however, in a woman with unilateral CVA pain and tenderness, fever, pyuria, and no vaginal symptoms.

Risk Factors for Occult Renal Infection or a Complicated Urinary Tract Infection	
Male sex	Functional or anatomic abnormality of the urinary tract
Elderly	Recent antimicrobial use
Presentation in emergency department	Symptoms for more than seven days at presentation
Hospital-acquired infection	Diabetes mellitus
Pregnancy	Immunosuppression
Indwelling urinary catheter	
Recent urinary tract instrumentation	
Childhood urinary tract infection	

II. Laboratory features

A. Pyuria is present in virtually all women with acute pyelonephritis; its absence strongly suggests an alternative diagnosis. Hematuria is common with urinary tract infection but not in urethritis or vaginitis. Most patients with acute pyelonephritis have leukocytosis and an elevated erythrocyte sedimentation rate and serum C-reactive protein.

B. Some patients with pyelonephritis may have colony counts of 10^3 to 10^4 CFU per mL. Blood cultures are positive in 10 to 20% of women with acute uncomplicated pyelonephritis.

C. A urinalysis should be performed to look for pyuria. White cell casts indicate a renal origin for the pyuria. Gram stain, usually performed on spun urine, may distinguish Gram negative from Gram positive infections. A pregnancy test should be performed if there is missed menses or lack of contraception.

D. Urine culture and antimicrobial susceptibility testing should be performed routinely in acute pyelonephritis.

E. Rapid methods for detection of bacteriuria, such as the nitrite test, should not be relied upon in the evaluation of patients with suspected pyelonephritis because tests lack adequate sensitivity for detection of "low count" urinary tract infection and common uropathogenic species. The nitrite test has a sensitivity of 35 to 80% and does not detect organisms unable to reduce nitrate to nitrite, such as enterococci and staphylococci.

F. Blood cultures are limited to those patients who warrant hospitalization.

III. **Treatment.** Microbiology of acute uncomplicated upper and lower urinary tract infection is rather limited with Escherichia coli accounting for 70 to 95% of infections and Staphylococcus saprophyticus 5 to 20%.

A. **Indications for admission to the hospital include:**
1. Inability to maintain oral hydration or take medications.
2. Patient noncompliance.
3. Uncertainty about the diagnosis.
4. Severe illness with high fevers, pain, and marked debility.
5. Outpatient therapy should generally be reserved for nonpregnant women with mild-to-moderate uncomplicated pyelonephritis who are compliant.

B. **Empiric antibiotic therapy**
1. Ampicillin and sulfonamides should not be used for empiric therapy because of the high rate of resistance. An increasing proportion of uropathogens demonstrate resistance to trimethoprim-sulfamethoxazole. In comparison, resistance to the fluoroquinolones and aminoglycosides is very low in uncomplicated UTIs.
2. **Oral agents.** In patients with acute uncomplicated pyelonephritis, an oral fluoroquinolone, such as ciprofloxacin (500 mg PO BID), levofloxacin (Levaquin [250 to 500 mg PO QD]), or gatifloxacin (Tequin [400 mg PO QD]), is recommended for outpatients as initial empiric treatment of infection caused by Gram negative bacilli. The newer fluoroquinolones, sparfloxacin, trovafloxacin and moxifloxacin, should be avoided because they may not achieve adequate concentrations in urine.
   a. Trimethoprim, trimethoprim-sulfamethoxazole or other agents can be used if the infecting strain is known to be susceptible. If enterococcus is suspected by the presence of small Gram positive cocci on Gram stain, amoxicillin (500 mg PO TID) should be added to the treatment regimen until the causative organism is identified.
   b. Cefixime (Suprax) and cefpodoxime proxetil (Vantin) also appear to be effective for the treatment of acute uncomplicated pyelonephritis. Cefixime is less effective against S. saprophyticus. Nitrofurantoin should not be used for the treatment of pyelonephritis since it does not achieve reliable tissue levels.

Parenteral Regimens for Empiric Treatment of Acute Uncomplicated Pyelonephritis	
Antibiotic, dose	**Interval**
Ceftriaxone (Rocephin), 1 g	q24h
Ciprofloxacin (Cipro), 200-400 mg	q12h

Antibiotic, dose	Interval
Levofloxacin (Levaquin), 250-500 mg	q24h
Ofloxacin (Floxin), 200-400 mg	q12 h
Gatifloxacin (Tequin), 400 mg	q24h
Gentamicin, 3-5 mg/kg (±ampicillin)	q24h
Gentamicin, 1 mg per kg (±ampicillin)	q8h
Ampicillin, 1-2 g (plus gentamicin)*	q6h
Aztreonam (Azactam), 1 g	q8-12h

*Recommended regimen if enterococcus suspected.

3. **Parenteral therapy.** For hospitalized patients, ceftriaxone (Rocephin [1 gram IV QD]) is recommended if enterococcus is not suspected. Aminoglycosides (3 to 5 mg/kg) given once daily provide a therapeutic advantage compared with beta lactams because of their marked and sustained concentration in renal tissue.
   a. Ciprofloxacin, ofloxacin, levofloxacin and gatifloxacin are also effective for the parenteral treatment of uncomplicated pyelonephritis but should be used orally if the patient is able to tolerate oral medications since the costs are lower and serum levels are equivalent.
   b. If enterococcus is suspected based upon the Gram stain, ampicillin (1 to 2 g IV Q6h) plus gentamicin (1.0 mg/kg IV Q8h) or piperacillin-tazobactam (3.375 g IV Q8h) are reasonable broad spectrum empiric choices. Once-daily dosing of aminoglycosides is not recommended for serious probable enterococcal infection since this regimen may not provide adequate synergy against the organism.
C. **Duration.** Patients with acute uncomplicated pyelonephritis can often be switched to oral therapy at 24 to 48 hours. Patients should be evaluated for complicated pyelonephritis if they fail to defervesce or if bacteremia persists. A 14-day regimen is recommended. In sicker patients, a longer duration of treatment may be required (14 to 21 days).
D. **Posttreatment follow-up cultures** in an asymptomatic patient are not indicated. In women whose pyelonephritis symptoms resolve but recur within two weeks, a repeat urine culture and antimicrobial susceptibility testing should be performed. If the initially infecting species is isolated again with the same susceptibility profile, a renal ultrasound or computed tomographic (CT) scan should be performed. Retreatment with a two-week regimen using another agent should be considered.
E. **Urologic evaluation**
   1. Routine urologic investigation of young healthy women with acute uncomplicated pyelonephritis is generally not recommended. Ultrasound or CT scan should be considered if the patient remains febrile or has not shown clinical improvement after 72 hours of treatment. CT scan or renal ultrasound should be performed after two recurrences of pyelonephritis.
IV. **Acute complicated pyelonephritis**
   A. **Clinical features.** In addition to flank pain, dysuria and fever, complicated urinary tract infections may also be associated with malaise, fatigue, nausea, or abdominal pain.

B. A urine Gram stain and culture should always be performed in patients with suspected complicated UTI. A colony count threshold of $>10^3$ CFU per mL should be used to diagnose symptomatic complicated infection except when urine cultures are obtained through a newly-inserted catheter in which case a level of $\geq 10^{(2)}$ CFU per mL is evidence of infection.

C. Microbiology. E. coli is still the predominant uropathogen, but other uropathogens, including Citrobacter sp, Enterobacter sp, Pseudomonas aeruginosa, enterococci, Staphylococcus aureus, and fungi account for a higher proportion of cases compared with uncomplicated urinary tract infections.

D. Treatment. Patients with complicated pyelonephritis, including pregnant women, should be managed as inpatients. Underlying anatomic (eg, stones, obstruction), functional (eg, neurogenic bladder), or metabolic (eg, poorly controlled diabetes) defects must be corrected.

  1. In contrast to uncomplicated UTI, S. aureus is relatively more likely to be found. For those patients with mild to moderate illness who can be treated with oral medication, a fluoroquinolone is the best choice for empiric therapy. Fluoroquinolones are comparable or superior to other broad spectrum regimens, including parenteral therapy. Sparfloxacin, trovafloxacin and moxifloxacin are not effective.

  2. Antimicrobial regimen can be modified when the infecting strain susceptibilities are known. Patients on parenteral regimens can be switched to oral treatment, generally a fluoroquinolone, after clinical improvement. Patients undergoing effective treatment with an antimicrobial to which the infecting pathogen is susceptible should have definite improvement within 24 to 48 hours and, if not, a repeat urine culture and imaging studies should be performed.

  3. At least 10 to 14 days of therapy is recommended. Urine culture should be repeated one to two weeks after the completion of therapy. Suppressive antibiotics may be considered with complicated pyelonephritis and a positive follow-up urine culture.

Parenteral Regimens for Empiric Treatment of Acute Complicated Pyelonephritis	
Antibiotic, dose	**Interval**
Cefepime (Maxipime) , 1 g	q12 hours
Ciprofloxacin (Cipro), 400 mg	q12 hours
Levofloxacin (Levaquin), 500 mg	q24 hours
Ofloxacin (Floxin), 400 mg	q12 hours
Gatifloxacin (Tequin), 400 mg	q24 hours
Gentamicin, 3-5 mg/kg (+ ampicillin)*	q24 hours
Gentamicin, 1 mg per kg (+ ampicillin)*	q8 hours
Ampicillin, 1-2 g (+ gentamicin)*	q6 hours
Ticarcillin-clavulante (Timentin), 3.2 g	q8 hours
Piperacilin-tazobactam (Zosyn), 3.375 g*	q6-8 hours
Imipenem-cilastatin, 250-500 mg	q6-8 hours
*Recommended regimen if enterococcus suspected	

References: See page 208.

Pubic Infections

I. Molluscum contagiosum

  A. This disease is produced by a virus of the pox virus family and is spread by sexual or close personal contact. Lesions are usually asymptomatic and multiple, with a central umbilication. Lesions can be spread by autoinoculation and last from 6 months to many years.

    B. **Diagnosis.** The characteristic appearance is adequate for diagnosis, but biopsy may be used to confirm the diagnosis.

    C. **Treatment.** Lesions are removed by sharp dermal curette, liquid nitrogen cryosurgery, or electrodesiccation.

II. **Pediculosis pubis (crabs)**

    A. Phthirus pubis is a blood sucking louse that is unable to survive more than 24 hours off the body. It is often transmitted sexually and is principally found on the pubic hairs. Diagnosis is confirmed by locating nits or adult lice on the hair shafts.

    B. **Treatment**

       1. **Permethrin cream (Elimite),** 5% is the most effective treatment; it is applied for 10 minutes and washed off.

       2. **Kwell shampoo,** lathered for at least 4 minutes, can also be used, but it is contraindicated in pregnancy or lactation.

       3. All contaminated clothing and linen should be laundered.

III. **Pubic scabies**

    A. This highly contagious infestation is caused by the Sarcoptes scabiei (0.2-0.4 mm in length). The infestation is transmitted by intimate contact or by contact with infested clothing. The female mite burrows into the skin, and after 1 month, severe pruritus develops. A multiform eruption may develop, characterized by papules, vesicles, pustules, urticarial wheals, and secondary infections on the hands, wrists, elbows, belt line, buttocks, genitalia, and outer feet.

    B. **Diagnosis** is confirmed by visualization of burrows and observation of parasites, eggs, larvae, or red fecal compactions under microscopy.

    C. **Treatment.** Permethrin 5% cream (Elimite) is massaged in from the neck down and remove by washing after 8 hours.

References: See page 208.

Pelvic Inflammatory Disease

Pelvic inflammatory disease (PID) is an acute infection of the upper genital tract structures in women, involving the uterus, oviducts, and ovaries. PID usually is a community-acquired infection initiated by a sexually transmitted agent. The estimated number of cases of PID in women 15 to 44 years of age in the United States was 168,837 in 2003.

I. **Clinical features**

    A. **Lower abdominal pain** is the cardinal presenting symptom in women with PID. The recent onset of pain that worsens during coitus or with jarring movement may be the only presenting symptom of PID; the onset of pain during or shortly after menses is particularly suggestive. The abdominal pain is usually bilateral and rarely of more than two weeks' duration.

    B. **Abnormal uterine bleeding** occurs in one-third or more of patients with PID. New vaginal discharge, urethritis, proctitis, fever, and chills can be associated signs. The presence of PID is less likely if symptoms referable to the bowel or urinary tract predominate.

    C. **Risk factors for sexually transmitted diseases:**

       1. Age less than 25 years

       2. Young age at first sex

       3. Nonbarrier contraception

       4. New, multiple, or symptomatic sexual partners

       5. Oral contraception

       6. Cervical ectopy

    D. **Factors that facilitate pelvic inflammatory disease:**

       1. Previous episode of PID

       2. Sex during menses

       3. Vaginal douching

       4. Bacterial vaginosis

       5. Intrauterine device

E. **Physical examination.** Only one-half of patients with PID have fever. Abdominal examination reveals diffuse tenderness greatest in the lower quadrants, which may or may not be symmetrical. Rebound tenderness and decreased bowel sounds are common. Marked tenderness in the right upper quadrant does not exclude PID, since 10% of these patients have perihepatitis (Fitz-Hugh Curtis syndrome).

F. **Pelvic examination.** Purulent endocervical discharge and/or acute cervical motion and adnexal tenderness with bimanual examination is strongly suggestive of PID. Significant lateralization of adnexal tenderness is uncommon in PID.

G. **Subclinical pelvic inflammatory disease.** Lower genital tract infection with gonorrhea, chlamydia, or bacterial vaginosis is a risk factor for subclinical PID, defined by the presence of neutrophils and plasma cells in endometrial tissue.

II. **Diagnostic considerations**

A. Laparoscopy is recommended for the following:
1. A sick patient with high suspicion of a competing diagnosis (appendicitis)
2. An acutely ill patient who has failed outpatient treatment for PID
3. Any patient not clearly improving after 72 hours of inpatient treatment for PID. Consent for laparotomy at the same procedure should be obtained in advance for these patients.

B. **Diagnostic criteria.** The index of suspicion for the clinical diagnosis of PID should be high, especially in adolescent women, even if they deny sexual activity. Empiric treatment is recommended for women with abdominal pain who have at least one of the following:
1. Cervical motion tenderness or uterine/adnexal tenderness
2. Oral temperature >101 F (>38.3 C)
3. Peripheral leukocytosis/left shift
4. Abnormal cervical or vaginal mucopurulent discharge
5. Presence of white blood cells (WBCs) on saline microscopy of vaginal secretions
6. Elevated erythrocyte sedimentation rate
7. Elevated C-reactive protein

III. **Differential diagnosis.** In addition to PID, the differential diagnosis of lower abdominal pain in a young woman includes the following conditions:

A. Gastrointestinal: Appendicitis, cholecystitis, constipation, gastroenteritis, inflammatory bowel disease

B. Renal: Cystitis, pyelonephritis, nephrolithiasis, urethritis

C. Obstetric/Gynecologic: Dysmenorrhea, ectopic pregnancy, intrauterine pregnancy complication, ovarian cyst, ovarian torsion, ovarian tumor.

Differential Diagnosis of Pelvic Inflammatory Disease	
Appendicitis	Irritable bowel syndrome
Ectopic pregnancy	Somatization
Hemorrhagic ovarian cyst	Gastroenteritis
Ovarian torsion	Cholecystitis
Endometriosis	Nephrolithiasis
Urinary tract Infection	

IV. **Diagnostic testing**

A. **Laboratory testing** for patients suspected of PID always begins with a pregnancy test to rule out ectopic pregnancy and complications of an intrauterine pregnancy. A urinalysis (preferably on a catheterized specimen) and a stool for occult blood should be obtained since abnormalities in either lessen the probability of PID. Although PID is usually an acute process, fewer than one-half of PID patients exhibit leukocytosis. A hematocrit of less than 0.30 makes PID less likely.

B. **Gram stain and microscopic examination** of vaginal discharge. If a cervical Gram stain is positive for Gram negative intracellular diplococci, the probability of PID greatly increases; if negative, it is of little use.

C. Increased white blood cells (WBC) in vaginal fluid is the most sensitive single laboratory test for PID (78% for $\geq$3 WBC per high power field. However, the specificity is only 39%.

D. **Recommended laboratory tests:**
1. Pregnancy test
2. Microscopic exam of vaginal discharge in saline
3. Complete blood counts
4. Nucleic acid amplification tests for chlamydia and gonococcus
5. Urinalysis
6. Fecal occult blood test
7. C-reactive protein (optional)
8. Ultrasounds are reserved for acutely ill patients with PID in whom a pelvic abscess is a consideration.

V. **Treatment and sequelae of pelvic inflammatory disease**

A. **Outpatient therapy.** The CDC recommends either oral ofloxacin (Floxin, 400 mg twice daily) or levofloxacin (Levaquin, 500 mg once daily) with or without metronidazole (Flagyl) 500 mg twice daily for 14 days. Metronidazole is added when anaerobic coverage is of concern. Beyond 48 hours of symptoms, the most frequent isolates are anaerobes.

B. An alternative is an initial single dose of ceftriaxone (Rocephin, 250 mg IM), cefoxitin (Mefoxin, 2 g IM plus probenecid 1 g orally), or another parenteral third-generation cephalosporin, followed by doxycycline (100 mg orally twice daily) with or without metronidazole for 14 days. The combination of amoxicillin-clavulanate and doxycycline is also an alternative that has achieved short-term clinical response. For patients younger than 18 years of age, one of the alternative regimens should be used since neither ofloxacin nor levofloxacin is approved for systemic use in this age group.

C. **For women younger than 18 years** treatment consists of an initial single dose of ceftriaxone (Rocephin, 250 mg IM) or cefoxitin (Mefoxin, 2 g IM plus probenecid 1 g orally), or another parenteral third-generation cephalosporin, followed by doxycycline (100 mg orally twice daily) with or without metronidazole for 14 days. For those who are unlikely to complete at least seven days of doxycycline, some providers suggest administration of azithromycin 1 g PO should be given at the time of parenteral administration of cephalosporin to ensure eradication of chlamydia.

D. **For women >18 years azithromycin (Zithromax)** 1 g PO should be given for Chlamydia coverage, and either cefixime (Suprax) 400 mg PO or ceftriaxone (Rocephin) 125 mg IM (for gonococcus coverage) given for one dose by directly observed therapy, followed by amoxicillin-clavulanate 875 mg PO twice daily for 7 to 10 days. For penicillin-allergic patients, a fluoroquinolone or spectinomycin may be used for initial single-dose gonococcus coverage, followed by doxycycline and metronidazole for 14 days.

E. Reevaluation two to three days after the initiation of therapy to assure accuracy of diagnosis and response to therapy is an extremely important aspect of outpatient treatment of PID.

F. **Inpatient therapy.** The CDC suggest either of the following regimens:
1. Cefotetan (Cefotan, 2 g IV every12h) or cefoxitin (Mefoxin, 2 g IV every 6h) plus doxycycline (100 mg IV or PO every 12h), or
2. Clindamycin (900 mg IV every 8h) plus gentamicin loading dose (2 mg/kg of body weight) followed by a maintenance dose (1.5 mg/kg) every 8 hours. Single daily dosing of gentamicin may be substituted.

3. **Alternative regimens:**
   a. Ofloxacin (Floxin, 400 mg IV every12h) or levofloxacin (Levoquin, 500 mg IV daily) with or without metronidazole (Flagyl, 500 mg IV every 8h), or
   b. Ampicillin-sulbactam (Unasyn, 3 g IV every 6h) plus doxycycline (100 mg IV or PO every12h).
   c. Ofloxacin has been studied as monotherapy for the treatment of PID; however, due to concerns regarding its lack of activity against anaerobic flora, some clinicians prefer to also add metronidazole. Ampicillin-sulbactam plus oral doxycycline is effective coverage against Chlamydia trachomatis, Neisseria gonorrhoeae, and anaerobes.
4. Parenteral administration of antibiotics should be continued for 24 hours after a clear clinical response, followed by doxycycline (100 mg PO BID) or clindamycin (450 mg PO QID) for a total of 14 days.

G. **Recommended regimens:**
   1. **Levofloxacin** (Levoquin, 500 mg IV Q24h) plus metronidazole (500 mg IV Q8h)
   2. A broad spectrum cephalosporin plus doxycycline with or without metronidazole
   3. Ertapenem (Invanz, 1 g IV Q24h)

H. For patients younger than 18 years of age, the second regimen should be used since levofloxacin is not approved for use in this age group when other effective alternatives are available.

I. Some providers prescribe azithromycin (Zithromax, 1 g PO once) as soon as the patient is tolerating oral intake if the patient is unlikely to comply with doxycycline administration. Parenteral therapy should continue until the pelvic tenderness is absent (two to five days).

J. **Treatment for PID** must be accompanied by a discussion of sexually transmitted infections, partner treatment, and future safe sex practices. Male sex partners of women with PID should be examined and empirically treated if they had sexual contact during the preceding 60 days. Other important components of the evaluation include:
   1. Serology for human immunodeficiency virus (HIV)
   2. Papanicolaou smear
   3. Hepatitis B surface antigen determination and initiation of the vaccine series for patients who are antigen negative and unvaccinated
   4. Hepatitis C virus serology
   5. Serologic tests for syphilis

References: See page 208.

Genital Chlamydia Trachomatis Infections

Chlamydia trachomatis is the most common sexually transmitted genital infection. Infants born to mothers through an infected birth canal can develop conjunctivitis and pneumonia. These syndromes are caused by the C. trachomatis serovars B and D through K. The L serovars cause lymphogranuloma venereum (LGV), a genital ulcer syndrome. Chlamydia trachomatis serovars A to C cause endemic trachoma, a common ocular infection in the developing world.

I. **Microbiology and epidemiology**
   A. C. trachomatis is a small gram-negative bacterium and an obligate intracellular parasite.
   B. Chlamydia cannot be cultured on artificial media; tissue culture has been required. Rapid screening tests are now available.
   C. 4,000,000 cases of C. trachomatis infection occur annually. C. trachomatis and Neisseria gonorrhoeae cause similar clinical syndromes, but chlamydia infections tend to have fewer acute symptoms and more significant long-term complications.

    D. Prevalence. The rates of chlamydia are highest in adolescent women. Between 18 and 26 years of age, the prevalence of chlamydial infection is 4.2%. The highest rates are in African American women (14%) and are higher in women than men.

    E. Risk factors for Chlamydia trachomatis infection:

       1. Adolescents and young adults

       2. Multiple sex partners or a partner with other partners during the last three months or a recent new sex partner

       3. Inconsistent use of barrier contraceptives

       4. Clinical evidence of mucopurulent cervicitis

       5. Cervical ectopy

       6. Unmarried status

       7. History of prior sexually transmitted disease

       8. Lower socioeconomic class or education not beyond high school.

II. Clinical manifestations

    A. The majority of women with C. trachomatis infection are asymptomatic; however, cervicitis or pelvic inflammatory disease may occur.

    B. Cervicitis. Cervical infection is the most common chlamydial syndrome in women. More than 50% of these women are asymptomatic. Vaginal discharge, poorly differentiated abdominal pain, or lower abdominal pain are the most frequent symptoms.

    C. Physical examination is often unremarkable, mucopurulent cervical discharge, cervical friability, cervical edema, and endocervical ulcers may be seen.

    D. Perihepatitis (Fitzhugh-Curtis syndrome). Patients with chlamydia infection occasionally develop perihepatitis, an inflammation of the liver capsule and adjacent peritoneal surfaces. Perihepatitis is more commonly seen in PID, occurring in 5% of cases.

    E. Pelvic inflammatory disease. 30% of women with chlamydia infection will develop PID if left untreated. While PID caused by N. gonorrhoeae infection may be more acutely symptomatic, PID due to C. trachomatis tends to cause higher rates of infertility.

    F. Pregnancy. Untreated chlamydia infection can increase the risk for premature rupture of the membranes and low birth weight. If the mother is untreated, 20 to 50% of newborns will develop conjunctivitis, and 10 to 20% will develop pneumonia.

III. Diagnosis

    A. Nucleic acid amplification (NAAT) uses polymerase chain reaction (PCR). These sensitive and specific tests have replaced poorly standardized cell culture methods as the "gold standard."

       1. Another advantage of NAATs is the ability to perform testing on urine as well as urethral specimens. Since urine collection is noninvasive, it is a preferred method.

       2. The PCR assay has a sensitivity and specificity of 83 and 99.5% for urine samples and 86 and 99.6% for cervical samples.

    B. Antigen detection requires a swab from the cervix or urethra. The sensitivity of this method is 80 to 95% compared to culture.

IV. Chlamydia screening

    A. Clinical practice guidelines strongly recommend routine chlamydia screening for sexually-active women below the age of 25.

V. Treatment. Chlamydiae are susceptible to the tetracyclines and the macrolides. Treatment efficacy with recommended regimens is >95%.

    A. Azithromycin (Zithromax, 1 g PO as a single dose) or doxycycline (100 mg PO BID for 7 days) are the two recommended regimens.

    B. Alternative regimens include seven days of erythromycin base (500 mg PO QID), erythromycin ethylsuccinate (800 mg PO), ofloxacin (300 mg PO BID), or levofloxacin (500 mg PO QD). Erythromycin is associated with significant gastrointestinal side effects; ofloxacin and levofloxacin are expensive alternatives.

Treatment of chlamydia trachomatis infection and related syndromes
Urethritis, cervicitis, conjunctivitis, or proctitis
Azithromycin (Zithromax) 1 g oral once **OR** Doxycycline 100 mg oral twice daily for seven days **Alternatives** Ofloxacin (Floxin) 300 mg oral twice daily for seven days Levofloxacin (Levaquin) 500 mg oral daily for seven days Erythromycin 500 mg oral four times daily for seven days
Infection in pregnancy
Azithromycin (Zithromax) 1 g oral once **OR** Amoxicillin 500 mg oral three times daily for seven days Alternatives Erythromycin 500 mg oral four times daily for seven days
Neonatal ophthalmia or pneumonia
Azithromycin 20 mg/kg oral once daily for three days Alternatives Erythromycin 12.5 mg/kg oral four times daily for 14 days§
Lymphogranuloma venereum
Doxycycline 100 mg oral twice daily for 21 days Alternatives Erythromycin 500 mg oral four times daily for 21 days

C. **Adjunctive measures:**
1. Presumptive treatment of partners
2. Evaluation for other STDs (syphilis serology, gonococcal testing)
3. HIV counseling and testing
4. Safer-sex counseling and condom provision
5. Contraception provision or referral
6. Test of cure. Testing for C. trachomatis following treatment with azithromycin or doxycycline is not recommended. Exceptions include:
   a. Patients with persisting symptoms or
   b. Those in whom compliance with the treatment regimen is suspected.
   c. Pregnant females
7. If a test for cure is performed, this should be done more than three weeks after the completion of therapy.
8. Repeat screening should be considered within the first three to four months after therapy is completed or at least when the patient has her next encounter with the healthcare system within the first 12 months because patients who have the disease once are at a higher risk for acquiring it again.

References: See page 208.

Vaginitis

Approximately 8-18% of women report an episode of vaginal symptoms each year. The etiology of vaginal complaints includes infection of the vagina, cervix, and upper genital tract, chemicals or irritants (eg, spermicides or douching), hormone deficiency, and rarely systemic diseases.

I. Clinical evaluation

A. Symptoms of vaginitis include vaginal discharge, pruritus, irritation, soreness, odor, dyspareunia and dysuria. Dyspareunia is a common feature of atrophic vaginitis. Abdominal pain is suggestive of pelvic inflammatory disease and suprapubic pain is suggestive of cystitis.

B. A new sexual partner increases the risk of acquiring sexually transmitted diseases, such as trichomonas, chlamydia, or Neisseria gonorrheae. Trichomoniasis often occurs during or immediately after the menstrual period; candida vulvovaginitis often occurs during the premenstrual period.

C. Antibiotics and high-estrogen oral contraceptive pills may predispose to candida vulvovaginitis; increased physiologic discharge can occur with oral contraceptives; pruritus unresponsive to antifungal agents suggests vulvar dermatitis.

II. Physical examination

A. The vulva usually appears normal in bacterial vaginosis. Erythema, edema, or fissure formation suggest candidiasis, trichomoniasis, or dermatitis.

B. Trichomonas is associated with a purulent discharge; candidiasis is associated with a thick, adherent, "cottage cheese-like" discharge; and bacterial vaginosis is associated with a thin, homogeneous, "fishy smelling" discharge. The cervix in women with cervicitis is usually erythematous and friable, with a mucopurulent discharge.

C. Abdominal or cervical motion tenderness is suggestive of PID.

III. Diagnostic studies

A. **Vaginal pH.** The pH of the normal vaginal secretions is 4.0 to 4.5. A pH above 4.5 suggests bacterial vaginosis or trichomoniasis (pH 5 to 6), and helps to exclude candida vulvovaginitis (pH 4 to 4.5).

B. **Saline microscopy** should look for candidal buds or hyphae, motile trichomonads, epithelial cells studded with adherent coccobacilli (clue cells), and polymorphonuclear cells (PMNs). The addition of 10% potassium hydroxide to the wet mount is helpful in diagnosing candida vaginitis. Culture for candida and trichomonas may be useful if microscopy is negative.

C. **Cervical culture.** A diagnosis of cervicitis, typically due to Neisseria gonorrhoeae or Chlamydia trachomatis, must always be considered in women with purulent vaginal discharge. The presence of high-risk behavior or any sexually transmitted disease requires screening for HIV, hepatitis B, and other STDs.

Clinical Manifestations of Vaginitis	
Candidal Vaginitis	Nonmalodorous, thick, white, "cottage cheese-like" discharge that adheres to vaginal walls Hyphal forms or budding yeast cells on wet-mount Pruritus Normal pH (<4.5)
Bacterial Vaginosis	Thin, dark or dull grey, homogeneous, malodorous discharge that adheres to the vaginal walls Elevated pH level (>4.5) Positive KOH (whiff test) Clue cells on wet-mount microscopic evaluation

Trichomonas Vaginalis	Copious, yellow-gray or green, homogeneous or frothy, malodorous discharge Elevated pH level (>4.5) Mobile, flagellated organisms and leukocytes on wet-mount microscopic evaluation Vulvovaginal irritation, dysuria
Atrophic Vaginitis	Vaginal dryness or burning

IV. Bacterial vaginosis

A. Incidence. Bacterial vaginosis is the most common cause of vaginitis in women of childbearing age, with prevalence of 5-60%.

B. Microbiology and risk factors. Bacterial vaginosis represents a change in vaginal flora characterized by a reduction of lactobacilli and an increase of Gardnerella vaginalis, Mobiluncus species, Mycoplasma hominis, anaerobic gram-negative rods, and Peptostreptococcus species. Risk factors for bacterial vaginosis include multiple or new sexual partners, early age of first coitus, douching, cigarette smoking, and use of an intrauterine contraceptive device.

C. Clinical features. Symptoms include a "fishy smelling" discharge that is more noticeable after unprotected intercourse. The discharge is off-white, thin, and homogeneous. Pruritus and inflammation are absent.

D. Complications
   1. Pregnant women appear to be at higher risk of preterm delivery.
   2. Bacterial vaginosis may cause plasma-cell endometritis, postpartum fever, post-hysterectomy vaginal-cuff cellulitis, and postabortal infection.
   3. Bacterial vaginosis is a risk factor for HIV acquisition and transmission.

E. Diagnosis. Three of the four criteria listed below are necessary for diagnosis.
   1. Homogeneous, grayish-white discharge
   2. Vaginal pH >4.5
   3. Positive whiff-amine test, defined as the presence of a fishy odor when 10% KOH is added to vaginal discharge samples
   4. Clue cells on saline wet mount (epithelial cells studded with coccobacilli)

F. Therapy. Treatment is indicated in women with symptomatic infection and those with asymptomatic infection prior to abortion or hysterectomy.
   1. Metronidazole or clindamycin administered either orally or intravaginally will result in a high rate of clinical cure (70-80%). Oral medication is more convenient.
   2. The oral regimen is 500 mg twice daily for 7 days. Topical vaginal therapy with 0.75% metronidazole gel (MetroGel, 5 g once daily for 5 days) is as effective as oral metronidazole.
   3. Single-dose therapy with 2 g of metronidazole achieves a similar immediate rate of clinical response.
   4. Side effects of metronidazole include a metallic taste, nausea, a disulfiram-like effect with alcohol, interaction with warfarin, and peripheral neuropathy.

G. Relapse
   1. Approximately 30% of patients have a recurrence within three months. Recurrence usually reflects a failure to eradicate the offending organisms. Management of symptomatic relapse includes prolonged therapy for 10 to 14 days.
   2. Most women with a history of recurrent infection benefit from suppressive therapy with metronidazole gel 0.75% for 10 days, followed by twice-weekly applications for three to six months.

V. Candida vulvovaginitis

A. Incidence. Candida vulvovaginitis accounts for one-third of vaginitis. Up to 75% of women report having had at least one episode of candidiasis.

The condition is rare before menarche. It is less common in postmenopausal women, unless they are taking estrogen replacement therapy.
B. Microbiology and risk factors. Candida albicans is responsible for 80-92% of vulvovaginal candidiasis.
  1. **Antibiotics.** A minority of women are prone to vulvovaginal candidiasis while taking antibiotics.
  2. **Intrauterine devices** have been associated with vulvovaginal candidiasis.
  3. **Pregnancy.** Symptomatic infection is more common in pregnancy.
C. Clinical features. Vulvar pruritus is the dominant feature. Women may also complain of dysuria (external rather than urethral), soreness, irritation, and dyspareunia. There is often little or no discharge. Physical examination often reveals erythema of the vulva and vaginal mucosa. The discharge is thick, adherent, and "cottage cheese-like."
D. Diagnosis
  1. The vaginal pH is typically 4 to 4.5, which distinguishes candidiasis from Trichomonas or bacterial vaginosis. The diagnosis is confirmed by finding the organism on a wet mount; adding 10% potassium hydroxide facilitates recognition of budding yeast and hyphae. Microscopy is negative in 50% of patients with vulvovaginal candidiasis.
  2. Empiric therapy is often considered in women with typical clinical features, a normal vaginal pH, and no other pathogens visible on microscopy. Culture should be performed in patients with persistent or recurrent symptoms.
E. Therapy
  1. Women with mild infection usually respond to treatment within a couple of days. More severe infections require a longer course of therapy and may take up to 14 days to fully resolve.
  2. **Uncomplicated infection.** Both oral and topical antimycotic drugs achieve comparable clinical cure rates that are in excess of 80%.
  3. Oral azole agents are more convenient. Side effects of single-dose fluconazole (150 mg) tend to be mild and infrequent, including gastrointestinal intolerance, headache, and rash.

Treatment regimens for yeast vaginitis*

1-day regimens
Clotrimazole vaginal tablets (Mycelex G), 500 mg hs**
Fluconazole tablets (Diflucan), 150 mg PO
Itraconazole capsules (Sporanox), 200 mg PO bid
Tioconazole 6.5% vaginal ointment (Vagistat-1), 4.6 g hs** [5 g]

3-day regimens
Butoconazole nitrate 2% vaginal cream (Femstat 3), 5 g hs [28 g]
Clotrimazole vaginal inserts (Gyne-Lotrimin 3), 200 mg hs**
Miconazole vaginal suppositories (Monistat 3), 200 mg hs**
Terconazole 0.8% vaginal cream (Terazol 3), 5 g hs
Terconazole vaginal suppositories (Terazol 3), 80 mg hs
Itraconazole capsules (Sporanox), 200 mg PO qd

5-day regimen
Ketoconazole tablets (Nizoral), 400 mg PO bid

7-day regimens
Clotrimazole 1% cream (Gyne-Lotrimin, Mycelex-7, Sweet'n Fresh Clotrimazole 7), 5 g hs**
Clotrimazole vaginal tablets (Gyne-Lotrimin, Mycelex-7, Sweet'n Fresh Clotrimazole-7), 100 mg hs**
Miconazole 2% vaginal cream (Femizol-M, Monistat 7), 5 g hs**
Miconazole vaginal suppositories (Monistat 7), 100 mg hs**
Terconazole 0.4% vaginal cream (Terazol 7), 5 g hs

14-day regimens
Nystatin vaginal tablets (Mycostatin), 100,000 U hs

*Suppositories can be used if inflammation is predominantly vaginal; creams if vulvar; a combination if both. Cream-suppository combination packs available: clotrimazole (Gyne-Lotrimin, Mycelex); miconazole (Monistat, M-Zole). Use 1-day or 3-day regimen if compliance is an issue. Miconazole nitrate may be used during pregnancy.

**Nonprescription formulation. If nonprescription therapies fail, use terconazole 0.4% cream or 80-mg suppositories at bedtime for 7 days.

4. **Complicated infections.** Factors that predispose to complicated infection include uncontrolled diabetes, immunosuppression, and a history of recurrent vulvovaginal candidiasis. Women with severe inflammation or complicated infection require seven to 14 days of topical therapy or two doses of oral therapy 72 hours apart.

Management options for complicated or recurrent yeast vaginitis

Extend any 7-day regimen to 10 to 14 days
Eliminate use of nylon or tight-fitting clothing
Consider discontinuing oral contraceptives
Consider eating 8 oz yogurt (with Lactobacillus acidophilus culture) per day
Improve glycemic control in diabetic patients
For long-term suppression of recurrent vaginitis, use ketoconazole, 100 mg (½ of 200-mg tablet) qd for 6 months

5. **Partner treatment** is not necessary since this is not a primary route of transmission.
6. **Pregnancy.** Topical azoles applied for seven days are recommended for treatment during pregnancy.

VI. **Trichomoniasis**
A. Trichomoniasis, the third most common cause of vaginitis, is caused by the flagellated protozoan, Trichomonas vaginalis. The disorder is virtually always sexually transmitted.
B. **Clinical features.** Trichomoniasis in women ranges from an asymptomatic state to a severe, acute, inflammatory disease. Signs and symptoms include a purulent, malodorous, thin discharge (70%) with associated burning, pruritus, dysuria, and dyspareunia. Physical examination reveals erythema of the vulva and vaginal mucosa; the classic green-yellow frothy discharge is observed in 10-30%. Punctate hemorrhages may be visible on the vagina and cervix in 2%.
C. **Complications.** Infection is associated with premature rupture of the membranes and prematurity; however, treatment of asymptomatic infection has not been shown to reduce these complications. Trichomoniasis is a risk factor for development of post-hysterectomy cellulitis. The infection facilitates transmission of the human immunodeficiency virus.
D. **Diagnosis**
1. The presence of motile trichomonads on wet mount is diagnostic of infection, but this occurs in only 50-70% of cases. Other findings include an elevated vaginal pH (>4.5) and an increase in polymorphonuclear leukocytes on saline microscopy.
E. **Culture on Diamond's medium** has a high sensitivity (95%) and specificity (>95%) and should be considered in patients with elevated vaginal pH, increased numbers of polymorphonuclear leukocytes and an absence of motile trichomonads and clue cells on wet mount.
F. **The OSOM Trichomonas Rapid Test for Trichomonas** antigens has a sensitivity of 88.3% and specificity of 98.8%. Results can be read in 10 minutes. The Affirm VP III Microbial Identification System (Becton Dickinson) test uses a nucleic acid probe and is read in 45 minutes.

G. **Cervical cytology.** Trichomonads are sometimes reported on conventional Papanicolaou (Pap) smears. Conventional Pap smears are
inadequate for diagnosis of trichomoniasis because this technique has
a sensitivity of only 60 to 70% and false positive results are common (at
least 8%). Asymptomatic women with trichomonads identified on
conventional Pap smear should be evaluated by wet mount and should
not be treated until the diagnosis is confirmed.

H. Treatment of asymptomatic women with trichomonads noted on liquid-
based cervical cytology is appropriate.

VII. **Treatment of Trichomonas vaginitis**

A. **Nonpregnant women**

1. The 5-nitroimidazole drugs (metronidazole or tinidazole) are the only
   class of drugs that provide curative therapy of trichomoniasis. Cure
   rates are 90 to 95%.
2. Treatment consists of a single oral dose of 2 grams (four 500 mg
   tablets) of either tinidazole (Fasigyn) or metronidazole (Flagyl). Cure
   rates with tinidazole are comparable to those of metronidazole, but
   better tolerated.
3. Similar cure rates are obtained with single and multiple dose regimens (82 to 88%). Side effects (eg, nausea, vomiting, headache,
   metallic taste, dizziness) appear to be dose related and occur less
   frequently with the lower doses of multiple dose, prolonged therapy
   (eg, metronidazole 500 mg twice daily for seven days. There is no
   multiple dose regimen for tinidazole).
4. Oral is preferred to vaginal therapy since systemic administration
   achieves therapeutic drug levels in the urethra and periurethral
   glands.
5. Patients should be advised to not consume alcohol for 24 hours after
   metronidazole treatment and 72 hours after tinidazole treatment
   because of the possibility of a disulfiram-like (Antabuse effect)
   reaction.
6. Follow-up is unnecessary for women who become asymptomatic
   after treatment.

B. **Male partners.** T vaginalis infection in men is often asymptomatic and
transient (spontaneous resolution within 10 days). Symptoms, when
present, consist of a clear or mucopurulent urethral discharge and/or
dysuria. Complications include prostatitis, balanoposthitis, epididymitis,
and infertility. Maximal cure rates are achieved when sexual partners
are treated simultaneously with the affected woman Neither partner
should resume intercourse until both partners have completed treatment, otherwise reinfection can occur.

C. **Pregnancy**

1. Metronidazole is the drug of choice for treatment of symptomatic
   trichomoniasis in pregnancy. Meta-analysis has not found any
   relationship between metronidazole exposure during the first trimester of pregnancy and birth defects. The Centers for Disease Control
   and Prevention no longer discourage the use of metronidazole in the
   first trimester.
2. In pregnant women, some clinicians prefer metronidazole 500 mg
   twice daily for five to seven days to the 2 g single dose regimen
   because of the lower frequency of side effects.
3. Asymptomatic infections during pregnancy should not be treated
   because treatment does not prevent, and may even increase, the
   risk of preterm delivery.

...easures
...ole (Fasigyn) 2 g PO in a single dose. Cure rates with tinidazole are compa-
...o those of metronidazole, but better tolerated.
Me... nidazole (Flagyl, Protostat), 2 g PO in a single dose, or metronidazole, 500 mg
PO bid X 7 days, or metronidazole, 375 mg PO bid X 7 days
Treat male sexual partners

Measures for treatment failure
Treatment sexual contacts
Re-treat with tinazole 2 gm PO or metronidazole, 500 mg PO bid X 7 days
If infection persists, confirm with culture and re-treat with metronidazole,
2-4 g PO qd X 3-10 days

VIII. Other causes of vaginitis and vaginal discharge
A. Atrophic vaginitis
1. Reduced endogenous estrogen causes thinning of the vaginal epithelium. Symptoms include vaginal soreness, postcoital burning, dyspareunia, and spotting. The vaginal mucosa is thin with diffuse erythema, occasional petechiae or ecchymoses, and few or no vaginal folds. There may be a serosanguineous or watery discharge with a pH of 5.0-7.0.
2. Treatment consists of topical vaginal estrogen. **Vaginal ring estradiol (Estring)**, a silastic ring impregnated with estradiol, is the preferred means of delivering estrogen to the vagina. The silastic ring delivers 6 to 9 µg of estradiol to the vagina daily. The rings are changed once every three months. Concomitant progestin therapy is not necessary.
3. **Conjugated estrogens (Premarin)**, 0.5 gm of cream, or one-eighth of an applicatorful daily into the vagina for three weeks, followed by twice weekly thereafter is also effective. Concomitant progestin therapy is not necessary.
4. **Estrace cream (estradiol)** can also by given by vaginal applicator at a dose of one-eighth of an applicator or 0.5 g (which contains 50 µg of estradiol) daily into the vagina for three weeks, followed by twice weekly thereafter. Concomitant progestin therapy is not necessary.
5. **Oral estrogen (Premarin)** 0.3 mg qd should also provide relief.
B. Desquamative inflammatory vaginitis
1. Chronic purulent vaginitis usually occurs perimenopausally, with diffuse exudative vaginitis, massive vaginal-cell exfoliation, purulent vaginal discharge, and occasional vaginal and cervical spotted rash.
2. Laboratory findings included an elevated pH, increased numbers of parabasal cells, the absence of gram-positive bacilli and their replacement by gram-positive cocci on Gram staining. Clindamycin 2% cream is usually effective.
C. Noninfectious vaginitis and vulvitis
1. Noninfectious causes of vaginitis include irritants (eg, minipads, spermicides, povidone-iodine, topical antimycotic drugs, soaps and perfumes) and contact dermatitis (eg, latex condoms and antimycotic creams).
2. Typical symptoms include pruritus, irritation, burning, soreness, and variable discharge. The diagnosis should be suspected in symptomatic women who do not have an otherwise apparent infectious cause.
3. Management of noninfectious vaginitis includes identifying and eliminating the offending agent. Sodium bicarbonate sitz baths and topical vegetable oils. Topical corticosteroids are not recommended.

References: See page 208.

Trichomonas Vaginitis

Trichomonas vaginalis is the causative agent of trichomoniasis, accounting for 35% of vaginitis. The prevalence of trichomoniasis in black, white, and Mexican-American women is 13.5, 1.2, and 1.5%, respectively.

I. Microbiology and risk factors
   A. Trichomonas is a flagellated protozoan, which may be found in the vagina, urethra, paraurethral glands, and Bartholins and Skene's glands.
   B. Trichomoniasis is virtually always sexually transmitted, although survival on fomites has been reported. It is associated with a high prevalence of coinfection with other sexually transmitted diseases.

II. Clinical features
   A. Trichomoniasis in women ranges from an asymptomatic carrier state to a severe, acute, inflammatory disease.
   B. **Signs and symptoms** include a purulent, malodorous, thin discharge (70% of cases) with burning, pruritus, dysuria, frequency, and dyspareunia. Postcoital bleeding can occur. The urethra is also infected in the majority of women.
   C. **Physical examination** often reveals erythema of the vulva and vaginal mucosa; green-yellow frothy discharge is observed in 10 to 30%. Punctate hemorrhages may be visible on the vagina and cervix ("strawberry cervix") in 2%.

Clinical Features of Vaginitis

Variable	Normal	Vulvovaginal candidiasis	Bacterial vaginosis	Trichomoniasis
Symptoms	None	Pruritus, soreness, change in discharge, dyspareunia	Malodorous discharge, no dyspareunia	Malodorous, purulent discharge, dyspareunia
Signs	-	Vulvar erythema, edema, fissure	Adherent discharge	Purulent discharge, vulvovaginal erythema
pH	4.0-4.5	4.0-4.5	>4.5	5.0-6.0
Saline microscopy	PMN:EC ratio <1; rods dominate; squames +++	PMN:EC ratio <1; rods dominate; squames +++; pseudohyphae (about 40%)	PMN:EC <1; loss of rods; increased cocccobacilli; clue cells (>90%)	PMN ++++; mixed flora; motile trichomonads (60%)
10% potassium hydroxide examination	Negative	Pseudohyphae (about 70%)	Negative	Negative
Miscellaneous	-	Culture if microscopy negative	Culture of no value	Culture if microscopy negative

Vari-able	Nor-mal	Vulvovaginal candidiasis	Bacterial vaginosis	Trichomoniasis
Differ-ential diag-nosis	Physi-ologic leukor-rhea	Contact irritant or allergic vulvitis, chemi-cal irritation, focal vulvitis (vulvodynia)		Purulent vaginitis, desquamative inflamma-tory vaginitis, atrophic vaginitis plus secondary infection, erosive lichen planus

III. Complications

A. Trichomoniasis is a risk factor for post-hysterectomy cellulitis, tubal infertility, and cervical neoplasia. Infection facilitates transmission of the human immunodeficiency virus (HIV).

B. **Trichomoniasis in pregnancy** is associated with premature rupture of the membranes and preterm delivery; however, treatment of asymptomatic infection has not been shown to reduce these compli-cations.

IV. Diagnosis

A. **Microscopy and pH.** The presence of motile trichomonads on wet mount is diagnostic of infection, but this occurs in only 50 to 70% of cases. Other findings include an elevated vaginal pH (>4.5) and an increase in polymorphonuclear leukocytes.

B. **Culture on Diamond's medium** has a high sensitivity (95%) and specificity (>95%) and should be considered in patients with elevated vaginal pH, increased numbers of polymorphonuclear leukocytes and an absence of motile trichomonads and clue cells on wet mount.

C. **OSOM Trichomonas Rapid Test for Trichomonas antigens** has a sensitivity of 88.3% and specificity of 98.8%. Results can be read in 10 minutes. The Affirm VP III Microbial Identification System (Becton Dickinson) test uses a nucleic acid probe and is read in 45 minutes.

D. **Cervical cytology.** Trichomonads are sometimes reported on Papanicolaou (Pap) smears. Pap smears are inadequate for diagno-sis of trichomoniasis because this technique has a sensitivity of only 60 to 70% and false positive results are common (at least 8%). Asymptomatic women with trichomonads identified on conventional Pap smear should be evaluated by wet mount and should not be treated until the diagnosis is confirmed.

E. Treatment of asymptomatic women with trichomonads noted on liquid-based cervical cytology is appropriate.

V. Treatment of Trichomonas vaginitis

A. **Nonpregnant women**

1. The 5-nitroimidazole drugs (metronidazole or tinidazole) are the only class of drugs that provide curative therapy of trichomoniasis. Cure rates are 90 to 95%.

2. Treatment consists of a single oral dose of 2 grams (four 500 mg tablets) of either tinidazole or metronidazole. Cure rates with tinidazole are comparable to those of metronidazole, but better tolerated.

3. Similar cure rates are obtained with single and multiple dose regimens (82 to 88%). Side effects (eg, nausea, vomiting, head-ache, metallic taste, dizziness) appear to be dose related and occur less frequently with the lower doses of multiple dose, pro-longed therapy (eg, metronidazole 500 mg twice daily for seven days. There is no multiple dose regimen for tinidazole).

4. Oral is preferred to vaginal therapy since systemic administration achieves therapeutic drug levels in the urethra and periurethral glands.

5. Patients should be advised to not consume alcohol for 24 hours after metronidazole treatment and 72 hours after tinidazole treat-ment because of the possibility of a disulfiram-like (Antabuse effect) reaction.

6. Follow-up is unnecessary for women who become asymptomatic after treatment.

B. Male partners. T vaginalis infection in men is often asymptomatic and transient. Symptoms, when present, consist of a clear or mucopurulent urethral discharge and/or dysuria. Complications include prostatitis, balanoposthitis, epididymitis, and infertility. Maximal cure rates are achieved when sexual partners are treated simultaneously with the affected woman. Neither partner should resume intercourse until both partners have completed treatment

C. Pregnancy

1. Metronidazole is the drug of choice for treatment of symptomatic trichomoniasis in pregnancy.

2. In pregnant women, some clinicians prefer metronidazole 500 mg twice daily for five to seven days to the 2 g single dose regimen because of the lower frequency of side effects.

3. Asymptomatic infections during pregnancy should not be treated because treatment does not prevent, and may even increase, the risk of preterm delivery.

References: See page 208.

Gynecologic Oncology

Cervical Cancer

Invasive cervical carcinoma is the third most common cancer in the United States. The International Federation of Gynecology and Obstetrics (FIGO) recently revised its staging criteria. Survival rates for women with cervical cancer improve when radiotherapy is combined with cisplatin-based chemotherapy.

I. **Clinical evaluation**
   A. Human papillomavirus is the most important factor contributing to the development of cervical intraepithelial neoplasia and cervical cancer. Other epidemiologic risk factors associated with cervical intraepithelial neoplasia and cervical cancer include history of sexual intercourse at an early age, multiple sexual partners, sexually transmitted diseases (including chlamydia), and smoking. Additional risk factors include a male partner or partners who have had multiple sexual partners; previous history of squamous dysplasias of the cervix, vagina, or vulva; and immunosuppression.
   B. The signs and symptoms of early cervical carcinoma include watery vaginal discharge, intermittent spotting, and postcoital bleeding. Diagnosis often can be made with cytologic screening, colposcopically directed biopsy, or biopsy of a gross or palpable lesion. In cases of suspected microinvasion and early-stage cervical carcinoma, cone biopsy of the cervix is indicated to evaluate the possibility of invasion or to define the depth and extent of microinvasion. Cold knife cone biopsy provides the most accurate evaluation of the margins.
   C. **Histology.** The two major histologic types of invasive cervical carcinomas are squamous cell carcinomas and adenocarcinomas. Squamous cell carcinomas comprise 80% of cases, and adenocarcinoma or adenosquamous carcinoma comprise approximately 15%.
II. **Staging of cervical cancer**
   A. Histologic confirmation of invasive cervical cancer should be followed by a careful staging evaluation.
   B. **Physical examination.** The cervix and entire vagina should be carefully inspected and palpated to identify overt tumors or subepithelial vaginal extension. Rectovaginal examination permits the best clinical assessment of tumor size and parametrial involvement. Palpation of the right upper quadrant and inguinal and supraclavicular lymph nodes is important to screen for metastatic disease.
   C. **Laboratory studies.** Laboratory studies should include a complete blood count and renal and liver function tests.

Pretreatment Assessment of Women with Histologic Diagnosis of Cervical Cancer

History
Physical examination
Complete blood count, blood urea nitrogen, creatinine, hepatic function
Chest radiography
Intravenous pyelography or computed tomography of abdomen with intravenous contrast
Consider the following: barium enema, cystoscopy, rectosigmoidoscopy

Staging of Carcinoma of the Cervix Uteri: FIGO Nomenclature

Stage 0 Carcinoma in situ, cervical intraepithelial neoplasia Grade III

Stage I The carcinoma is strictly confined to the cervix (extension to the corpus would be disregarded).

Ia	Invasive carcinoma that can be diagnosed only by microscopy. All macroscopically visible lesions-even with superficial invasion-are allotted to Stage Ib carcinomas. Invasion is limited to a measured stromal invasion with a maximal depth of 5.0 mm and a horizontal extension of not more than 7.0 mm. Depth of invasion should not be more than 5.0 mm taken from the base of the epithelium of the original tissue-superficial or glandular. The involvement of vascular spaces-venous or lymphatic-should not change the stage allotment.
Ia1	Measured stromal invasion of not more than 3.0 mm in depth and extension of not more than 7.0 mm
Ia2	Measured stromal invasion of more than 3.0 mm and not more than 5.0 mm with an extension of not more than 7.0 mm
Ib	Clinically visible lesions limited to the cervix uteri or preclinical cancers greater than Stage Ia
Ib1	Clinically visible lesions not more than 4.0 cm
Ib2	Clinically visible lesions more than 4.0 cm

Stage II Cervical carcinoma invades beyond the uterus, but not to the pelvic wall or to the lower third of the vagina

IIa	No obvious parametrial involvement
IIb	Obvious parametrial involvement

Stage III The carcinoma has extended to the pelvic wall. On rectal examination, there is no cancer-free space between the tumor and the pelvic wall. The tumor involves the lower third of the vagina. All cases with hydronephrosis or nonfunctioning kidney are included, unless they are known to be due to other causes.

IIIa	Tumor involves lower third of the vagina, with no extension to the pelvic wall
IIIb	Extension to the pelvic wall or hydronephrosis or nonfunctioning kidney

Stage IV The carcinoma has extended beyond the true pelvis, or has involved (biopsy proved) the mucosa of the bladder or rectum. Bullous edema, as such, does not permit a case to be allotted to Stage IV.

IVa	Spread of the growth to adjacent organs (bladder or rectum or both)
IVb	Spread to distant organs

Guidelines for Clinical Staging of Invasive Cervical Carcinoma

Examinations should include inspection, palpation, colposcopy, endocervical curettage, hysteroscopy, cystoscopy, proctoscopy, intravenous pyelography, and X-ray examination of lungs and skeleton.

Conization of the cervix is considered a clinical examination.

Suspected bladder or rectal involvement should be confirmed histologically.

If there is a question about the most appropriate stage, the earlier stage should be assigned.

III. **FIGO staging systems**
   A. The International Federation of Gynecologists and Obstetricians (FIGO) staging system is based upon clinical evaluation. This examination should be performed under anesthesia whenever necessary.

B. Based upon FIGO guidelines, the following examinations are appropriate to establish the stage of disease: palpation and inspection of the primary tumor, palpation of groin and supraclavicular lymph nodes, colposcopy, endocervical curettage, conization, hysteroscopy, cystoscopy, proctoscopy, intravenous pyelogram (IVP), and radiographic examination of the lungs and skeleton.

C. Chest X-rays are indicated in all patients with cervical cancer, and imaging of the urinary tract (IVP, magnetic resonance or computed tomography urogram) should be carried out in all patients with more than microscopic cervical cancer. Suspected rectal or bladder involvement requires confirmation by biopsy.

IV. **Optional evaluation procedures.** Although they are not used to assign disease stage in the FIGO classification, optional staging examinations, including computed tomography (CT), magnetic resonance imaging (MRI), positron emission tomography (PET), lymphangiography, ultrasonography, or laparoscopy, may be of value for planning treatment, particularly the extent of the radiation therapy (RT) field or scope of surgery.

A. MRI is the preferred modality to provide information about tumor size, degree of stromal penetration, nodal metastasis, and local tissue extension. Positive findings should be histologically confirmed by fine needle aspiration under CT guidance.

V. **Surgical evaluation.** Although cervical cancer is staged clinically, the results of surgical staging can be used for treatment planning. The staging procedure can be performed through a laparotomy (transperitoneal or extraperitoneal) or laparoscopically. Surgical staging allows for a complete pelvic and paraaortic lymphadenectomy. Nodal tissue obtained at the time of surgery can detect microscopic disease. Staging offers an opportunity to resect bulky metastatic lymph nodes and allows for individualization of the radiation field. In premenopausal women, oophoropexy can be done at the same time to protect the ovaries from radiation damage.

VI. **Treatment of microinvasive cervical cancer.** According to the FIGO criteria, patients with stage Ia 1 carcinoma could be treated with simple hysterectomy without nodal dissection or conization in selected cases. Those patients with invasion >3 mm and no greater than 5 mm (stage Ia2) should undergo radical hysterectomy and pelvic lymphadenectomy. Although lymphatic-vascular invasion should not alter the FIGO stage, it is an important factor in treatment decisions. The risk of recurrence with lymphatic-vascular involvement is 3.1% if the extent of invasion is 3 mm or less and 15.7% if it is greater than 3 mm and no greater than 5 mm. Therefore, the presence of lymphatic-vascular invasion would suggest the need for more radical treatment.

VII. **Treatment of early-stage (Ib-IIa) carcinoma**

A. Both treatment strategies for stage Ib and early-stage IIa invasive carcinoma include 1) a primary surgical approach with radical hysterectomy and pelvic lymphadenectomy or 2) primary radiation therapy with external beam radiation and either high-dose-rate or low-dose-rate brachytherapy. The 5-year survival rate is 87-92% using either approach.

B. Radical surgery leaves the vagina in more functional condition, while radiation therapy results in a reduction in length, caliber, and lubrication of the vagina. In premenopausal women, ovarian function can be preserved with surgery. The surgical approach also provides the opportunity for pelvic and abdominal exploration and provides better clinical and pathologic information with which to individualize treatment.

VIII. **Adjuvant therapy following primary surgery in early-stage carcinoma**

A. Patients with histologically documented extracervical disease (pelvic nodal involvement, positive margins, or parametrial extension) are treated with concurrent pelvic radiation therapy and cisplatin-based chemotherapy. The use of combined adjuvant chemotherapy and radiation therapy in these high-risk patients following primary surgery significantly improves relapse-free survival and overall survival rates when compared with radiation therapy alone.

B. Following radical hysterectomy, a subset of node-negative patients who have a constellation of primary risk factors (large tumors, depth of stromal infiltration, and lymphovascular space involvement) may be defined as having intermediate risk for relapse. For these patients, adjuvant pelvic radiation therapy provides clear therapeutic benefit, with significantly improved relapse-free survival rates when compared with those who had no further therapy.

IX. **Treatment of late-stage carcinoma (IIb or later).** Cisplatin is usually administered weekly as a single agent because of its ease of delivery and favorable toxicity profile. Women with locally advanced cervical cancer in North America should receive cisplatin-based chemotherapy concurrent with radiation therapy.

X. **Long term monitoring.** Approximately 35% of patients will have persistent or recurrent disease. A common approach includes examinations and Pap tests every 3-4 months for the first 3 years, decreasing to twice yearly in the fourth and fifth years, with and chest X-rays annually for up to 5 years.

References: See page 208.

Endometrial Cancer

Uterine cancer is the most common malignant neoplasm of the female genital tract and the fourth most common cancer in women. About 6,000 women in the United States die of this disease each year. It is more frequent in affluent and white, especially obese, postmenopausal women of low parity. Hypertension and diabetes mellitus are also predisposing factors.

I. **Risk factors**

A. Any characteristic that increases exposure to unopposed estrogen increases the risk for endometrial cancer. Conversely, decreasing exposure to estrogen limits the risk. Unopposed estrogen therapy, obesity, anovulatory cycles and estrogen-secreting neoplasms all increase the amount of unopposed estrogen and thereby increase the risk for endometrial cancer. Smoking seems to decrease estrogen exposure, thereby decreasing the cancer risk, and oral contraceptive use increases progestin levels, thus providing protection.

Risk Factors for Endometrial Cancer

Unopposed estrogen exposure
Median age at diagnosis: 59 years
Menstrual cycle irregularities, specifically menorrhagia and menometrorrhagia
Postmenopausal bleeding
Chronic anovulation
Nulliparity
Early menarche (before 12 years of age)
Late menopause (after 52 years of age)
Infertility
Tamoxifen (Nolvadex) use
Granulosa and thecal cell tumors
Ovarian dysfunction
Obesity
Diabetes mellitus
Arterial hypertension with or without atherosclerotic heart disease
History of breast or colon cancer

B. **Hormone replacement therapy.** Unopposed estrogen treatment of menopause is associated with an eightfold increased incidence of endometrial cancer. The addition of progestin decreases this risk dramatically.

II. Clinical evaluation

A. Ninety% of patients with endometrial cancer have abnormal vaginal bleeding, usually presenting as menometrorrhagia in a perimenopausal woman or menstrual-like bleeding in a woman past menopause. Perimenopausal women relate a history of intermenstrual bleeding, excessive bleeding lasting longer than seven days or an interval of less than 21 days between menses. Heavy, prolonged bleeding in patients known to be at risk for anovulatory cycles should prompt histologic evaluation of the endometrium. The size, contour, mobility and position of the uterus should be noted.

B. Patients who report abnormal vaginal bleeding and have risk factors for endometrial cancer should have histologic evaluation of the endometrium. Premenopausal patients with amenorrhea for more than six to 12 months should be offered endometrial sampling, especially if they have risk factors associated with excessive estrogen exposure. Postmenopausal women with vaginal bleeding who either are not on hormonal replacement therapy or have been on therapy longer than six months should be evaluated by endometrial sampling.

C. **Endometrial sampling**

1. In-office sampling of the endometrial lining may be accomplished with a Novak or Kevorkian curet, the Pipelle endometrial-suction curet, or the Vabra aspirator. Before having an in-office biopsy, the patient should take a preoperative dose of a nonsteroidal anti-inflammatory drug (NSAID). With the patient in the lithotomy position, a speculum is inserted in the vaginal canal. The cervix should be cleansed with a small amount of an antiseptic solution. After 1 mL of a local anesthetic is infused into the anterior lip of the cervix, a tenaculum is placed. The paracervical block is then performed using 1 or 2% lidocaine (Xylocaine) without epinephrine.

2. The cannula is then placed in the uterus and placement is confirmed with the help of the centimeter markings along the cannula. The inner sleeve is pulled back while the cannula is held within the cavity. This generates a vacuum in the cannula that can be used to collect endometrial tissue for diagnosis. Moving the cannula in and out of the cavity no more than 2 to 3 cm with each stroke while turning the cannula clockwise or counterclockwise is helpful in obtaining specimens from the entire cavity.

III. Treatment of endometrial cancer

A. The treatment of endometrial cancer is usually surgical, such as total abdominal hysterectomy, bilateral salpingo-oophorectomy and evaluation for metastatic disease, which may include pelvic and para-aortic lymphadenectomy, peritoneal cytologic examination and peritoneal biopsies. The extent of the surgical procedure is based on the stage of disease, which can be determined only at the time of the operation.

Staging for Carcinoma of the Corpus Uteri	
Stage*	**Description**
IA (G1, G2, G3)	Tumor limited to endometrium
IB (G1, G2, G3)	Invasion of less than one half of the myometrium
IC (G1, G2, G3)	Invasion of more than one half of the myometrium
IIA (G1, G2, G3)	Endocervical gland involvement

Stage*	Description
IIB (G1, G2, G3)	Cervical stromal involvement
IIIA (G1, G2, G3)	Invasion of serosa and/or adnexa and/or positive peritoneal cytologic results
IIIB (G1, G2, G3)	Metastases to vagina
IIIC (G1, G2, G3)	Metastases to pelvic and/or para-aortic lymph nodes
IVA (G1, G2, G3)	Invasion of bladder and/or bowel mucosa
IVB	Distant metastases including intra-abdominal and/or inguinal lymph nodes

*--Carcinoma of the corpus is graded (G) according to the degree of histologic differentiation: G1 = 5% or less of a solid growth pattern; G2 = 6 to 50% of a solid growth pattern; G3 = more than 50% of a solid growth pattern.

   B. For most patients whose cancers have progressed beyond stage IB grade 2, postoperative radiation therapy is recommended. Because tumor response to cytotoxic chemotherapy has been poor, chemotherapy is used only for palliation.
   C. Endometrial hyperplasia with atypia should be treated with hysterectomy except in extraordinary cases. Progestin treatment is a possibility in women younger than 40 years of age who refuse hysterectomy or who wish to retain their childbearing potential, but an endometrial biopsy should be performed every three months. Treatment of atypical hyperplasia and well-differentiated endometrial cancer with progestins in women younger than 40 years of age results in complete regression of disease in 94% and 75%, respectively.
   D. Patients found to have hyperplasia without atypia should be treated with progestins and have an endometrial biopsy every three to six months.
IV. **Serous and clear cell adenocarcinomas**
   A. These cancers are considered in a separate category from endometrioid adenocarcinomas. They have a worse prognosis overall. Patients with serous carcinomas have a poorer survival. The 3 year survival is 40% for stage I disease.
   B. Serous and clear cell carcinomas are staged like ovarian cancer. A total abdominal hysterectomy and bilateral salpingo-oophorectomy, lymph node biopsy, and omental biopsy/omentectomy are completed. Washings from the pelvis, gutters and diaphragm are obtained, and the diaphragm is sampled and peritoneal biopsies completed.
References: See page 208.

Ovarian Cancer

Ovarian cancer is the second most common gynecologic malignancy, but the most common cause of death among women who develop gynecologic cancer, and it is the fifth most common cancer in females. The majority (90%) of primary ovarian tumors derive from epithelial cells, although they can also arise from germ cell tumors, sex cord-stromal tumors, and mixed cell type tumors.

I. Clinical manifestations

A. Most ovarian cancers are diagnosed between the ages of 40 and 65. Symptoms of early stage disease are often vague. Acute symptoms due to ovarian rupture or torsion are unusual. As a result, 75 to 85% of cases of ovarian cancer are advanced at the time of diagnosis. More advanced disease is typically associated with abdominal distention, nausea, anorexia, or early satiety due to the presence of ascites and omental or bowel metastases.

B. Most women have nonspecific symptoms, such as lower abdominal discomfort or pressure, gas, bloating, constipation, irregular menstrual cycles/abnormal vaginal bleeding, low-back pain, fatigue, nausea, indigestion, urinary frequency, or dyspareunia.

II. Physical examination

A. Palpation of an asymptomatic adnexal mass during a routine pelvic examination is the usual presentation for ovarian cancer. The presence of a solid, irregular, fixed pelvic mass on pelvic examination is highly suggestive of an ovarian malignancy. However, endometriomas and tubo-ovarian abscesses are benign tumors that may be fixed, while cystadenofibromas and tubo-ovarian abscesses are benign masses that feel irregular. The diagnosis of malignancy is almost certain if a fixed, irregular pelvic mass is associated with an upper abdominal mass or ascites.

Differential Diagnosis of Adnexal Masses in Women	
Extraovarian mass Ectopic pregnancy Hydosalpinx or tuboovarian abscess Paraovarian cyst Peritoneal inclusion cyst	Pedunculated fibroid Diverticular abscess Appendiceal abscess
Ovarian mass Simple or hemorrhagic physiologic cysts (eg, follicular, corpus luteum) Endometrioma	Theca lutein cysts Benign or malignant neoplasms (eg, epithelial, germ cell, sex-cord) Metastatic carcinoma (eg, breast, colon, endometrium)

III. Diagnostic evaluation

A. The finding of a pelvic mass usually requires surgery for definitive histologic diagnosis. Tumor markers (eg, serum CA 125) and ultrasound examination can help distinguish between malignant and benign pelvic masses.

B. A complete pelvic examination and assessment of cervical cytology should be performed preoperatively. Routine hematologic and biochemical assessments should be obtained prior to surgery. Ultrasonography for diagnosis of ovarian malignancy has a sensitivity of 62 to 100% and a specificity of 77 to 95%.

C. It is reasonable to pursue a period of observation in a premenopausal woman with an adnexal mass if the mass is not clinically suspicious on ultrasonography. Adnexal masses that are mobile, purely cystic, unilateral, less than 8 to 10 cm in diameter, and have smooth internal and external contours by ultrasound are highly unlikely to be malignant and can be followed for two months; the majority of physiologic cysts will regress during this time.

D. Exploration is indicated if there is no resolution within two months. However, women who have solid, fixed, irregularly shaped, or large masses should undergo surgery. A mass that increases in size or does not regress must be presumed to be neoplastic and should be removed surgically.

    E. The threshold for surgical intervention is lower in postmenopausal women; those with cysts >3 cm should undergo exploratory surgery, laparotomy, or laparoscopy.

    F. Tumor markers. CA 125: The preoperative evaluation of a woman with suspected ovarian cancer should include measurement of the CA 125 concentration. The serum CA 125 (normal <35 U/mL) is elevated (>65 U/mL) in 80% of women with epithelial ovarian cancer. It is also increased in patients with other malignancies, including endometrial cancer and certain pancreatic cancers; in endometriosis, uterine leiomyoma, and pelvic inflammatory disease; and in approximately 1% of healthy women.

IV. Staging

    A. Surgery is necessary for diagnosis, accurate staging and optimal cytoreduction, and is crucial for the successful treatment of EOC. Ovarian malignancies are surgically staged according to the 2002 revised American Joint Committee on Cancer (AJCC) and International Federation of Gynecologic Oncologists (FIGO) joint staging system, as long as the patient is an appropriate surgical candidate.

Definitions of the Stages in Primary Carcinoma of the Ovary	
Stage	**Definition**
I	Growth is limited to the ovaries
IA	Growth is limited to one ovary; no ascites present containing malignant cells; no tumor on the external surface; capsule is intact
IB	Growth is limited to both ovaries; no ascites present containing malignant cells; no tumor on the external surfaces; capsules are intact
IC	Tumor is classified as either stage IA or IB but with tumor on the surface of one or both ovaries; or with ruptured capsule(s); or with ascites containing malignant cells present or with positive peritoneal washings
II	Growth involves one or both ovaries with pelvic extension
IIA	Extension and/or metastases to the uterus and/or tubes
IIB	Extension to other pelvic tissues
IIC	Tumor is either stage IIA or IIB but with tumor on the surface of one or both ovaries; or with capsule(s) ruptured; or with ascites containing malignant cells present or with positive peritoneal washings

Stage	Definition
III	Tumor involves one or both ovaries with peritoneal implants outside the pelvis and/or positive retroperitoneal or inguinal nodes; superficial liver metastasis equals stage III; tumor is limited to the true pelvis but with histologically proven malig-
IIIA	nant extension to small bowel or omentum
IIIB	Tumor is grossly limited to the true pelvis with negative nodes but with histologically confirmed microscopic seeding of abdominal peritoneal surfaces
IIIC	Tumor involves one or both ovaries with histologically con-firmed implants of abdominal peritoneal surfaces, none ex-ceeding 2 cm in diameter; nodes are negative
	Abdominal implants >2 cm in diameter and/or positive retroperitoneal or inguinal nodes
IV	Growth involves one or both ovaries with distant metastases; if pleural effusion is present, there must be positive cytology findings to assign a case to stage IV; parenchymal liver me-tastasis equals stage IV

B. Procedure
   1. The staging procedure is usually approached through a laparotomy incision. Any free fluid in the cul-de-sac is submitted for cytologic evaluation. Washings of the peritoneal cavity are ob-tained by instilling and removing 50 to 100 mL of saline. The affected adnexa should be removed intact and a frozen section obtained to determine or confirm the diagnosis. Thorough surgical staging should be carried out in the absence of obvious stage IV disease. Preservation of the uterus and a normal appearing contralateral adnexa is an option in women desirous of maintaining future fertility.
   2. All intraperitoneal surfaces should be carefully inspected and suspicious areas or adhesions should be biopsied. If there is no evidence of disease, multiple intraperitoneal biopsies should be performed, including from the cul-de-sac, both gutters, bladder peritoneum, and bowel mesentery.
   3. The diaphragm is evaluated by either biopsy or cytologic smear. A complete omentectomy should be performed.
   4. The retroperitoneal spaces are explored to dissect the pelvic and paraaortic lymph nodes. Any enlarged lymph nodes should be resected and submitted separately for histopathologic evaluation.
   5. For patients with advanced disease, optimal cytoreduction (debulking) should be attempted at the time of initial surgery. The majority of women with EOC (except for those with stage I dis-ease) will require surgery and chemotherapy.

V. Treatment of ovarian cancer
   A. Cytoreductive surgery improves response to chemotherapy and survival of women with advanced ovarian cancer. Operative manage-ment is designed to remove as much tumor as possible. When a malignant tumor is present, a thorough abdominal exploration, total abdominal hysterectomy, bilateral salpingo-oophorectomy, lymphadenectomy, omentectomy, and removal of all gross cancer are standard therapy.
   B. Adjuvant therapy
   1. Patients with stage IA or IB disease (who have been completely surgically staged) and who have borderline, well- or moderately

differentiated tumors do not benefit from additional chemotherapy because their prognosis is excellent with surgery alone.

2. Chemotherapy improves survival and is an effective means of palliation of ovarian cancer. In patients who are at increased risk of recurrence (stage I G3 and all IC-IV), chemotherapy is recommended. Sequential clinical trials of chemotherapy agents demonstrate that cisplatin (or carboplatin) given in combination with paclitaxel is the most active combination identified.

References: See page 208.

Breast Cancer

One of 8 women will develop breast cancer. The risk of breast cancer increases with age; approximately half of new cases occur in women aged 65 years or older. Two% of 40- to 49-year-old women in the United States develop breast cancer during the fifth decade of their lives, and 0.3% die from breast cancer. Breast cancer is the most common malignancy in American women, and the second most lethal malignancy in women, following lung cancer.

I. Risk Factors
   A. Major risk factors for breast cancer include: 1) early menarche, 2) nulliparity, 3) delayed childbirth, 4) increasing age, 5) race, and 6) family history.

Risk Factors for Breast Cancer

Major Risk Factors
Early menarche
Nulliparity
Delayed childbirth
Increasing age
Race
Family history

Other Risk Factors

Late menopause	A history of breast cancer
Obesity	Exposure to ionizing radiation
Weight gain	Higher bone mineral density
Increased intra-abdominal fat (android body habitus)	Smoking
	Alcohol consumption
Lack of regular exercise	Elevated insulin-like growth factor- I (IGF- I) levels
Elevated serum estradiol	Increased mammographic density
Elevated free testosterone levels	Oral contraceptives
A previous premalignant breast biopsy	
Radial scars in benign breast biopsies	

Familial Risk Factors for Breast Cancer
More than 50% of women in family have breast cancer
Breast cancer present in more than I generation
Multiple occurrences of breast cancer (>3) in close relatives
Onset at less than age 45 years
History of bilateral breast cancer
High rate of co-existing ovarian cancer
BRCA1 gene mutation

   B. Nulliparity and increased age at first pregnancy are associated with an increased risk for breast cancer. Nulliparity alone accounts for 16% of new cases of breast cancer each year. The relative risk for breast cancer increases with advancing age.
   C. Race is an independent risk factor. While white women are at an increased risk for breast cancer, African American women with breast cancer have higher fatality rates and a later stage at diagnosis.

D. A family history of breast cancer, especially in first-degree relatives, increases the risk.

E. A history of breast cancer increases a woman's risk for subsequent breast cancers. If the woman has no family history of breast cancer, then the initial occurrence was sporadic, and the incidence for developing a second breast cancer is 1% per year. If the initial occurrence was hereditary, the incidence for developing a second breast cancer is 3% per year. Approximately 10% of women with breast cancer will develop a second primary breast cancer.

F. **Familial or Genetic Risk Factors.** A mutation in a tumor-suppresser gene occurs in 1 of 400 women and is located on chromosome 17q. Carriers of a BRCA1 mutation have an 85% lifetime risk of developing breast cancer. In addition, the risk of colon and ovarian cancers is also increased (40% to 50%) in these groups. The 70% of breast cancer patients who do not have inherited mutations on BRCA1 have mutations on BRCA2. The cumulative lifetime risk of breast cancer in a woman with the BRCA2 mutation is 87%.

G. **Conclusions.** Seventy-five% of women with newly diagnosed breast cancer demonstrate no specific, identifiable risk factor. Most premenopausal breast cancer cases are genetically determined. In contrast, many post-menopausal cases are environmentally related.

II. **Screening Guidelines**

A. **Breast Self-Examination.** All women older than age 20 years should perform regular monthly breast self-examinations. Menstruating women should examine their breasts in the first 7 to 10 days of the menstrual cycle.

Breast Screening Criteria		
Age	Clinical Breast Examination	Mammography
30-39	Every 1-3 years	None
40-49	Annual	Optional 1-2 years
≥ 50	Annual	Annual
Women aged 50 to 69 years should be offered mammography and receive a clinical breast examination every 1 to 2 years.		

B. **Clinical Breast Examination (CBE)** is recommended every 1 to 3 years for women aged 30 to 39 years and annually for those aged 40 years and older.

C. **Mammography** alone is 75% sensitive, and, when combined with CBE, the screening sensitivity for detecting breast cancer increases to 88%. Screening guidelines from the US Preventive Services Task Force suggest mammography alone or with CBE every 1 to 2 years for women aged 50 to 69 years. Recent evidence suggests a benefit from annual mammography with or without CBE for women aged 40 to 49 years.

III. **History and physical examination**

A. In the woman with a suspicious breast mass, risk factors and a family history of breast cancers should be assessed. A personal history of radiation to the chest or breast, breast masses, biopsies, history of collagen vascular disease, and menstrual and gynecologic history are also important. Symptoms of nipple discharge, pain, skin changes, or rashes may occur.

B. On physical examination, the breast mass should be palpated for size, position, adherence of the tumor to the skin or chest wall, density, fluctuance, and tenderness. In addition, both breasts and axillae should be examined for other tumors and any lymph nodes. A search for supraclavicular lymph nodes should also be conducted.

   C. Any evidence of skin changes, ulceration, peau d'orange (thickening of skin to resemble an orange skin), or lymphedema is suspicious for locally advanced cancer.
   D. Immediate mammography should be obtained. A white blood count, hematocrit, and erythrocyte sedimentation rate may be needed if cancer is found.

IV. **Diagnosis**
   A. The definitive diagnosis is made by pathological evaluation of tissue.
   B. A combination of clinical breast examination, mammography, and fine-needle aspiration and biopsy may be sufficient to make a diagnosis. If all studies are "benign," there is a >99% chance that a benign breast lesion is present.
   C. Open biopsy in the operating room or wire-localization of a suspicious lesion noted on mammography may be necessary if fine-needle aspiration and biopsy is nondiagnostic. Biopsy by stereo tactic technique in radiology also may be used to obtain tissue for diagnosis of the suspicious area.

V. **Definition and classification of breast cancer for staging**
   A. The definition for staging and the classification of stages for breast cancer follow the system of the International Union Against Cancer. This system is based on the tumor, nodes, and metastases (TNM) nomenclature.

Definitions for Breast Cancer Staging	
Tumor	
TIS	Carcinoma in situ (intraductal carcinoma, lobular)
T0	No evidence of primary tumor
T1	Tumor ≤2 cm in greatest dimension
T2	Tumor >2 cm but <5 cm in greatest dimension
T3	Tumor >5 cm in greatest dimension
T4	Tumor of any size with direct extension into chest wall or skin
Nodes	
N0	No regional lymph node metastases
N1	Metastases to movable ipsilateral axillary node(s)
N2	Metastases to ipsilateral axillary lymph node(s), fixed to one another or other structures

Metastases	
M0	No distant metastases
M I	Metastases to movable ipsilateral axillary node(s); metastases to ipsilateral axillary lymph node(s); fixed to one another or other structures; or metastases to ipsilateral internal mammary lymph node(s); distant metastases

Classification of Breast Cancer Staging	
Stage	Description*
0	TIS, N0, M0
I	TI, N0, M0
IIA	T0, NI, M0
IIB	T2, NI, M0, or T3, N0, M0
IIIA	T0, N2, M0, or TI, N2, M0, or T2, N2, M0, or T3, NI, or N2, M0
IIIB	T4, any N, M0 or any T, N3
IV	Any T, any N, MI
*Tumor/nodes/metastases	

    B. The HER-2 gene (c-erbB-2, HER-2/neu) has been identified, and the HER-2 receptor is correlated with aggressive biological behavior of the cancer and a poor clinical outcome.

    C. The staging of breast cancer dictates not only the prognosis but also directs treatment modality recommendations. The prognosis for women is based on their age, tumor type, initial tumor size, presence of nodes and staging, and hormone-re-ceptor status. The overall 10-year survival rates for the more common breast cancer stages are >90% for stage 0, >75% for stage I, >50% for stage IIA, and approximately 50% for stage IIB.

VI. Treatment of breast cancer

    A. Treatment choices for ductal carcinoma in situ, a stage 0 cancer, include 1) mastectomy, 2) lumpectomy followed by radiation therapy, or 3) lumpectomy followed by radiation therapy and then tamoxifen if the tumor is estrogen-receptor test positive.

    B. Surgical Treatment

        1. Conservative therapy and radiation result in at least as good a prognosis as radical mastectomy. Skin-sparing mastectomy involves removing all the breast tissue, the nipple, and the areolar complex. Reconstruction is then completed with a natural-appearing breast. This procedure is considered for those women with ductal carcinoma in situ or T1 or T2 invasive carcinomas. The recurrence rate for this procedure is comparable with a modified radical mastectomy.

        2. Local excision of the tumor mass (lumpectomy) followed by lymph node staging and subsequent adjuvant hormone therapy, chemotherapy, or radiation therapy is an accepted treatment. Long-term studies have found that recurrence rates are similar when lumpectomy was compared with radiation therapy and mastectomy.

C. **Radiation Therapy.** External beam radiation therapy has proven effective in preventing recurrence of breast cancer and for palliation of pain. The risk of relapse after radiation therapy ranges from 4% to 10%. Lumpectomy can now be performed followed by implantation of high-dose brachytherapy catheters.

D. **Anti-Hormonal Therapy**. Hormonal therapy is indicated for those tumors that test positive for hormone receptors. Tamoxifen has both estrogenic and anti-estrogenic effects. In women who are older than 50 years with breast cancers that test positive for hormone receptors, tamoxifen use produces a 20% increase in 5-year survival rates. The response rate in advanced cases increases to 35%.

E. **Chemotherapy**
   1. Chemotherapy is used in women at risk for metastatic disease. Cytotoxic agents used include methotrexate, fluorouracil, cyclophosphamide (Cytoxan, Neosar), doxorubicin, mitoxantrone (Novantrone), and paclitaxel (Taxol). In the management of stage 0 disease, chemotherapy is not used initially.
   2. Stage I and stage II disease are treated with chemotherapy based on the relative risk of systemic recurrence. This risk is often based on the woman's age, axillary lymph node involvement, tumor size, hormone receptor status, histologic tumor grade, and cellular aggressiveness. Systemic chemotherapy is recommended for women with stage I disease who have node-negative cancers and a tumor size >1 cm in diameter.
   3. Women with stage IIA breast cancer are treated with adjuvant chemotherapy with or without tamoxifen. Some women with positive lymph nodes are placed on chemotherapy, including doxorubicin, fluorouracil, and methotrexate.
   4. In women with stage III breast cancer, similar agents are selected. Doxorubicin is particularly useful in treating inflammatory breast cancer. In women with stage IIIB cancer, chemotherapy is usually administered before primary surgery or radiation therapy.

References: See page 208.

Obstetrics

Prenatal Care

Prenatal care should make an early, accurate estimation of gestational age, identify patients at risk for complications, and monitor the health status of both mother and fetus on an ongoing basis. Patient education and communication are also important components of prenatal care.

I. **Prenatal history and physical examination**. Women at increased risk of maternal medical complications, pregnancy complications, or fetal abnormalities should be identified.
   A. **Diagnosis of pregnancy**
      1. **Amenorrhea** is usually the first sign of conception. Other symptoms include breast fullness and tenderness, skin changes, nausea, vomiting, urinary frequency, and fatigue.
      2. **Pregnancy tests.** Urine pregnancy tests may be positive within days of the first missed menstrual period. Serum beta human chorionic gonadotropin (HCG) is accurate up to a few days after implantation.
      3. **Fetal movements** ("quickening") are first felt by the patient at 17-19 weeks.
      4. **Ultrasound** will visualize a gestational sac at 5-6 weeks and a fetal pole with movement and cardiac activity by 7-8 weeks. Ultrasound can estimate fetal age accurately if completed before 24 weeks.
      5. **Estimated date of confinement.** The mean duration of pregnancy is 40 weeks from the LMP. Estimated date of confinement (EDC) can be calculated by Nägele's rule: Add 7 days to the first day of the LMP, then subtract 3 months.
   B. **Contraceptive history.** Recent oral contraceptive usage often causes postpill amenorrhea, and may cause erroneous pregnancy dating.
   C. **Gynecologic and obstetric history**
      1. Gravidity is the total number of pregnancies. Parity is expressed as the number of term pregnancies, preterm pregnancies, abortions, and live births.
      2. The character and length of previous labors, type of delivery, complications, infant status, and birth weight are recorded.
      3. Assess prior cesarean sections and determine type of C-section (low transverse or classical), and determine reason it was performed.
   D. **Medical and surgical history** and prior hospitalizations are documented.
   E. **Medications** and allergies are recorded.
   F. **Family history** of medical illnesses, hereditary illness, or multiple gestation is sought.
   G. **Social history.** Cigarettes, alcohol, or illicit drug use.
   H. **Review of systems.** Abdominal pain, constipation, headaches, vaginal bleeding, dysuria or urinary frequency, or hemorrhoids.

Basic Prenatal Medical History	

Endocrine disorder
    Thyroid
    Adrenal
    Diabetes
	Autoimmune disorder
	    Systemic lupus erythematosus
	    Rheumatoid arthritis

Cardiovascular disease
   Hypertension
   Arrhythmia
   Congenital anomalies
   Rheumatic Fever
   Thromboembolic disease
	History of blood transfusion
	Pulmonary disease
	   Asthma
	   Tuberculosis

Kidney disease
   Pyelonephritis
   Urinary tract infections
   Anomalies
	Breast disorders
	Infectious diseases
	   Herpes
	   Gonorrhea
	   Chlamydia
	   Syphilis
	   HIV

Neurologic or muscular disorders
   Seizure disorder
   Aneurysm
   Arteriovenous malformation
	Gynecologic history
	   Abnormal PAP smear
	   Genital tract disease or procedures

Gastrointestinal disease
   Hepatitis
   Gall bladder disease
   Inflammatory bowel disease
	Surgical procedures
	Allergies
	Medications
	Substance abuse
	   Alcohol
	   Cigarettes
	   Illicit drugs

Current Pregnancy History

Medications taken Alcohol use Cigarette use Illicit drug use Exposure to radiation	Vaginal bleeding Nausea, vomiting, weight loss Infections Exposure to toxic substances

Initial Prenatal Assessment of past Obstetrical History

Date of delivery Gestational age at delivery Location of delivery Sex of child Birth weight Mode of delivery	Type of anesthesia Length of labor Outcome (miscarriage, stillbirth, ectopic, etc.) Details (eg, type of cesarean section scar, forceps, etc.) Complications (maternal, fetal child)

I. **Physical examination**
   1. Baseline blood pressure, weight, and height should be recorded as part of the examination. Funduscopic examination, thyroid, breast, lungs, and heart are examined.
   2. An extremity and neurologic exam are completed, and the presence of a cesarean section scar is sought.
   3. **Fetal heart tones** can be detected as early as 9-12 weeks from the last menstrual period (LMP) by Doppler. The normal fetal heart rate is 120-160 beats per minute. Transvaginal ultrasound can visualize fetal cardiac motion as early as 5.5 to 6.0 weeks.
   4. **Pelvic examination**
      a. Pap smear, culture for gonorrhea, and Chlamydia testing are completed routinely. Adnexa are palpated for masses.

    b. Estimation of gestational age by uterine size
        (1) The nongravid uterus is 3 x 4 x 7 cm. The uterus begins to change in size at 5-6 weeks.
        (2) Gestational age is estimated by uterine size: 8 weeks = 2 x normal size; 10 weeks = 3 x normal; 12 weeks = 4 x normal.
        (3) At 12 weeks the fundus becomes palpable at the symphysis pubis.
        (4) At 16 weeks, the uterus is midway between the symphysis pubis and the umbilicus.
        (5) At 20 weeks, the uterus is at the umbilicus. After 20 weeks, there is a correlation between the number of weeks of gestation and the number of centimeters from the pubic symphysis to the top of the fundus.
        (6) Uterine size that exceeds the gestational dating by 3 or more weeks suggests multiple gestation, molar pregnancy, or (most commonly) an inaccurate date for LMP.
        Ultrasonography will confirm inaccurate dating or intrauterine growth failure.

II. Initial visit laboratory testing

  A. Routine. A standard panel of laboratory tests should be obtained on every pregnant woman at the first prenatal visit. Chlamydia screening is recommended for all pregnant women.

Initial Prenatal Laboratory Examination

Blood type and antibody screen	Urinary infection screen
Rhesus type	Hepatitis B surface antigen
Hematocrit or hemoglobin	HIV counseling and testing
TSH, free T4	Chlamydia
PAP smear	Gonorrhea
Rubella status (immune or nonimmune)	
Syphilis screen	

  B. Human immunodeficiency virus
    1. HIV testing is recommended for all pregnant women.
    2. Retesting in the third trimester (around 36 weeks of gestation) is recommended for women at high risk for acquiring HIV infection.

  C. At-risk women should receive additional tests:
    1. Gonorrhea, tuberculosis and red cell indices to screen for thalassemia (eg, MCV <80), hemoglobin electrophoresis to detect hemoglobinopathies (eg, sickle cell, thalassemias)
    2. Hexosaminidase A for Tay Sachs screening (serum test in nonpregnant and leukocyte assay in pregnant individuals), DNA analysis for Canavan's disease, cystic fibrosis carrier testing, serum phenylalanine level, toxoplasmosis screen, and Hepatitis C antibodies.
    3. Testing for sexually transmitted diseases (eg, HIV, syphilis, hepatitis B surface antigen, chlamydia, gonorrhea) should be repeated in the third trimester in any woman at high risk for acquiring these infections; all women under age 25 years should be retested for Chlamydia trachomatis late in pregnancy.

  D. CBC, AB blood typing and Rh factor, antibody screen, rubella, VDRL/RPR, hepatitis B surface Ag.

  E. Pap smear, urine pregnancy test, urinalysis. Cervical culture for gonorrhea and chlamydia.

  F. Tuberculosis skin testing, HIV counseling/testing.

  G. Hemoglobin electrophoresis is indicated in risks groups, such as sickle hemoglobin in African patients, B-thalassemia in Mediterranean patients, and alpha-thalassemia in Asian patients. Tay-Sachs carrier testing is indicated in Jewish patients.

III. Initial patient education

A. Frequency of prenatal visits, recommendations for nutrition, weight gain, exercise, rest, and sexual activity, routine pregnancy monitoring (eg, weight, urine dipstick, blood pressure, uterine growth, fetal activity and heart rate), listeria precautions, toxoplasmosis precautions (eg, hand washing, eating habits, cat care) should be discussed. Pregnant women should continue wearing three-point seat belts during pregnancy. The lap belt is placed across the hips and below the uterus; the shoulder belt goes between the breasts and lateral to the uterus.

B. Abstinence from alcohol, cigarettes, illicit drugs should be assessed. Information on the safety of commonly used nonprescription drugs, signs and symptoms to be reported should be discussed, as appropriate for gestational age (eg, vaginal bleeding, ruptured membranes, contractions, decreased fetal activity).

C. Headache and backache. Acetaminophen (Tylenol) 325-650 mg every 3-4 hours is effective. Aspirin is contraindicated.

D. Nausea and vomiting. First-trimester morning sickness may be relieved by eating frequent, small meals, getting out of bed slowly after eating a few crackers, and by avoiding spicy or greasy foods. Promethazine (Phenergan) 12.5-50 mg PO q4-6h prn or diphenhydramine (Benadryl) 25-50 mg tid-qid is useful.

E. Constipation. A high-fiber diet with psyllium (Metamucil), increased fluid intake, and regular exercise should be advised. Docusate (Colace) 100 mg bid may provide relief.

IV. Nutrition, vitamins, and weight gain

A. All pregnant women should be encouraged to eat a well-balanced diet. Folic acid is recommended in the preconceptional and early prenatal period to prevent neural tube defects (NTDs). A standard prenatal multivitamin satisfies the requirements of most pregnant women.

B. Nutritional recommendations for pregnant women are based upon the prepregnancy body mass index (BMI). A weight gain of 12.5 to 18 kg (28 to 40 lb) for underweight women (BMI<19.8), 7 to 11.5 kg (15 to 25 lb) for overweight women (BMI ≥26), and 11.5 to 16 kg (25 to 35 lb) for women of average weight (BMI 19.8 to 26.0) is recommended.

V. Clinical assessment at first trimester prenatal visits

A. Routine examination at each subsequent visit consists of measurement of blood pressure and weight, measurement of the uterine fundus to assess fetal growth, auscultation of fetal heart tones, and determination of fetal presentation and activity. The urine is typically screened for protein and glucose at each visit.

B. At 9 to 12 weeks the fetal heart usually can be heard by of gestation using a Doppler instrument. Transvaginal ultrasound can determine fetal viability as early as 5.5 to 6.5 weeks.

C. Aneuploidy testing with full integrated test. The full integrated test consists of ultrasound measurement of nuchal translucency thickness combined with a pregnancy-associated plasma protein-A at 10 to 13 weeks.

Frequency of Prenatal Care Visits in Low-Risk Pregnancies	
<28 weeks	Every month
28-36 weeks	Every 2 weeks
36-delivery	Every 1 week until delivery

VI. Clinical assessment at second trimester visits
   A. Questions for each follow-up visit
   1. **First detection of fetal movement (quickening)** should occur at around 17 weeks in a multigravida and 19 weeks in a primigravida. **Fetal movement** should be documented at each visit after 17 weeks.
   2. **Vaginal bleeding or symptoms of preterm labor** should be sought.
   B. Fetal heart rate is documented at each visit.

VII. Second-trimester laboratory
   A. Maternal serum testing at 15-18 weeks: Quadruple markers should be obtained at 15 to 18 weeks, measuring alpha-fetoprotein (AFP), unconjugated estriol (uE3), hCG, and inhibin A. **Genetic amniocentesis** should be offered to patients who screen positive, and it should be offered if a birth defect has occurred in the mother, father, or in previous offspring.
   B. Screening ultrasound. Ultrasound measurement of crown-rump length at 7 to 14 weeks is the most accurate technique for estimation of gestational age; it is accurate within three to five days.
   C. At 24-28 weeks, a one-hour Glucola (blood glucose measurement 1 hour after 50-gm oral glucose) is obtained to screen for gestational diabetes. Those with a particular risk (eg, previous gestational diabetes or fetal macrosomia), require earlier testing. If the 1 hour test result is >140 mg/dL, a 3-hour glucose tolerance test is necessary.
   D. Second trimester education. Discomforts include backache, round ligament pain, constipation, and indigestion.

VIII. Clinical assessment at third trimester visits
   A. Fetal movement is documented. Vaginal bleeding or symptoms of preterm labor should be sought. Preeclampsia symptoms (blurred vision, headache, rapid weight gain, edema) are sought.
   B. Fetal heart rate is documented at each visit.
   C. At 26-30 weeks, repeat hemoglobin and hematocrit are obtained to determine the need for iron supplementation.
   D. At 28-30 weeks, an antibody screen is obtained in Rh-negative women, and D immune globulin (RhoGAM) is administered if negative.
   E. At 36 weeks, repeat serologic testing for syphilis is recommended for high risk groups.
   F. Sexually transmitted disease. Testing for sexually transmitted diseases (eg, HIV, syphilis, hepatitis B surface antigen, chlamydia, gonorrhea) should be repeated in the third trimester in any woman at high risk for acquiring these infections; all women under age 25 years should be retested for Chlamydia trachomatis late in pregnancy.
   G. Screening for group B streptococcus colonization at 35-37 weeks. All pregnant women should be screened for group B beta-hemolytic streptococcus (GBS) colonization with swabs of both the lower vagina and rectum at 35 to 37 weeks of gestation. The only patients who are excluded from screening are those with GBS bacteriuria earlier in the current pregnancy or those who gave birth to a previous infant with invasive GBS disease. These latter patients are not included in the screening recommendation because they should receive intrapartum antibiotic prophylaxis regardless of the colonization status.
   H. Influenza immunization is recommended for women in the second and third trimesters and for high-risk women prior to influenza season regardless of stage of pregnancy.
   I. Third trimester education
   1. **Signs of labor.** The patient should call physician when rupture of membranes or contractions have occurred every 5 minutes for one hour.
   2. **Danger signs.** Preterm labor, rupture of membranes, bleeding, edema, signs of preeclampsia.

3. **Common discomforts.** Cramps, edema, frequent urination.
J. **At 36 weeks,** a cervical exam may be completed. Fetal position should be assessed by palpation (Leopold's Maneuvers).

References: See page 208.

Normal Labor

Labor consists of the process by which uterine contractions expel the fetus. A term pregnancy is 37 to 42 weeks from the last menstrual period (LMP).

I. **Obstetrical History and Physical Examination**
A. **History of the present labor**
1. **Contractions.** The frequency, duration, onset, and intensity of uterine contractions should be determined. Contractions may be accompanied by a "bloody show" (passage of blood-tinged mucus from the dilating cervical os). Braxton Hicks contractions are often felt by patients during the last weeks of pregnancy. They are usually irregular, mild, and do not cause cervical change.
2. **Rupture of membranes.** Leakage of fluid may occur alone or in conjunction with uterine contractions. The patient may report a large gush of fluid or increased moisture. The color of the liquid should be determine, including the presence of blood or meconium.
3. **Vaginal bleeding** should be assessed. Spotting or blood-tinged mucus is common in normal labor. Heavy vaginal bleeding may be a sign of placental abruption.
4. **Fetal movement.** A progressive decrease in fetal movement from baseline, should prompt an assessment of fetal well-being with a nonstress test or biophysical profile.
B. **History of present pregnancy**
1. **Estimated date of confinement** (EDC) is calculated as 40 weeks from the first day of the LMP.
2. **Fetal heart tones** are first heard with a Doppler instrument 10-12 weeks from the LMP.
3. **Quickening** (maternal perception of fetal movement) occurs at about 17 weeks.
4. **Uterine size** before 16 weeks is an accurate measure of dates.
5. **Ultrasound** measurement of fetal size before 24 weeks of gestation is an accurate measure of dates.
6. **Prenatal history.** Medical problems during this pregnancy should be reviewed, including urinary tract infections, diabetes, or hypertension.
7. **Antepartum testing.** Nonstress tests, contraction stress tests, biophysical profiles.
8. **Review of systems.** Severe headaches, scotomas, hand and facial edema, or epigastric pain (preeclampsia) should be sought. Dysuria, urinary frequency or flank pain may indicate cystitis or pyelonephritis.
C. **Obstetrical history.** Past pregnancies, durations and outcomes, preterm deliveries, operative deliveries, prolonged labors, pregnancy-induced hypertension should be assessed.
D. **Past medical history** of asthma, hypertension, or renal disease should be sought.
II. **Physical examination**
A. Vital signs are assessed.
B. **Head.** Funduscopy should seek hemorrhages or exudates, which may suggest diabetes or hypertension. Facial, hand and ankle edema suggest preeclampsia.
C. **Chest.** Auscultation of the lungs for wheezes and crackles may indicate asthma or heart failure.
D. **Uterine Size.** Until the middle of the third trimester, the distance in centimeters from the pubic symphysis to the uterine fundus should

correlate with the gestational age in weeks. Toward term, the measurement becomes progressively less reliable because of engagement of the presenting part.

E. **Estimation of fetal weight** is completed by palpation of the gravid uterus.

F. **Leopold's maneuvers** are used to determine the position of the fetus.
1. **The first maneuver** determines which fetal pole occupies the uterine fundus. The breech moves with the fetal body. The vertex is rounder and harder, feels more globular than the breech, and can be moved separately from the fetal body.
2. **Second maneuver.** The lateral aspects of the uterus are palpated to determine on which side the fetal back or fetal extremities (the small parts) are located.
3. **Third maneuver.** The presenting part is moved from side to side. If movement is difficult, engagement of the presenting part has occurred.
4. **Fourth maneuver.** With the fetus presenting by vertex, the cephalic prominence may be palpable on the side of the fetal small parts.

G. **Pelvic examination.** The adequacy of the bony pelvis, the integrity of the fetal membranes, the degree of cervical dilatation and effacement, and the station of the presenting part should be determined.

H. **Extremities.** Severe lower extremity or hand edema suggests preeclampsia. Deep-tendon hyperreflexia and clonus may signal impending seizures.

I. **Laboratory tests**
1. Prenatal labs should be documented, including CBC, blood type, Rh, antibody screen, serologic test for syphilis, rubella antibody titer, urinalysis, culture, Pap smear, cervical cultures for gonorrhea and Chlamydia, and hepatitis B surface antigen (HbsAg).
2. During labor, the CBC, urinalysis and RPR are repeated. The HBSAG is repeated for high-risk patients. A clot of blood is placed on hold.

J. **Fetal heart rate.** The baseline heart rate, variability, accelerations, and decelerations are recorded.

III. **Normal labor**

A. Labor is characterized by uterine contractions of sufficient frequency, intensity, and duration to result in effacement and dilatation of the cervix.

B. **The first stage of labor** starts with the onset of regular contractions and ends with complete dilatation (10 cm). This stage is further subdivided into the latent and an active phases.
1. The latent phase starts with the onset of regular uterine contractions and is characterized by slow cervical dilatation to 4 cm. The latent phase is variable in length.
2. The active phase follows and is characterized by more rapid dilatation to 10 cm. During the active phase of labor, the average rate of cervical dilatation is 1.5 cm/hour in the multipara and 1.2 cm/hour in the nullipara.

C. **The second stage of labor** begins with complete dilatation of the cervix and ends with delivery of the infant. It is characterized by voluntary and involuntary pushing. The average second stage of labor is one-half hour in a multipara and 1 hour in the primipara.

D. **The third stage of labor** begins with the delivery of the infant and ends with the delivery of the placenta.

E. **Intravenous fluids**. IV fluid during labor is usually Ringer's lactate or 0.45% normal saline with 5% dextrose. Intravenous fluid infused rapidly or given as a bolus should be dextrose-free because maternal hyperglycemia can occur.

F. **Activity.** Patients in the latent phase of labor are usually allowed to walk.

G. **Narcotic and analgesic drugs**
1. Nalbuphine (Nubain) 5 to 10 mg SC or IV q2-3h.

2. Butorphanol (Stadol) 2 mg IM q3-4h or 0.5-1.0 mg IV q1.5-2.0h **OR**
3. Meperidine (Demerol) 50 to 100 mg IM q3-4h or 10 to 25 mg IV q1.5-3.0 h **OR**
4. Narcotics should be avoided if their peak action will not have diminished by the time of delivery. Respiratory depression is reversed with naloxone (Narcan): Adults, 0.4 mg IV or IM and neonates, 0.01 mg/kg.

Labor History and Physical

Chief compliant: Contractions, rupture of membranes.
HPI: ___ year old Gravida (number of pregnancies) Para (number of deliveries).
Gestational age, last menstrual period, estimated date of confinement. Contractions (onset, frequency, intensity), rupture of membranes (time, color). Vaginal bleeding (consistency, quantity, bloody show); fetal movement.
Fetal Heart Rate Strip: Baseline rate, accelerations, reactivity, decelerations, contraction frequency.
Dates: First day of last menstrual period, estimated date of confinement. Ultrasound dating.
Prenatal Care: Date of first exam, number of visits; has size been equal to dates? infections, hypertension, diabetes.
Obstetrical History: Dates of prior pregnancies, gestational age, route (C-section with indications and type of uterine incision), weight, complications, length of labor, hypertension.
Gynecologic History: Menstrual history (menarche, interval, duration), herpes, gonorrhea, chlamydia, abortions; oral contraceptives.
Past Medical History: Illnesses, asthma, hypertension, diabetes, renal disease, surgeries.
Medications: Iron, prenatal vitamins.
Allergies: Penicillin, codeine?
Social History: Smoking, alcohol, drug use.
Family History: Hypertension, diabetes, bleeding disorders.
Review of Systems: Severe headaches, scotomas, blurred vision, hand and face edema, epigastric pain, pruritus, dysuria, fever.

Physical Exam
General Appearance:
Vitals: BP, pulse, respirations, temperature.
HEENT: Funduscopy, facial edema, jugular venous distention.
Chest: Wheezes, rhonchi.
Cardiovascular: Rhythm, S1, S2, murmurs.
Abdomen: Fundal height, Leopold's maneuvers (lie, presentation). Estimated fetal weight (EFW), tenderness, scars,
Cervix: Dilatation, effacement, station, position, status of membranes, presentation. Vulvar herpes lesions.
Extremities: Cyanosis, clubbing, edema.
Neurologic: Deep tender reflexes, clonus.
Prenatal Labs: Obtain results of one hour post glucola, RPR/VDRL, rubella, blood type, Rh, CBC, Pap, PPD, hepatitis B₃Ag, UA, C and S.
Current Labs: Hemoglobin, hematocrit, glucose, UA; urine dipstick for protein.
Assessment: Intrauterine pregnancy (IUP) at 40 weeks, admitted with the following problems:
Plan: Anticipated type of labor and delivery. List plan for each problem.

H. Epidural anesthesia

1. Contraindications include infection in the lumbar area, clotting defect, active neurologic disease, sensitivity to the anesthetic, hypovolemia, and septicemia.
2. Risks include hypotension, respiratory arrest, toxic drug reaction, and rare neurologic complications. An epidural has no significant effect on the progress of labor.
3. Before the epidural is initiated, the patient is hydrated with 500-1000 mL of dextrose-free intravenous fluid.

Labor and Delivery Admitting Orders

Admit: Labor and Delivery
Diagnoses: Intrauterine pregnancy at ____ weeks.
Condition: Satisfactory
Vitals: q1 hr per routine
Activity: May ambulate as tolerated.
Nursing: I and O. Catheterize prn; external or internal monitors.
Diet: NPO except ice chips.
IV Fluids: Lactated Ringers with 5% dextrose at 125 cc/h.
Medications:
Epidural at 4-5 cm.
Oxytocin (Pitocin) 6 mU per minute IV, increase dose by 6 mU per minute every 15 minutes until contractions occur every 3 minutes.
Nalbuphine (Nubain) 5-10 mg IV/SC q2-3h prn **OR**
Butorphanol (Stadol) 0.5-1 mg IV q1.5-2h prn **OR**
Meperidine (Demerol) 25-75 mg slow IV q1.5-3h prn pain **AND**
Promethazine (Phenergan) 25-50 mg, IV q3-4h prn nausea **OR**
Hydroxyzine (Vistaril) 25-50 mg IV q3-4h prn
Fleet enema PR prn constipation.
Labs: CBC, dipstick urine protein, blood type and Rh, antibody screen, VDRL, HBsAg, rubella, type and screen (C-section).

I. **Intrapartum antibiotic prophylaxis for group B streptococcus is recommended for the following:**

1. Pregnant women with a positive screening culture unless a planned Cesarean section is performed in the absence of labor or rupture of membranes
2. Pregnant women who gave birth to a previous infant with invasive GBS disease
3. Pregnant women with documented GBS bacteriuria during the current pregnancy
4. Pregnant women whose culture status is unknown (culture not performed or result not available) and who also have delivery at <37 weeks of gestation, amniotic membrane rupture for >18 hours, or intrapartum temperature >100.4°F (>38°C)
5. The recommended IAP regimen is penicillin G (5 million units IV initial dose, then 2.5 million units IV Q4h). In women with non-immediate-type penicillin-allergy, cefazolin (Ancef, 2 g initial dose, then 1 g Q8h) is recommended. Clindamycin (900 mg IV Q8h) or erythromycin (500 mg IV Q6h) are recommended for patients at high risk for anaphylaxis to penicillins as long as their GBS isolate is documented to be susceptible to both clindamycin and erythromycin.

IV. **Normal spontaneous vaginal delivery**

A. **Preparation.** As the multiparous patient approaches complete dilatation or as the nulliparous patient begins to crown the fetal scalp, preparations are made for delivery.
B. **Maternal position.** The mother is usually placed in the dorsal lithotomy position with left lateral tilt.

C. **Delivery of a fetus in an occiput anterior position**
  1. **Delivery of the head**
     a. The fetal head is delivered by extension as the flexed head passes through the vaginal introitus.
     b. Once the fetal head has been delivered, external rotation to the occiput transverse position occurs.
     c. The oropharynx and nose of the fetus are suctioned with the bulb syringe. A finger is passed into the vagina along the fetal neck to check for a nuchal cord. If one is present, it is lifted over the vertex. If this cannot be accomplished, the cord is doubly clamped and divided.
     d. If shoulder dystocia is anticipated, the shoulders should be delivered immediately.
  2. **Episiotomy** consists of incision of the perineum, enlarging the vaginal orifice at the time of delivery. If indicated, an episiotomy should be performed when 3-4 cm of fetal scalp is visible.
     a. With adequate local or spinal anesthetic in place, a medial episiotomy is completed by incising the perineum toward the anus and into the vagina.
     b. Avoid cutting into the anal sphincter or the rectum. A short perineum may require a mediolateral episiotomy.
     c. Application of pressure at the perineal apex with a towel-covered hand helps to prevent extension of the episiotomy.
  3. **Delivery of the anterior shoulder** is accomplished by gentle downward traction on the fetal head. The posterior shoulder is delivered by upward traction.
  4. **Delivery of the body.** The infant is grasped around the back with the left hand, and the right hand is placed, near the vagina, under the baby's buttocks, supporting the infant's body. The infant's body is rotated toward the operator and supported by the operator's forearm, freeing the right hand to suction the mouth and nose. The baby's head should be kept lower than the body to facilitate drainage of secretions.
  5. **Suctioning** of the nose and oropharynx is repeated.
  6. **The umbilical cord** is doubly clamped and cut, leaving 2-3 cm of cord.

D. **Delivery of the placenta**
  1. The placenta usually separates spontaneously from the uterine wall within 5 minutes of delivery. Gentle fundal massage and gentle traction on the cord facilitates delivery of the placenta.
  2. The placenta should be examined for missing cotyledons or blind vessels. The cut end of the cord should be examined for 2 arteries and a vein. The absence of one umbilical artery suggests a congenital anomaly.
  3. Prophylaxis against excessive postpartum blood loss consists of external fundal massage and oxytocin (Pitocin) 20 units in 1000 mL of IV fluid at 100 drops/minute after delivery of the placenta. Oxytocin can cause marked hypotension if administered as a IV bolus.
  4. After delivery of the placenta, the birth canal is inspected for lacerations.

Delivery Note

1. Note the age, gravida, para, and gestational age.
2. Time of birth, type of birth (spontaneous vaginal delivery), position (left occiput anterior).
3. Bulb suctioned, sex, weight, APGAR scores, nuchal cord, and number of cord vessels.
4. Placenta expressed spontaneously intact. Describe episiotomy degree and repair technique.
5. Note lacerations of cervix, vagina, rectum, perineum.
6. Estimated blood loss:
7. Disposition: Mother to recovery room in stable condition. Infant to nursery in stable condition.

Routine Postpartum Orders

Transfer: To recovery room, then postpartum ward when stable.
Vitals: Check vitals, bleeding, fundus q15min x 1 hr or until stable, then q4h.
Activity: Ambulate in 2 hours if stable
Nursing Orders: If unable to void, straight catheterize; sitz baths prn with 1:1000 Betadine prn, ice pack to perineum prn, record urine output.
Diet: Regular
IV Fluids: D5LR at 125 cc/h. Discontinue when stable and taking PO diet.
Medications:
  Oxytocin (Pitocin) 20 units in 1 L D5LR at 100 drops/minute or 10 U IM.
  FeSO4 325 mg PO bid-tid.
Symptomatic Medications:
  Acetaminophen/codeine (Tylenol #3) 1-2 tab PO q3-4h prn **OR**
  Oxycodone/acetaminophen (Percocet) 1 tab q6h prn pain.
  Milk of magnesia 30 mL PO q6h prn constipation.
  Docusate Sodium (Colace) 100 mg PO bid.
  Dulcolax suppository PR prn constipation.
  A and D cream or Lanolin prn if breast feeding.
  Breast binder or tight brazier and ice packs prn if not to breast feed.
Labs: Hemoglobin/hematocrit in AM. Give rubella vaccine if titer <1:10.

Active Management of Labor

The active management of labor refers to active control over the course of labor. There are three essential elements to active management are careful diagnosis of labor by strict criteria, constant monitoring of labor, and prompt intervention (eg, amniotomy, high dose oxytocin) if progress is unsatisfactory.

I. **Criteria for active management of labor:**
   A. Nulliparous
   B. Term pregnancy
   C. Singleton infant in cephalic presentation
   D. No pregnancy complications
   E. Experiencing spontaneous onset of labor.
II. **Diagnosis of labor**
   A. The diagnosis of labor is made only when contractions are accompanied by any one of the following:
      1. Bloody show
      2. Rupture of the membranes
      3. Full cervical effacement
   B. Women who meet these criteria are admitted to the labor unit.
III. **Management of labor**
   A. **Rupture of membranes.** Intact fetal membranes are artificially ruptured one hour after the diagnosis of labor is made to permit assessment of the quantity of fluid and the presence of meconium. Rupture of the membranes may accelerate labor.

B. Progress during the first stage of labor
   1. Satisfactory progress in the first stage of labor is confirmed by cervical dilatation of at least 1 cm per hour after the membranes have been ruptured.
   2. In the absence of medical contraindications, labor that fails to progress at the foregoing rate is treated with oxytocin.
   3. **Progress during the second stage of labor** is measured by fetal descent and rotation.
      a. The second stage of labor is divided into two phases: the first phase is the time from full dilatation until the fetal head reaches the pelvic floor; the second phase extends from the time the head reaches the pelvic floor to delivery of the infant.
      b. The first phase of the second stage is characterized by descent of the fetal head. If the fetal head is high in the pelvis at full dilatation, the woman often has no urge to push and should not be encouraged to do so. Oxytocin treatment may be useful if the fetal head fails to descend after a period of observation.
C. Administration of oxytocin. Oxytocin is administered for treatment of failure of labor to progress, unless its use is contraindicated. Oxytocin may only be administered if the following conditions are met:
   1. Fetal membranes are ruptured
   2. Absence of meconium in amniotic fluid
   3. Singleton fetus in a vertex position
   4. No evidence of fetal distress

High Dose Oxytocin (Pitocin) Regimen

Begin oxytocin 6 mU per minute IV
Increase dose by 6 mU per minute every 15 minutes
Maximum dose: 40 mU per minute

D. Failure to progress (dystocia) is diagnosed when the cervix fails to dilate at least 1 cm per hour during the first stage of labor or when the fetal head fails to descend during the second stage of labor. Three possible causes for failure to progress are possible (excluding malpresentations and hydrocephalus):
   1. Inefficient uterine action
   2. Occiput-posterior position
   3. Cephalopelvic disproportion.
E. Inefficient uterine action is the most common cause of dystocia in the nulliparous gravida, especially early in labor. Secondary arrest of labor after previously satisfactory progress may be due to an occiput-posterior position or cephalopelvic disproportion. It is often difficult for the clinician to differentiate among these entities, thus oxytocin is administered in all cases of failure to progress (unless a contraindication exists).
F. In the first stage, progressive cervical dilatation of at least 1 cm per hour should occur within one hour of establishing efficient uterine contractions (five to seven contractions within 15 minutes) with oxytocin. The second stage is considered prolonged if it extends longer than two hours in women without epidural anesthesia and longer than three hours in women with epidural anesthesia despite adequate contractions and oxytocin augmentation.
References: See page 208.

Perineal Lacerations and Episiotomies

I. First-degree laceration

A. A first degree perineal laceration extends only through the vaginal and perineal skin.

B. **Repair:** Place a single layer of interrupted 3-O chromic or Vicryl sutures about 1 cm apart.

II. Second-degree laceration and repair of midline episiotomy

A. A second degree laceration extends deeply into the soft tissues of the perineum, down to, but not including, the external anal sphincter capsule. The disruption involves the bulbocavernosus and transverse perineal muscles.

B. **Repair**

1. Proximate the deep tissues of the perineal body by placing 3-4 interrupted 2-O or 3-O chromic or Vicryl absorbable sutures. Reapproximate the superficial layers of the perineal body with a running suture extending to the bottom of the episiotomy.

2. Identify the apex of the vaginal laceration. Suture the vaginal mucosa with running, interlocking, 3-O chromic or Vicryl absorbable suture.

3. Close the perineal skin with a running, subcuticular suture. Tie off the suture and remove the needle.

III. Third-degree laceration

A. This laceration extends through the perineum and through the anal sphincter.

B. **Repair**

1. Identify each severed end of the external anal sphincter capsule, and grasp each end with an Allis clamp.

2. Proximate the capsule of the sphincter with 4 interrupted sutures of 2-O or 3-O Vicryl suture, making sure the sutures do not penetrate the rectal mucosa.

3. Continue the repair as for a second degree laceration as above. Stool softeners and sitz baths are prescribed post-partum.

IV. Fourth-degree laceration

A. The laceration extends through the perineum, anal sphincter, and extends through the rectal mucosa to expose the lumen of the rectum.

B. **Repair**

1. Irrigate the laceration with sterile saline solution. Identify the anatomy, including the apex of the rectal mucosal laceration.

2. Approximate the rectal submucosa with a running suture using a 3-O chromic on a GI needle extending to the margin of the anal skin.

3. Place a second layer of running suture to invert the first suture line, and take some tension from the first layer closure.

4. Identify and grasp the torn edges of the external anal sphincter capsule with Allis clamps, and perform a repair as for a third-degree laceration. Close the remaining layers as for a second-degree laceration.

5. A low-residue diet, stool softeners, and sitz baths are prescribed post-partum.

References: See page 208.

Antepartum Fetal Heart Rate Assessment

The health of the fetus may be assessed by the fetal heart rate (FHR). This assessment involves identification of two types of FHR patterns: those that may be associated with adverse fetal or neonatal outcomes (ie, nonreassuring patterns) and those that are indicative of fetal well-being (ie, reassuring patterns). The primary goal is to recognize fetuses in whom timely intervention will prevent death. A secondary goal is to avoid fetal neurologic injury.

I. Pathophysiology

A. Effect of gestational age on FHR. Advancing gestational age is associated with slowing of the baseline heart rate. At 20 weeks of gestation the average FHR is 155 beats/min, while at 30 weeks it is 144 beats/min.

B. FHR variability is rarely present before 24 weeks of gestation, while the absence of variability is abnormal after 28 weeks of gestation since the parasympathetic nervous system is developed by the third trimester.

C. Advancing gestational age is also associated with increased frequency and amplitude of FHR accelerations. Fifty% of normal fetuses demonstrate accelerations with fetal movements at 24 weeks; this proportion rises to over 95% at 30 weeks of gestation. Before 30 weeks, however, accelerations are typically only 10 beats per minute for 10 seconds rather than the 15 beats per minute sustained for 15 seconds noted after 30 weeks.

D. Nonreactivity of the nonstress test is characterized by loss of accelerations of the FHR caused by worsening of hypoxemia.

E. Persistent bradycardia or repetitive late decelerations results from myocardial depression caused by prolonged and/or severe hypoxemia. Variability is also lost. Ultimately there is a loss of fetal biophysical activities, such as breathing, movement, and body tone. At this stage, the fetus may be acidotic.

II. Fetal heart rate patterns

A. Reassuring patterns. The FHR pattern recorded by an electronic FHR monitor is typically interpreted as reassuring or nonreassuring. The presence of a reassuring pattern indicates that there is no fetal acidemia at the time of testing. A reassuring fetal heart rate pattern has the following components:

1. A baseline fetal heart rate of 110 to 160 bpm
2. Absence of FHR decelerations
3. Age appropriate FHR accelerations
4. Normal FHR variability (6 to 25 bpm)

B. FHR accelerations usually indicate that the fetus is not acidotic. FHR accelerations and mild variable decelerations are indicative of a normally functioning autonomic nervous system.

C. Early decelerations are shallow symmetrical decelerations in which the nadir of the deceleration occurs simultaneously with the peak of the contraction. Early decelerations and mild bradycardia (FHR as low as 100 bpm) with normal variability are caused by fetal head compression and are not associated with fetal acidosis or poor neonatal outcome.

D. Persistent tachyarrhythmias may cause fetal hydrops if present for many hours to days. Persistent bradyarrhythmias are often associated with fetal heart disease (eg, cardiac conduction defects due to anatomic derangements or autoantibody (SSA, anti-Ro) induced cardiomyopathy related to lupus), but seldom result in hypoxemia or acidosis in fetal life.

E. Nonreassuring FHR patterns are nonspecific and require further evaluation. The false positive rate for predicting adverse outcome is high. The fetus may not be acidotic initially; however, continuation or worsening of the clinical situation may result in fetal acidosis. Nonreassuring patterns include:

1. **Abnormal variability** refers to variability that is absent (amplitude undetectable), minimal (amplitude 0 to 5 bpm), or marked (amplitude over 25 bpm).
2. **Late decelerations** are a smooth U-shaped fall in FHR beginning after the contraction has started, and ending after the contraction has ended. The decline in FHR is gradual (>30 seconds from the onset of the deceleration to its nadir), as is the return to baseline. The nadir of the deceleration occurs after the peak of the contraction. Mild late decelerations are a central nervous system response

to hypoxia, while severe late decelerations can have a component of myocardial depression. Late decelerations with absent variability are especially predictive of fetal acidosis.

3. **Sinusoidal heart rate** is a pattern of regular variability resembling a sine wave with a fixed periodicity of three to five cycles per minute and an amplitude of 5 to 40 bpm. Sinusoidal pattern is a response to moderate fetal hypoxemia, often caused by fetal anemia.

4. **Variable decelerations** are a variable onset of abrupt slowing of the FHR in association with uterine contractions and are shaped like a U, V, or W.
   a. **Severe variable decelerations** have a late component, with delayed return to baseline until after the contraction, during which the fetal pH falls. They may also display loss of variability or rebound tachycardia and last longer than 60 seconds or fall to less than 70 bpm.
   b. **Mild or moderate variable decelerations** do not have a late component, are of short duration and depth, and end by rapid return to a normal baseline FHR. They are usually intermittent, rather than persistent. This pattern is not associated with acidosis or low Apgar scores .

5. **Saltatory pattern** refers to excessive variability, with amplitude >25 bpm and cycles of three to six times per minute. The pattern is probably related to mild, compensated fetal hypoxemia and increased alpha-adrenergic activity.

F. **Ominous patterns.** Fetal distress is defined as a pathological condition of the fetus that is likely to cause fetal or neonatal death or damage if left uncorrected. It is often associated with fetal acidemia and hypoxemia.

1. There are only a few patterns associated with true fetal distress; these FHR patterns can be a useful noninvasive means of assessing for fetal acidemia and hypoxemia.
   a. **Undulating baseline** refers to a regular pattern of alternating tachycardia and bradycardia, often with reduced variability between the wide swings in heart rate.
   b. **Diminished or absent variability associated with baseline FHR abnormalities.** The absence of FHR variability is thought to be a result of cerebral hypoxemia and acidosis, and signifies failure of fetal compensatory mechanisms to maintain adequate oxygenation of the brain.
   c. **Severe bradycardia with diminished variability** appears as a smooth FHR below 100 bpm for a prolonged period of time (ie, at least 10 minutes). It is ominous when it occurs in the absence of hypothermia, complete heart block, or use of certain drugs (eg, beta-adrenergic blockers, paracervical block).
   d. **Tachycardia** with diminished variability appears as a smooth FHR above 160 bpm. It is especially ominous when it occurs with late decelerations or severe variable decelerations. Tachycardia with normal variability and no decelerations, tachycardia is unlikely to be related to hypoxemia or acidosis. Possible causes include fever, thyrotoxicosis, arrhythmia, maternal tachycardia, and drugs.
   e. **Fetal neurological injury.** The most common FHR abnormality is a persistent nonreactive heart rate, and a persistent fixed baseline with minimal or absent variability.

National Institutes of Health guidelines for interpretation of fetal heart tracings

Variability

Absent = amplitude undetectable
Minimal = amplitude 0 to 5 bpm
Moderate = amplitude 6 to 25 bpm
Marked = amplitude over 25 bpm
There is no distinction between shortterm and longterm variability

Baseline rate

Bradycardia = below 110 bpm
Normal = 110 to 160 bpm
Tachycardia = over 160 bpm
The baseline rate is the mean bpm (rounded to 0 or 5) over a 10 minute interval, excluding periodic changes, periods of marked variability, and segments that differ by more than 25 bpm. The baseline must continue for 2 minutes during the interval, otherwise it is considered indeterminate.

Acceleration

An abrupt increase in the FHR. Before 32 weeks of gestation, accelerations should last >10 sec and peak >10 bpm above baseline. As of 32 weeks gestation, accelerations should last $\geq$15 sec and peak $\geq$15 bpm above baseline.
A prolonged acceleration is $\geq$2 minutes but less than 10 minutes. An acceleration of 10 minutes or more is considered a change in baseline.

Late deceleration

A gradual decrease and return to baseline of the FHR associated with a uterine contraction. The deceleration is delayed in timing, with the nadir of the deceleration occurring after the peak of the contraction.

Early deceleration

A gradual decrease and return to baseline of the FHR associated with a uterine contraction. The deceleration's onset, nadir, and termination are coincident with the onset, peak, and termination of the contraction.

Variable deceleration

An abrupt decrease in FHR below the baseline. The decrease is $\geq$15 bpm, lasting $\geq$15 secs and <2 minutes from onset to return to baseline. The onset, depth, and duration of variable decelerations commonly vary with successive uterine contractions.

Prolonged deceleration

A decrease in FHR below the baseline of 15 bpm, lasting 2 minutes but <10 minutes from onset to return to baseline. A prolonged deceleration of 10 minutes or more is considered a change in baseline.

III. **Overview of antepartum FHR monitoring**
   A. Antepartum FHR monitoring is performed in pregnancies in which the risk of fetal demise is known to be increased.
   B. **Nonstress test (NST)** is the most common cardiotocographic method of antepartum fetal assessment. There are no direct maternal or fetal risks from nonstress testing.

1. Testing may be initiated when the fetal neurological maturity enables FHR accelerations to occur, typically at 26 to 28 weeks, and the fetus is believed to be at increased risk of death. Testing is performed at daily to weekly intervals. The presence of a reassuring pattern indicates that there is no fetal hypoxemia.
2. The test is reactive if there are two or more fetal heart rate accelerations reaching a peak of 15 bpm above the baseline rate, and lasting for 15 seconds in a 20-minute period. A reactive test is reassuring of fetal well-being. Reactivity prior to 32 weeks may be defined as two accelerations of at least 10 beats per minute, lasting 10 seconds or more, over a 20-minute interval.
3. A nonreactive NST is defined as one that does not show such accelerations over a 40-minute period. Nonreactivity may be a sign of fetal hypoxemia or acidosis and is nonreassuring. Fetuses with a nonreactive NST have a mean umbilical vein pH of 7.28, while those with low biophysical profile (BPP) scores have a mean pH of 7.16.
4. **Management of the fetus with a nonreactive NST.** At term, delivery is usually indicated since fetal hypoxemia cannot be definitively excluded when the NST is nonreactive. A nonreassuring NST in a preterm gestation poses a greater dilemma. Ancillary tests may prove useful in avoiding a premature iatrogenic delivery, since the false positive rate of an isolated nonreactive NST is 50 to 60%. Some options include:
   a. Vibroacoustic stimulation.
   b. Biophysical profile or Doppler velocimetry.
   c. Modify factors potentially causing abnormal test results, such as correction of diabetic ketoacidosis or maternal hypotension.
5. **Vibroacoustic stimulation** is useful for decreasing the number of nonreactive NSTs related to quiet fetal sleep cycles. This test is performed by placing an artificial larynx on the maternal abdomen and delivering a short burst of sound to the fetus. The procedure shortens the duration of time needed to produce an acceleration.

C. **Contraction stress test (CST)** is usually performed using oxytocin. A dilute solution of oxytocin is infused until three contractions occur within 10 minutes. Relative contraindications include preterm labor, patients at high risk of preterm delivery, preterm premature rupture of membranes, placenta previa, and previous classical cesarean delivery or extensive uterine surgery.

D. **CST interpretation:**
   1. A positive (nonreassuring) test is defined by the presence of late decelerations following 50% or more of the contractions (such a test is considered positive even if the contraction frequency is less than three in 10 minutes).
   2. A negative (reassuring) test has no late or significant variable decelerations.
   3. An equivocal-suspicious pattern consists of intermittent late or significant variable decelerations, while an equivocal-hyperstimulatory pattern refers to fetal heart rate decelerations occurring with contractions more frequent than every two minutes or lasting longer than 90 seconds.
   4. An unsatisfactory test is one in which the tracing is uninterpretable or contractions are fewer than three in 10 minutes.
   5. The CST is also interpreted as described above in women who are having spontaneous contractions of adequate frequency.

E. A positive (nonreassuring) CST may indicate decreased fetal reserve and correlates with a 20 to 40% incidence of abnormal FHR patterns during labor. An equivocal-suspicious test with repetitive variable decelerations is also associated with abnormal FHR patterns in labor, which are often related to cord compression due to oligohydramnios.

IV. **Delivery**. After weighing the potential risks of fetal hypoxemia versus the maternal and neonatal risks associated with iatrogenic preterm birth, preterm delivery may be indicated for nonreactive nonstress test results that are persistent and have been confirmed by additional tests of fetal well-being (eg, BPP).

A. At term, additional testing can be omitted since the neonatal risk from delivery is small.

B. Depending on the FHR pattern, induction of labor with continuous FHR and contraction monitoring may be attempted in the absence of obstetrical contraindications. Repetitive late decelerations or severe variable decelerations generally mandate expeditious delivery by cesarean.

References: See page 208.

Antepartum Fetal Surveillance

I. Antepartum fetal surveillance techniques

A. Antepartum fetal surveillance should be initiated in pregnancies when the risk of fetal demise is known to be increased. These problems can include antiphospholipid syndrome, chronic hypertension, renal disease, systemic lupus erythematosus, or type 1 diabetes mellitus. Monitoring should also be initiated in pregnancy-related conditions such as preeclampsia, intrauterine growth restriction (IUGR), multiple gestation, or postterm pregnancy.

B. Antepartum fetal surveillance can include the nonstress test (NST), BPP, oxytocin challenge test (OCT), or modified BPP.

C. Nonstress test

1. A NST is performed using an electronic fetal monitor. Testing is generally begun at 32 to 34 weeks. Testing is performed at daily to weekly intervals as long as the indication for testing persists.

2. The test is reactive if there are two or more fetal heart rate accelerations of 15 bpm above the baseline rate lasting for 15 seconds in a 20 minute period. A nonreactive NST does not show such accelerations over a 40 minute period. Nonreactivity may be related to fetal immaturity, a sleep cycle, drugs, fetal anomalies, or fetal hypoxemia.

3. If the NST is nonreactive, it is considered nonreassuring and further evaluation or delivery of the fetus is indicated. At term, delivery rather than further evaluation is usually warranted. A nonreassuring NST preterm usually should be assessed with ancillary tests, since the false positive rate of an isolated NST may be 50 to 60%.

D. Fetal movement assessment ("kick counts")

1. A decrease in the maternal perception of fetal movement often precedes fetal death by several days.

2. The woman lies on her side and counts distinct fetal movements. Perception of 10 distinct movements in a period of up to 2 hours is considered reassuring. Once 10 movements have been perceived, the count may be discontinued. In the absence of a reassuring count, non stress testing is recommended.

Indications for Antepartum Fetal Surveillance	
Maternal	**Pregnancy complications**
Antiphospholipid syndrome	Preeclampsia
Poorly controlled hyperthyroidism	Decreased fetal movement
Hemoglobinopathies	Oligohydramnios
Cyanotic heart disease	Polyhydramnios
Systemic lupus erythematosus	Intrauterine growth restriction
Chronic renal disease	Postterm pregnancy
Type I diabetes mellitus	Isoimmunization
Hypertensive disorders	Previous unexplained fetal demise
	Multiple gestation

Components of the Biophysical Profile		
Parameter	**Normal (score = 2)**	**Abnormal (score = 0)**
Nonstress test	$\geq$2 accelerations $\geq$15 beats per minute above baseline during test lasting $\geq$15 seconds in 20 minutes	<2 accelerations
Amniotic fluid volume	Amniotic fluid index >5 or at least 1 pocket measuring 2 cm x 2 cm in perpendicular planes	AFI <5 or no pocket >2 cm x 2 cm
Fetal breathing movement	Sustained FBM ($\geq$30 seconds)	Absence of FBM or short gasps only <30 seconds total
Fetal body movements	>3 episodes of either limb or trunk movement	<3 episodes during test
Fetal tone	Extremities in flexion at rest and >1 episode of extension of extremity, hand or spine with return to flexion	Extension at rest or no return to flexion after movement

A total score of 8 to 10 is reassuring; a score of 6 is suspicious, and a score of 4 or less is ominous.
Amniotic fluid index = the sum of the largest vertical pocket in each of four quadrants on the maternal abdomen intersecting at the umbilicus.

E. **Ancillary tests**
   1. **Vibroacoustic stimulation** is performed by placing an artificial larynx on the maternal abdomen and delivering a short burst of sound to the fetus. The procedure can shorten the duration of time needed to produce reactivity and the frequency of nonreactive NSTs.
   2. **Oxytocin challenge test**
      a. The oxytocin challenge test (OCT) is done by intravenously infusing dilute oxytocin until three contractions occur within ten minutes. The test is interpreted as follows:
         (1) A positive test is defined by the presence of late decelerations following 50% or more of the contractions
         (2) A negative test has no late or significant variable decelerations
         (3) An equivocal-suspicious pattern consists of intermittent late or significant variable decelerations, while an equivocal-hyperstimulatory pattern refers to fetal heart rate decelerations occurring with contractions more frequent than every two minutes or lasting longer than 90 seconds
      b. An unsatisfactory test is one in which the tracing is uninterpretable or contractions are fewer than three in 10 minutes
      c. A positive test indicates decreased fetal reserve and correlates with a 20 to 40% incidence of abnormal FHR patterns during labor. An equivocal-suspicious test with repetitive variable decelerations is also associated with abnormal FHR patterns in labor, which are often related to cord compression due to oligohydramnios.
   3. **Fetal biophysical profile**
      a. The fetal biophysical profile score refers to the sonographic assessment of fetal movement, fetal tone, fetal breathing,

amniotic fluid volume and nonstress testing. Each of these five parameters is given a score of 0 or 2 points. Fetal BPS is a noninvasive, highly accurate means for predicting the presence of fetal asphyxia.

b. Criteria

  (1) A normal variable is assigned a score of two and an abnormal variable a score of zero. The maximal score is 10/10 and the minimal score is 0/10.

  (2) Amniotic fluid volume is based upon an ultrasound-based objective measurement of the largest visible pocket. The selected largest pocket must have a transverse diameter of at least one centimeter.

c. Clinical utility

  (1) The fetal BPS is noninvasive and highly accurate for predicting the presence of fetal asphyxia. The probability of fetal acidemia is virtually zero when the score is normal (8 to 10). The false negative rate (ie, fetal death within one week of a last test with a normal score) is exceedingly low. The likelihood of fetal compromise and death rises as the score falls.

  (2) The risk of fetal demise within one week of a normal test result is 0.8 per 1000 women tested. The positive predictive value of the BPS for evidence of true fetal compromise is only 50%, with a negative predictive value >99.9%.

d. Indications and frequency of testing

  (1) ACOG recommends antepartum testing in the following situations:

    (a) Women with high-risk factors for fetal asphyxia should undergo antepartum fetal surveillance with tests (eg, BPS, nonstress test).

    (b) Testing may be initiated as early as 26 weeks of gestation when clinical conditions suggest early fetal compromise is likely. Initiating testing at 32 to 34 weeks of gestation is appropriate for most pregnancies at increased risk of stillbirth.

    (c) A reassuring test (eg, BPS of 8 to 10) should be repeated periodically (weekly or twice weekly) until delivery when the high-risk condition persists.

    (d) Any significant deterioration in the clinical status (eg, worsening preeclampsia, decreased fetal activity) requires fetal reevaluation.

    (e) Severe oligohydramnios (no vertical pocket >2 cm or amniotic fluid index <5) requires either delivery or close maternal and fetal surveillance.

    (f) Induction of labor may be attempted with abnormal antepartum testing as long as the fetal heart rate and contractions are monitored continuously and are reassuring. Cesarean delivery is indicated if there are repetitive late decelerations.

  (2) The minimum gestational age for testing should reflect the lower limit that intervention with delivery would be considered. This age is now 24 to 25 weeks.

  (3) Modified biophysical profile. Assessment of amniotic fluid volume and nonstress testing appear to be as reliable a predictor of long-term fetal well-being as the full BPS. The rate of stillbirth within one week of a normal modified BPS is the same as with the full BPS, 0.8 per 1000 women tested.

Guidelines for Antepartum Testing		
Indication	**Initiation**	**Frequency**
Post-term pregnancy	41 weeks	Twice a week
Preterm rupture of membranes	At onset	Daily
Bleeding	26 weeks or at onset	Twice a week
Oligohydramnios	26 weeks or at onset	Twice a week
Polyhydramnios	32 weeks	Weekly
Diabetes	32 weeks	Twice a week
Chronic or pregnancy-induced hypertension	28 weeks	Weekly. Increase to twice-weekly at 32 weeks.
Steroid-dependent or poorly controlled asthma	28 weeks	Weekly
Sickle cell disease	32 weeks (earlier if symptoms)	Weekly (more often if severe)
Impaired renal function	28 weeks	Weekly
Substance abuse	32 weeks	Weekly
Prior stillbirth	At 2 weeks before prior fetal death	Weekly
Multiple gestation	32 weeks	Weekly
Congenital anomaly	32 weeks	Weekly
Fetal growth restriction	26 weeks	Twice a week or at onset
Decreased fetal movement	At time of complaint	Once

F. **Perinatal outcome.** An abnormal NST result should be interpreted with caution. Further assessment of fetal condition using the NST, OCT, or BPP should usually be performed to help determine whether the fetus is in immediate jeopardy.

G. **Management of abnormal test results**
   1. Maternal reports of decreased fetal movement should be evaluated by an NST, CST, BPP, or modified BPP. These results, if normal, usually are sufficient to exclude imminent fetal jeopardy. A nonreactive NST or an abnormal modified BPP generally should be followed by additional testing (either a CST or a full BPP). In many circumstances, a positive CST result generally indicates that delivery is appropriate.
   2. A BPP score of 6 is considered equivocal; in the term fetus, this score generally should prompt delivery, whereas in the preterm fetus, it should result in a repeat BPP in 24 hours. In the interim, maternal corticosteroid administration should be considered for

pregnancies of less than 34 weeks of gestation. Repeat equivocal scores should result either in delivery or continued intensive surveillance. A BPP score of 4 usually indicates that delivery is warranted.
3. Preterm delivery is indicated for nonreassuring antepartum fetal testing results that have been confirmed by additional testing. Depending on the fetal heart rate pattern, induction of labor with continuous FHR and contraction monitoring may be attempted in the absence of obstetrical contraindications. Repetitive late decelerations or severe variable decelerations usually require cesarean delivery.

References: See page 208.

Intrapartum Fetal Heart Rate Assessment

Fetal heart rate (FHR) patterns are indirect indicators of the fetal cardiac and medullary responses to blood volume changes, academia, and hypoxemia. The FHR is determined using a Doppler ultrasound device belted to the maternal abdomen. A pressure transducer simultaneously monitors the frequency, timing, and duration of uterine contractions.

I. Intrapartum FHR monitoring
   A. Internal measurement of FHR is an invasive procedure; thus, its use is restricted to the intrapartum period. A bipolar spiral electrode is inserted transcervically to penetrate the fetal scalp.

II. Further evaluation of nonreassuring tests
   A. Transient episodes of hypoxemia, such as during a contraction or temporary cord compression, are generally well-tolerated by the fetus. Repeated or prolonged episodes, especially if severe, may lead to fetal acidosis and subsequent hypoxic-ischemic encephalopathy (defined as metabolic acidosis pH <7, base deficit $\geq$12 mmol/L and Apgar score 0 to 3 for >5 minutes, and evidence of neurologic sequelae).
   B. One goal of intrapartum fetal surveillance is to distinguish the fetus with a nonreassuring FHR tracing who is hypoxemic, but well compensated, from one who is acidotic and at risk for neurologic impairment or death. Further evaluation using ancillary tests are useful for this purpose.
      1. **FHR response to stimulation.** The examiner stimulates the fetal vertex with the examining finger during vaginal examination. If a FHR acceleration is elicited, absence of acidosis (ie, fetal pH >7.20) is likely. Vibroacoustic stimulation is a less invasive technique. When accelerations are induced by scalp stimulation, acidosis is present in less than 10% of fetuses, and when no accelerations occur, acidosis is present in about 50% of fetuses.
      2. **Fetal scalp blood sampling.** An amnioscope with a light source is used to expose the fetal scalp. The scalp is smeared with silicone gel so that a droplet of blood forms when the scalp is punctured with a 2-mm blade. The blood is collected in long, heparinized capillary tubes. The test requires that the cervix be dilated at least 2 to 3 cm.
      3. Capillary blood collected from the fetal scalp correlates well with fetal arterial values. However, scalp edema can result in erroneous results. A scalp pH value of <7.20 is used to identify fetal acidosis.
      4. Technical skill and parturient discomfort have precluded use of fetal blood sampling in many labor and delivery units. Furthermore, the test has poor sensitivity and positive predictive value (PPV) for predicting umbilical arterial pH <7.0.

III. Management of nonreassuring FHR patterns
   A. Determine the cause of the abnormality: Abruptio placenta, cord prolapse, maternal medication (eg, butorphanol, opiates, betamimetics).

B. **Change maternal position** from side to side, into Trendelenburg, or to knee-elbow. This may dislodge an occult cord prolapse. The supine position should be avoided because of markedly reduced cardiac output due to uterine compression of the vena cava.

C. **Give an intravenous fluid bolus of nonglucose crystalloid** (eg, 1000 mL), unless there is volume overload. This may improve placental blood flow if the patient is intravascularly hypovolemic from prolonged lack of intake, vomiting, or sympathetic blockade.

D. **Discontinue oxytocin.** Blood flow to the placenta is reduced during contractions. Iatrogenic hyperstimulation is a leading cause of nonreassuring FHR tracings.

E. **Perform a vaginal examination to check for a prolapsed umbilical cord** or rapid cervical dilatation and descent of the fetal head.

F. **If neuraxial anesthesia** was recently administered, check for maternal hypotension and ask the anesthesiologist to evaluate the patient and administer ephedrine. Reduced perfusion of the placenta from sympathetic blockade can occur without marked changes in maternal blood pressure.

G. **Administer oxygen** by mask (10 L/min) to the mother to improve fetal oxygenation.

H. **Tocolysis with subcutaneous terbutaline** 0.25 mg should be initiated if uterine hypercontractility is present (not secondary to oxytocin).

I. **Amnioinfusion** if there are persistent variable decelerations.

J. **Ancillary tests to determine the fetal condition** should be completed if the nonreassuring pattern does not resolve within a few minutes.

   1. **Digital or vibroacoustic stimulation** should be administered it accelerations are not observed. Presence of accelerations almost always assures the absence of fetal acidosis.

   2. If accelerations cannot be elicited, further evaluation by fetal scalp sampling for pH, lactate concentration, or fetal ECG is indicated to help clarify the fetal acid-base status. If accelerations cannot be elicited, then variability should be evaluated. If variability is decreased in the setting of repetitive decelerations, delivery should be accomplished.

K. **Determine whether operative intervention** (cesarean or instrumental vaginal delivery) is needed.

L. **Expeditious delivery** is indicated for persistent nonreassuring FHR patterns associated with acidosis or if the presence of acidosis cannot be excluded.

Management of Variant Fetal Heart Rate Patterns

FHR Pattern	Diagnosis	Action
Normal rate normal variability, accelerations, no decelerations	Fetus is well oxygenated	None
Normal variability, accelerations, mild nonreassuring pattern (bradycardia, late decelerations, variable decelerations)	Fetus is still well oxygenated centrally	Conservative management.
Normal variability, ± accelerations, moderate-severe nonreassuring pattern (bradycardia, late decelerations, variable decelerations)	Fetus is still well oxygenated centrally, but the FHR suggests hypoxia	Continue conservative management. Consider stimulation testing. Prepare for rapid delivery if pattern worsens

FHR Pattern	Diagnosis	Action
Decreasing variability, ± accelerations, moderate-severe nonreassuring patterns (bradycardia, late decelerations, variable decelerations)	Fetus may be on the verge of decompensation	Deliver if spontaneous delivery is remote, or if stimulation supports diagnosis of decompensation. Normal response to stimulation may allow time to await a vaginal delivery
Absent variability, no accelerations, moderate/severe nonreassuring patterns (bradycardia, late decelerations, variable decelerations)	Evidence of actual or impending asphyxia	Deliver. Stimulation or in-utero management may be attempted if delivery is not delayed

References: See page 208.

Brief Postoperative Cesarean Section Note

Pre-op diagnosis:
1. 23 year old G_1P_0, estimated gestational age = 40 weeks
2. Dystocia
3. Non-reassuring fetal tracing

Post-op diagnosis: Same as above
Procedure: Primary low segment transverse cesarean section
Attending Surgeon, Assistant:
Anesthesia: Epidural
Operative Findings: Weight and sex of infant, APGARs at 1 min and 5 min; normal uterus, tubes, ovaries
Cord pH:
Specimens: Placenta, cord blood (type and Rh).
Estimated Blood Loss: 800 cc; no blood replaced.
Fluids, blood and urine output:
Drains: Foley to gravity.
Complications: None
Disposition: Patient sent to recovery room in stable condition.

Cesarean Section Operative Report

Preoperative Diagnosis:
1. 23 year old G_1P_0, estimated gestational age = 40 weeks
2. Dystocia
3. Non-reassuring fetal tracing

Postoperative Diagnosis: Same as above
Title of Operation: Primary low segment transverse cesarean section
Surgeon:
Assistant:
Anesthesia: Epidural
Findings At Surgery: Male infant in occiput posterior presentation. Thin meconium with none below the cords, pediatrics present at delivery, APGAR's 6/8, weight 3080 g. Normal uterus, tubes, and ovaries.
Description of Operative Procedure:
  After assuring informed consent, the patient was taken to the operating room and spinal anesthesia was initiated. The patient was placed in the dorsal, supine position with left lateral tilt. The abdomen was prepped and draped in sterile fashion.

A Pfannenstiel skin incision was made with a scalpel and carried through to the level of the fascia. The fascial incision was extended bilaterally with Mayo scissors. The fascial incision was then grasped with the Kocher clamps, elevated, and sharply and bluntly dissected superiorly and inferiorly from the rectus muscles.

The rectus muscles were then separated in the midline, and the peritoneum was tented up, and entered sharply with Metzenbaum scissors. The peritoneal incision was extended superiorly and inferiorly with good visualization of the bladder.

A bladder blade was then inserted, and the vesicouterine peritoneum was identified, grasped with the pick-ups, and entered sharply with the Metzenbaum scissors. This incision was then extended laterally, and a bladder flap was created. The bladder was retracted using the bladder blade. The lower uterine segment was incised in a transverse fashion with the scalpel, then extended bilaterally with bandage scissors. The bladder blade was removed, and the infants head was delivered atraumatically. The nose and mouth were suctioned and the cord clamped and cut. The infant was handed off to the pediatrician. Cord gases and cord blood were sent.

The placenta was then removed manually, and the uterus was exteriorized, and cleared of all clots and debris. The uterine incision was repaired with 1-O chromic in a running locking fashion. A second layer of 1-O chromic was used to obtain excellent hemostasis. The bladder flap was repaired with a 3-O Vicryl in a running fashion. The cul-de-sac was cleared of clots and the uterus was returned to the abdomen. The peritoneum was closed with 3-0 Vicryl. The fascia was reapproximated with O Vicryl in a running fashion. The skin was closed with staples.

The patient tolerated the procedure well. Needle and sponge counts were correct times two. Two grams of Ancef was given at cord clamp, and a sterile dressing was placed over the incision.

Estimated Blood Loss (EBL): 800 cc; no blood replaced (normal blood loss is 500-1000 cc).

Specimens: Placenta, cord pH, cord blood specimens.

Drains: Foley to gravity.

Fluids: Input - 2000 cc LR; Output - 300 cc clear urine.

Complications: None.

Disposition: The patient was taken to the recovery room then postpartum ward in stable condition.

Postoperative Management after Cesarean Section

I. **Post Cesarean Section Orders**
   A. **Transfer:** to post partum ward when stable.
   B. **Vital signs:** q4h x 24 hours, I and O.
   C. **Activity:** Bed rest x 6-8 hours, then ambulate; if given spinal, keep patient flat on back x 8h. Incentive spirometer q1h while awake.
   D. **Diet:** NPO x 8h, then sips of water. Advance to clear liquids, then to regular diet as tolerated.
   E. **IV Fluids:** IV D5 LR or D5 ½ NS at 125 cc/h. Foley to gravity; discontinue after 12 hours. I and O catheterize prn.
   F. **Medications**
      1. Cefazolin (Ancef) 1 gm IVPB x one dose at time of cesarean section.
      2. Nalbuphine (Nubain) 5 to 10 mg SC or IV q2-3h **OR**
      3. Meperidine (Demerol) 50-75 mg IM q3-4h prn pain.
      4. Hydroxyzine (Vistaril) 25-50 mg IM q3-4h prn nausea.
      5. Prochlorperazine (Compazine) 10 mg IV q4-6h prn nausea **OR**
      6. Promethazine (Phenergan) 25-50 mg IV q3-4h prn nausea
   G. **Labs:** CBC in AM.

II. Postoperative Day #1

A. Assess pain, lungs, cardiac status, fundal height, lochia, passing of flatus, bowel movement, distension, tenderness, bowel sounds, incision.

B. Discontinue IV when taking adequate PO fluids.

C. Discontinue Foley, and I and O catheterize prn.

D. Ambulate tid with assistance; incentive spirometer q1h while awake.

E. Check hematocrit, hemoglobin, Rh, and rubella status.

F. **Medications**
1. Acetaminophen/codeine (Tylenol #3) 1-2 PO q4-6h prn pain **OR**
2. Oxycodone/acetaminophen (Percocet) 1 tab q6h prn pain.
3. FeSO4 325 mg PO bid-tid.
4. Multivitamin PO qd, Colace 100 mg PO bid. Mylicon 80 mg PO qid prn bloating.

III. Postoperative Day #2

A. If passing gas and/or bowel movement, advance to regular diet.

B. Laxatives: Dulcolax supp prn or Milk of magnesia 30 cc PO tid prn. Mylicon 80 mg PO qid prn bloating.

IV. Postoperative Day #3

A. If transverse incision, remove staples and place steri-strips on day 3. If a vertical incision, remove staples on post op day 5.

B. Discharge home on appropriate medications; follow up in 2 and 6 weeks.

Laparoscopic Bilateral Tubal Ligation Operative Report

Preoperative Diagnosis: Multiparous female desiring permanent sterilization.
Postoperative Diagnosis: Same as above
Title of Operation: Laparoscopic bilateral tubal ligation with Falope rings
Surgeon:
Assistant:
Anesthesia: General endotracheal
Findings At Surgery: Normal uterus, tubes, and ovaries.
Description of Operative Procedure

After informed consent, the patient was taken to the operating room where general anesthesia was administered. The patient was examined under anesthesia and found to have a normal uterus with normal adnexa. She was placed in the dorsal lithotomy position and prepped and draped in sterile fashion. A bivalve speculum was placed in the vagina, and the anterior lip of the cervix was grasped with a single toothed tenaculum. A uterine manipulator was placed into the endocervical canal and articulated with the tenaculum. The speculum was removed from the vagina.

An infraumbilical incision was made with a scalpel, then while tenting up on the abdomen, a Verres needle was admitted into the intraabdominal cavity. A saline drop test was performed and noted to be within normal limits. Pneumoperitoneum was attained with 4 liters of carbon dioxide. The Verres needle was removed, and a 10 mm trocar and sleeve were advanced into the intraabdominal cavity while tenting up on the abdomen. The laparoscope was inserted and proper location was confirmed. A second incision was made 2 cm above the symphysis pubis, and a 5 mm trocar and sleeve were inserted into the abdomen under laparoscopic visualization without complication.

A survey revealed normal pelvic and abdominal anatomy. A Falope ring applicator was advanced through the second trocar sleeve, and the left Fallopian tube was identified, followed out to the fimbriated end, and grasped 4 cm from the cornual region. The Falope ring was applied to a knuckle of tube and good blanching was noted at the site of application. No bleeding was observed from the mesosalpinx. The Falope ring applicator was reloaded, and a Falope ring was applied in a similar fashion to the opposite tube. Carbon dioxide was allowed to escape from the abdomen.

The instruments were removed, and the skin incisions were closed with #3-O Vicryl in a subcuticular fashion. The instruments were removed from the vagina,

and excellent hemostasis was noted. The patient tolerated the procedure well, and sponge, lap and needle counts were correct times two. The patient was taken to the recovery room in stable condition.
Estimated Blood Loss (EBL): <10 cc
Specimens: None
Drains: Foley to gravity
Fluids: 1500 cc LR
Complications: None
Disposition: The patient was taken to the recovery room in stable condition.

Postpartum Tubal Ligation Operative Report

Preoperative Diagnosis: Multiparous female after vaginal delivery, desiring permanent sterilization.
Postoperative Diagnosis: Same as above
Title of Operation: Modified Pomeroy bilateral tubal ligation
Surgeon:
Assistant:
Anesthesia: Epidural
Findings At Surgery: Normal fallopian tubes bilaterally
Description of Operative Procedure:
    After assuring informed consent, the patient was taken to the operating room and spinal anesthesia administered. A small, transverse, infraumbilical skin incision was made with a scalpel, and the incision was carried down through the underlying fascia until the peritoneum was identified and entered. The left fallopian tube was identified, brought into the incision and grasped with a Babcock clamp. The tube was then followed out to the fimbria. An avascular midsection of the fallopian tube was grasped with a Babcock clamp and brought into a knuckle. The tube was doubly ligated with an O-plain suture and transected. The specimen was sent to pathology. Excellent hemostasis was noted, and the tube was returned to the abdomen. The same procedure was performed on the opposite fallopian tube.
    The fascia was then closed with O-Vicryl in a single layer. The skin was closed with 3-O Vicryl in a subcuticular fashion. The patient tolerated the procedure well. Needle and sponge counts were correct times 2.
Estimated Blood Loss (EBL): <20 cc
Specimens: Segments of right and left tubes
Drains: Foley to gravity
Fluids: Input - 500 cc LR; output - 300 cc clear urine
Complications: None
Disposition: The patient was taken to the recovery room in stable condition.

Prevention of D Isoimmunization

The morbidity and mortality of Rh hemolytic disease can be significantly reduced by identification of women at risk for isoimmunization and by administration of D immunoglobulin. Administration of D immunoglobulin [RhoGAM, Rho(D) immunoglobulin, RhIg] is very effective in the preventing isoimmunization to the D antigen.

I. **Prenatal testing**
    A. Routine prenatal laboratory evaluation includes ABO and D blood type determination and antibody screen.
    B. At 28-29 weeks of gestation woman who are D negative but not D isoimmunized should be retested for D antibody. If the test reveals that no D antibody is present, prophylactic D immunoglobulin [RhoGAM, Rho(D) immunoglobulin, RhIg] is indicated.
    C. If D antibody is present, D immunoglobulin will not be beneficial, and specialized management of the D isoimmunized pregnancy is undertaken to manage hemolytic disease of the fetus and hydrops fetalis.

II. Routine administration of D immunoglobulin

A. Abortion. D sensitization may be caused by abortion. D sensitization occurs more frequently after induced abortion than after spontaneous abortion, and it occurs more frequently after late abortion than after early abortion. D sensitization occurs following induced abortion in 4-5% of susceptible women. All unsensitized, D-negative women who have an induced or spontaneous abortion should be treated with D immunoglobulin unless the father is known to be D negative.

B. Dosage of D immunoglobulin is determined by the stage of gestation. If the abortion occurs before 13 weeks of gestation, 50 mcg of D immunoglobulin prevents sensitization. For abortions occurring at 13 weeks of gestation and later, 300-mcg is given.

C. Ectopic pregnancy can cause D sensitization. All unsensitized, D-negative women who have an ectopic pregnancy should be given D immunoglobulin. The dosage is determined by the gestational age, as described above for abortion.

D. Amniocentesis

1. D isoimmunization can occur after amniocentesis. D immunoglobulin, 300 mcg, should be administered to unsensitized, D-negative, susceptible patients following first- and second-trimester amniocentesis.

2. Following third-trimester amniocentesis, 300 mcg of D immunoglobulin should be administered. If amniocentesis is performed and delivery is planned within 48 hours, D immunoglobulin can be withheld until after delivery, when the newborn can be tested for D positivity. If the amniocentesis is expected to precede delivery by more than 48 hours, the patient should receive 300 mcg of D immunoglobulin at the time of amniocentesis.

E. Antepartum prophylaxis

1. Isoimmunized occurs in 1-2% of D-negative women during the antepartum period. D immunoglobulin, administered both during pregnancy and postpartum, can reduce the incidence of D isoimmunization to 0.3%.

2. Antepartum prophylaxis is given at 28-29 weeks of gestation. Antibody-negative, Rh-negative gravidas should have a repeat assessment at 28 weeks. D Immunoglobulin (RhoGAM, RhIg), 300 mcg, is given to D-negative women. However, if the father of the fetus is known with certainty to be D negative, antepartum prophylaxis is not necessary.

F. Postpartum D immunoglobulin

1. D immunoglobulin is given to the D negative mother as soon after delivery as cord blood findings indicate that the baby is Rh positive.

2. A woman at risk who is inadvertently not given D immunoglobulin within 72 hours after delivery should still receive prophylaxis at any time up until two weeks after delivery. If prophylaxis is delayed, it may not be effective.

3. A quantitative Kleihauer-Betke analysis should be performed in situations in which significant maternal bleeding may have occurred (eg, after maternal abdominal trauma, abruptio placentae, external cephalic version). If the quantitative determination is thought to be more than 30 mL, D immune globulin should be given to the mother in multiples of one vial (300 mcg) for each 30 mL of estimated fetal whole blood in her circulation, unless the father of the baby is known to be D negative.

G. Abruptio placentae, placenta previa, cesarean delivery, intrauterine manipulation, or manual removal of the placenta may cause more than 30 mL of fetal-to-maternal bleeding. In these conditions, testing for excessive bleeding (Kleihauer-Betke test) or inadequate D immunoglobulin dosage (indirect Coombs test) is necessary.

References: See page 208.

Complications of Pregnancy

Nausea and Vomiting of Pregnancy and Hyperemesis Gravidarum

Nausea and vomiting to affects about 70% to 85% of pregnant women. Symptoms of nausea and vomiting of pregnancy (NVP) are most common during the first trimester; however, some women have persistent nausea for their entire pregnancy. Hyperemesis often occurs in association with high levels of human chorionic gonadotropin (hCG), such as with multiple pregnancies, trophoblastic disease, and fetal anomalies such as triploidy.

Conditions that Predispose to Excessive Nausea and Vomiting

Viral gastroenteritis
Gestational trophoblastic disease
Hepatitis
Urinary tract infection
Multifetal gestation
Gallbladder disease
Migraine

I. **Treatment of nausea and vomiting of pregnancy**
   A. Patients should avoid odors or foods that seem to be aggravating the nausea. Useful dietary modifications include avoiding fatty or spicy foods, and stopping iron supplements. Frequent small meals also may improve symptoms. Recommendations include bland and dry foods, high-protein snacks, and crackers at the bedside to be taken first thing in the morning.
   B. Cholecystitis, peptic ulcer disease, or hepatitis can cause nausea and vomiting and should be excluded. Gastroenteritis, appendicitis, pyelonephritis, and pancreatitis also should be excluded. Obstetric explanations for nausea and vomiting may include multiple pregnancies or a hydatidiform mole.
   C. Non-pharmacologic remedies are adequate for up to 90% of patients with NVP. However, about 10% will require medication and about 1% have severe enough vomiting that they require hospitalization.
   D. **Vitamin therapy.** Pyridoxine is effective as first-line therapy and is recommended up to 25 mg three times daily. Pyridoxine serum levels do not appear to correlate with the prevalence or degree of nausea and vomiting. Multivitamins also are effective for prevention of NVP. Premesis Rx is a prescription tablet with controlled-release vitamin B6, 75 mg, so it can be given once a day. It also contains vitamin B12 (12 mcg), folic acid (1 mg), and calcium carbonate (200 mg).
   E. **Over-the-Counter Therapy.** If pyridoxine alone is not efficacious, an alternative is to combine over-the-counter doxylamine 25 mg (Unisom) and pyridoxine 25 mg. One could combine the 25 mg of pyridoxine three times daily with doxylamine 25 mg, 1 tablet every bedtime, and ½ tablet morning and afternoon. There is no evidence that doxylamine is a teratogen.

Drug Therapy for Nausea and Vomiting of Pregnancy	
Generic name (trade name)	**Dosage**
Antihistamines	
Doxylamine (Unisom)	25 mg ½ tab BID, 1 tab qhs
Dimenhydrinate (Dramamine)	25 to 100 mg po/im/iv every 4 to 6 hr
Diphenhydramine (Benadryl)	25 to 50 mg po/im/iv every 4 to 6 hr
Trimethobenzamide (Tigan)	250 mg po every 6 to 8 hr or 200 mg im/pr every 6 to 8 hr
Meclizine (Antivert)	12.5 to 25 mg BID/TID
Phenothiazines	
Promethazine (Phenergan)	12.5 to 25 mg po/iv/pr every 4 to 6 hr
Prochlorperazine (Compazine)	5 to 10 mg po/iv every 6 to 8 hr or 25 mg pr every 6 to 8 hr
Prokinetic agents	
Metoclopramide (Reglan)	10 to 20 mg po/iv every 6 hr
Serotonin (5-HT$_3$) antagonists	
Ondansetron (Zofran)	8 mg po/iv every 8 hr
Corticosteroids	
Methylprednisolone (Medrol)	16 mg po TID for 3 days then ½ dose every 3 days for 2 wks

F. Pharmacologic Therapy
   1. Prescribed medication is the next step if dietary modifications and vitamin B6 therapy with doxylamine are ineffective. The phenothiazines are safe and effective, and promethazine (Phenergan) often is tried first. One of the disadvantages of the phenothiazines is their potential for dystonic effects.
   2. **Metoclopramide (Reglan)** is the antiemetic drug of choice in pregnancy in several European countries. There was no increased risk of birth defects.
   3. **Ondansetron (Zofran)** has been compared with promethazine (Phenergan), and the two drugs are equally effective, but ondansetron is much more expensive. No data have been published on first trimester teratogenic risk with ondansetron.

II. Hyperemesis gravidarum
   A. Hyperemesis gravidarum occurs in the extreme 0.5% to 1% of patients who have intractable vomiting. Patients with hyperemesis have abnormal electrolytes, dehydration with high urine-specific gravity, ketosis and acetonuria, and untreated have weight loss >5% of body weight. Intravenous hydration is the first line of therapy for patients with severe

nausea and vomiting. Administration of vitamin B1 supplements may be necessary to prevent Wernicke's encephalopathy.

References: See page 208.

Spontaneous Abortion

Abortion is defined as termination of pregnancy resulting in expulsion of an immature, nonviable fetus. A fetus of <20 weeks gestation or a fetus weighing <500 gm is considered an abortus. Spontaneous abortion occurs in 15% of all pregnancies.

I. **Threatened abortion** is defined as vaginal bleeding occurring in the first 20 weeks of pregnancy, without the passage of tissue or rupture of membranes.
   A. Symptoms of pregnancy (nausea, vomiting, fatigue, breast tenderness, urinary frequency) are usually present.
   B. Speculum exam reveals blood coming from the cervical os without amniotic fluid or tissue in the endocervical canal.
   C. The internal cervical os is closed, and the uterus is soft and enlarged appropriate for gestational age.
   D. **Differential diagnosis**
      1. **Benign and malignant lesions.** The cervix often bleeds from an ectropion of friable tissue. Hemostasis can be accomplished by applying pressure for several minutes with a large swab or by cautery with a silver nitrate stick. Atypical cervical lesions are evaluated with colposcopy and biopsy.
      2. **Disorders of pregnancy**
         a. **Hydatidiform mole** may present with early pregnancy bleeding, passage of grape-like vesicles, and a uterus that is enlarged in excess of that expected from dates. An absence of heart tones by Doppler after 12 weeks is characteristic. Hyperemesis, preeclampsia, or hyperthyroidism may be present. Ultrasonography confirms the diagnosis.
         b. **Ectopic pregnancy** should be excluded when first trimester bleeding is associated with pelvic pain. Orthostatic light-headedness, syncope or shoulder pain (from diaphragmatic irritation) may occur.
            (1) Abdominal tenderness is noted, and pelvic examination reveals cervical motion tenderness.
            (2) Serum beta-HCG is positive.
   E. **Laboratory tests**
      1. **Complete blood count.** The CBC will not reflect acute blood loss.
      2. **Quantitative serum beta-HCG level** may be positive in nonviable gestations since beta-HCG may persist in the serum for several weeks after fetal death.
      3. **Ultrasonography** should detect fetal heart motion by 7 weeks gestation or older. Failure to detect fetal heart motion after 9 weeks gestation should prompt consideration of curettage.
   F. **Treatment of threatened abortion**
      1. Bed rest with sedation and abstinence from intercourse.
      2. The patient should report increased bleeding (>normal menses), cramping, passage of tissue, or fever. Passed tissue should be saved for examination.
II. **Inevitable abortion** is defined as a threatened abortion with a dilated cervical os. Menstrual-like cramps usually occur.
   A. **Differential diagnosis**
      1. **Incomplete abortion** is diagnosed when tissue has passed. Tissue may be visible in the vagina or endocervical canal.
      2. **Threatened abortion** is diagnosed when the internal os is closed and will not admit a fingertip.

    3. **Incompetent cervix** is characterized by dilatation of the cervix without cramps.
  B. **Treatment of inevitable abortion**
    1. Surgical evacuation of the uterus is necessary.
    2. D immunoglobulin (RhoGAM) is administered to Rh-negative, unsensitized patients to prevent isoimmunization. Before 13 weeks gestation, the dosage is 50 mcg IM; at 13 weeks gestation, the dosage is 300 mcg IM.

III. **Incomplete abortion** is characterized by cramping, bleeding, passage of tissue, and a dilated internal os with tissue present in the vagina or endocervical canal. Profuse bleeding, orthostatic dizziness, syncope, and postural pulse and blood pressure changes may occur.
  A. **Laboratory evaluation**
    1. **Complete blood count.** CBC will not reflect acute blood loss.
    2. **Rh typing**
    3. **Blood typing and cress-matching.**
    4. **Karyotyping** of products of conception is completed if loss is recurrent.
  B. **Treatment**
    1. **Stabilization.** If the patient has signs and symptoms of heavy bleeding, at least 2 large-bore IV catheters (<16 gauge) are placed. Lactate Ringer's or normal saline with 40 U oxytocin/L is given IV at 200 mL/hour or greater.
    2. Products of conception are removed from the endocervical canal and uterus with a ring forceps. Immediate removal decreases bleeding. Curettage is performed after vital signs have stabilized.
    3. **Suction dilation and curettage**
      a. Analgesia consists of meperidine (Demerol), 35-50 mg IV over 3-5 minutes until the patient is drowsy.
      b. The patient is placed in the dorsal lithotomy position in stirrups, prepared, draped, and sedated.
      c. A weighted speculum is placed intravaginally, the vagina and cervix are cleansed, and a paracervical block is placed.
      d. Bimanual examination confirms uterine position and size, and uterine sounding confirms the direction of the endocervical canal.
      e. Mechanical dilatation is completed with dilators if necessary. Curettage is performed with an 8 mm suction curette, with a single-tooth tenaculum on the anterior lip of the cervix.
    4. **Post-curettage.** After curettage, a blood count is ordered. If the vital signs are stable for several hours, the patient is discharged with instructions to avoid coitus, douching, or the use of tampons for 2 weeks. Ferrous sulfate and ibuprofen are prescribed for pain.
    5. **Rh-negative**, unsensitized patients are given IM RhoGAM.
    6. **Methylergonovine (Methergine)**, 0.2 mg PO q4h for 6 doses, is given if there is continued moderate bleeding.

IV. **Complete abortion**
  A. A complete abortion is diagnosed when complete passage of products of conception has occurred. The uterus is well contracted, and the cervical os may be closed.
  B. **Differential diagnosis**
    1. **Incomplete abortion**
    2. **Ectopic pregnancy.** Products of conception should be examined grossly and submitted for pathologic examination. If no fetal tissue or villi are observed grossly, ectopic pregnancy must be excluded by ultrasound.
  C. **Management of complete abortion**
    1. Between 8 and 14 weeks, curettage is necessary because of the high probability that the abortion was incomplete.
    2. D immunoglobulin (RhoGAM) is administered to Rh-negative, unsensitized patients.

> 3. Beta-HCG levels are obtained weekly until zero. Incomplete abortion is suspected if beta-HCG levels plateau or fail to reach zero within 4 weeks.

V. Missed abortion is diagnosed when products of conception are retained after the fetus has expired. If products are retained, a severe coagulopathy with bleeding often occurs.

    A. Missed abortion should be suspected when the pregnant uterus fails to grow as expected or when fetal heart tones disappear.

    B. Amenorrhea may persist, or intermittent vaginal bleeding, spotting, or brown discharge may be noted.

    C. Ultrasonography confirms the diagnosis.

    D. Management of missed abortion

        1. CBC with platelet count, fibrinogen level, partial thromboplastin time, and ABO blood typing and antibody screen are obtained.

        2. Evacuation of the uterus is completed after fetal death has been confirmed. Dilation and evacuation by suction curettage is appropriate when the uterus is less than 12-14 weeks gestational size.

        3. D immunoglobulin (RhoGAM) is administered to Rh-negative, unsensitized patients.

References: See page 208.

Urinary Tract Infections in Pregnancy

Urinary tract infection (UTI) is common in pregnancy. Although asymptomatic bacteriuria occurs with similar frequency in pregnant and nonpregnant women, bacteriuria progresses to symptomatic infection more frequently during pregnancy.

I. Incidence

    A. The prevalence of asymptomatic bacteriuria in pregnant and nonpregnant women is 5 to 9%. If asymptomatic bacteriuria is not treated, pyelonephritis will develop in 20 to 40% of pregnant patients. This rate of progression to symptomatic disease is three- to fourfold higher than in nonpregnant women.

    B. Microbiology. Escherichia coli is responsible for 60 to 90% of cases of asymptomatic bacteriuria, cystitis, and pyelonephritis.

    C. Asymptomatic Bacteriuria refers to the isolation of $\geq$100,000 CFU of a single organism/mL from a midstream-voided specimen in a woman without UTI symptoms. It occurs in 5 to 9% of pregnancies, usually developing in the first month of gestation.

II. Diagnosis

    A. A single clean-catch midstream urine culture detects 80% of patients with asymptomatic bacteriuria; two such cultures approach the sensitivity of catheterization (96%). A positive urine culture is $\geq 10^5$ CFU/mL. Isolation of more than one species or the presence of lactobacillus or propiobacterium indicates a contaminated specimen.

    B. Screening for asymptomatic bacteriuria is standard practice at the first prenatal visit.

III. Treatment of asymptomatic bacteriuria

    A. Amoxicillin-clavulanate (Augmentin) 500 mg PO BID for three days.

    B. Nitrofurantoin (Macrodantin) 50 mg PO QID for seven days.

    C. Cefixime (Suprax) 250 mg PO QD for three days.

    D. Fosfomycin (Monural) 3 g PO as a single dose.

    E. Relapse typically occurs in the first two weeks after treatment. Such infections should be treated with two weeks of oral antibiotics.

    F. Suppressive therapy is recommended for women with persistent bacteriuria (ie, >2 positive urine cultures). Nitrofurantoin (Macrodantin) 50 to 100 mg orally at bedtime, for the duration of the pregnancy is one option, or cephalexin (Keflex) 250 to 500 mg orally at bedtime. A culture for test of cure is obtained one week after completion of therapy and then repeated monthly until completion of the pregnancy.

IV. **Cystitis** occurs in 0.3 to 1.3% of pregnant women. Bacteria are confined to the lower urinary tract in these patients.

    A. Acute cystitis should be considered in any gravida with frequency, urgency, dysuria, hematuria, or suprapubic pain in the absence of fever and flank pain. Urine culture with a CFU count $\geq 10^2$/mL should be considered positive on a midstream urine specimen with pyuria.

    B. **Empiric treatment regimens:**
        1. Nitrofurantoin (Macrodantin) 100 mg BID
        2. Cephalexin (Keflex) 500 mg BID to QID

    C. Each of these drugs is given for three to seven days.

    D. Other regimens which have a broader spectrum of activity include amoxicillin-clavulanate (Augmentin) 500 mg BID or 250 mg TID, trimethoprim-sulfamethoxazole (Bactrim) 1 DS BID but not in the third trimester of pregnancy, cefpodoxime proxetil (Vantin) 100 mg BID, and cefixime (Suprax) 400 mg QD. All of these drugs can be used for three to seven days. Fluoroquinolones should be avoided in pregnancy.

    E. Monthly urine cultures should be performed beginning one to two weeks after completion of treatment.

V. **Pyelonephritis** complicates 1 to 2% of all pregnancies. Risk factors include asymptomatic bacteriuria, previous pyelonephritis, renal and collecting system anomalies, and renal calculi.

    A. **Presentation** consists of fever, chills, and costovertebral angle tenderness. Other symptoms include dysuria, nausea, vomiting, and respiratory distress.

    B. **Urinalysis** reveals one or two bacteria per high-power field in an unspun catheterized specimen or 20 bacteria per HPF in a spun specimen; white cell casts confirm the diagnosis. Urine culture and antimicrobial susceptibility testing should be performed.

    C. **Blood cultures** are positive in 10 to 20% of patients.

    D. **Outpatient treatment**, with one of the above regimens, may be considered in the absence of underlying medical conditions, anatomic abnormalities, pregnancy complications, or signs of sepsis.

    E. **Inpatient treatment**
        1. Fluoroquinolones should not be used because of adverse effects on growing cartilage. Parenteral beta lactams or gentamicin are the preferred antibiotics. Symptoms that persist for more than 48 hours, despite intravenous antibiotic therapy, require further evaluation with a renal ultrasound to assess for perinephric abscess or renal calculi.
        2. Intravenous treatment should continue until the patient is afebrile for 48 hours. Inpatient therapy is followed by oral antibiotics to complete 10 to 14 days of treatment.

Parenteral Regimens for Empiric Treatment of Acute Pyelonephritis in Pregnancy	
Antibiotic, dose	**Interval**
Ceftriaxone, 1 g	Q24 hours
Gentamicin, 1 mg/kg (+ ampicillin)	Q8 hours
Ampicillin, 1-2 g (plus gentamicin)*	Q6 hours

Antibiotic, dose	Interval
Ticarcillin-clavulanate (Timentin) 3.2 g	Q8 hours
Piperacillin-tazobactam 3.375 g*	Q8-12 hours
Imipenem-cilastatin, 250-500 mg	Q6-8 hours
* Recommended regimen if enterococcus suspected	

     3. Low-dose antimicrobial prophylaxis, such as nitrofurantoin
        (Macrodantin) 50 to 100 mg PO QHS or cephalexin (Keflex) 250 to
        500 mg PO QHS, and periodic urinary surveillance for infection are
        recommended for the remainder of the pregnancy.

References: See page 208.

Trauma During Pregnancy

Trauma is the leading cause of nonobstetric death in women of reproductive age. Six% of all pregnancies are complicated by some type of trauma.

I. Mechanism of injury
   A. Blunt abdominal trauma
      1. Blunt abdominal trauma secondary to motor vehicle accidents is the
         leading cause of nonobstetric-related fetal death during pregnancy,
         followed by falls and assaults. Uterine rupture or laceration,
         retroperitoneal hemorrhage, renal injury and upper abdominal
         injuries may also occur after blunt trauma.
      2. Abruptio placentae occurs in 40-50% of patients with major trau-
         matic injuries and in up to 5% of patients with minor injuries.
      3. Clinical findings in blunt abdominal trauma. Vaginal bleeding,
         uterine tenderness, uterine contractions, fetal tachycardia, late
         decelerations, fetal acidosis, and fetal death.
      4. Detection of abruptio placentae. Beyond 20 weeks of gestation,
         external electronic monitoring can detect uterine contractile activity.
         The presence of vaginal bleeding and tetanic or hypertonic contrac-
         tions is presumptive evidence of abruptio placentae.
      5. Uterine rupture
        a. Uterine rupture is an infrequent but life-threatening complication.
          It usually occurs after a direct abdominal impact.
        b. Findings of uterine rupture range from subtle (uterine tenderness,
          nonreassuring fetal heart rate pattern) to severe, with rapid onset
          of maternal hypovolemic shock and death.
      6. Direct fetal injury is an infrequent complication of blunt trauma.
        a. The fetus is more frequently injured as a result of hypoxia from
          blood loss or abruption.
        b. In the first trimester the uterus is well protected by the maternal
          pelvis; therefore, minor trauma usually does not usually cause
          miscarriage in the first trimester.
   B. Penetrating trauma
      1. Penetrating abdominal trauma from gunshot and stab wounds
         during pregnancy has a poor prognosis.
      2. Perinatal mortality is 41-71%. Maternal mortality is less than 5%.
II. Major trauma in pregnancy
   A. Initial evaluation of major abdominal trauma in pregnant patients
     does not differ from evaluation of abdominal trauma in a nonpregnant
     patient.

B. **Maintain airway, breathing, and circulatory volume.** Two large-bore (14-16-gauge) intravenous lines are placed.

C. **Oxygen** should be administered by mask or endotracheal intubation. Maternal oxygen saturation should be kept at >90% (an oxygen partial pressure [pO_2] of 60 mm Hg).

D. **Volume resuscitation**
   1. Crystalloid in the form of lactated Ringer's or normal saline should be given as a 3:1 replacement for the estimated blood loss over the first 30-60 minutes of acute resuscitation.
   2. O-negative packed red cells are preferred if emergent blood is needed before the patient's own blood type is known.
   3. A urinary catheter should be placed to measure urine output and observe for hematuria.

E. **Deflection of the uterus** off the inferior vena cava and abdominal aorta can be achieved by placing the patient in the lateral decubitus position. If the patient must remain supine, manual deflection of the uterus to the left and placement of a wedge under the patient's hip or backboard will tilt the patient.

F. **Secondary survey.** Following stabilization, a more detailed secondary survey of the patient, including fetal evaluation, is performed.

III. **Minor trauma in pregnancy**

A. **Clinical evaluation**
   1. Pregnant patients who sustain seemingly minimal trauma require an evaluation to exclude significant injuries. Common "minor" trauma include falls, especially in the third trimester, blows to the abdomen, and "fender benders" motor vehicle accidents.
   2. The patient should be questioned about seat belt use, loss of consciousness, pain, vaginal bleeding, rupture of membranes, and fetal movement.
   3. **Physical examination**
      a. Physical examination should focus on upper abdominal tenderness (liver or spleen damage), flank pain (renal trauma), uterine pain (placental abruption, uterine rupture), and pain over the symphysis pubis (pelvic fracture, bladder laceration, fetal skull fracture).
      b. A search for orthopedic injuries should be completed.

B. **Management of minor trauma**
   1. The minor trauma patient with a fetus that is less than 20 weeks gestation (not yet viable), with no significant injury can be safely discharged after documentation of fetal heart rate. Patients with potentially viable fetuses (over 20 weeks of gestation) require fetal monitoring, laboratory tests and ultrasonographic evaluation.
   2. A complete blood count, urinalysis (hematuria), blood type and screen (to check Rh status), and coagulation panel, including measurement of the INR, PTT, fibrinogen and fibrin split products, should be obtained. The coagulation panel is useful if any suspicion of abruption exists.
   3. **The Kleihauer-Betke (KB) test**
      a. This test detects fetal red blood cells in the maternal circulation. A KB stain should be obtained routinely for any pregnant trauma patient whose fetus is over 12 weeks.
      b. Regardless of the patient's blood type and Rh status, the KB test can help determine if fetomaternal hemorrhage has occurred.
      c. The KB test can also be used to determine the amount of Rho(D) immunoglobulin (RhoGAM) required in patients who are Rh-negative.
      d. A positive KB stain indicates uterine trauma, and any patient with a positive KB stain should receive at least 24 hours of continuous uterine and fetal monitoring and a coagulation panel.
   4. **Ultrasonography** is less sensitive for diagnosing abruption than is the finding of uterine contractions on external tocodynamometry.

Absence of sonographic evidence of abruption does not completely exclude an abruption.

5. Patients with abdominal pain, significant bruising, vaginal bleeding, rupture of membranes, or uterine contractions should be admitted to the hospital for overnight observation and continuous fetal monitor.
6. Uterine contractions and vaginal bleeding are suggestive of abruption. Even if vaginal bleeding is absent, the presence of contractions is still a concern, since the uterus can contain up to 2 L of blood from a concealed abruption.
7. Trauma patients with no uterine contraction activity, usually do not have abruption, while patients with greater than one contraction per 10 minutes (6 per hour) have a 20% incidence of abruption.

References: See page 208.

Gestational Diabetes Mellitus

Gestational diabetes (GDM) occurs when pancreatic function is not sufficient to overcome the insulin resistance caused by diabetogenic hormones during pregnancy. Diabetogenic hormones secreted by the placenta include growth hormone, corticotropin-releasing hormone, placental lactogen, and progesterone.

I. **Pathophysiology**
   A. Gestational diabetes mellitus is defined as glucose intolerance with onset during pregnancy. Most women with GDM have glucose intolerance that begins in pregnancy, but some may have type 2 diabetes that was not diagnosed before pregnancy.
   B. **Adverse effects of GDM and hyperglycemia:**
      1. Preeclampsia
      2. Polyhydramnios
      3. Fetal macrosomia
      4. Birth trauma
      5. Operative delivery
      6. Perinatal mortality
      7. Neonatal metabolic complications (hypoglycemia, hyperbilirubinemia, hypocalcemia, erythremia)
   C. There is a 10% per year risk development of maternal diabetes mellitus after a pregnancy with gestational diabetes.
II. **Prevalence rates** are higher in African, Hispanic, Native American, and Asian women than white women. The prevalence of GDM is 1.4% of pregnancies.

Risk Factors for Gestational Diabetes

- A family history of diabetes, especially in first degree relatives
- Prepregnancy weight of 110% of ideal body weight (pregravid weight more than 90 kg) or more or weight gain in early adulthood.
- Age >25 years
- A previous large baby (>9 pounds [4.1 kg])
- History of abnormal glucose tolerance
- Hispanic, African, Native American, South or East Asian, and Pacific Island ancestry
- A previous unexplained perinatal loss or birth of a malformed child
- The mother was large at birth (>9 pounds [4.1 kg])
- Polycystic ovary syndrome
- Glycosuria at the first prenatal visit
- Current use of glucocorticoids
- Pregnancy-related hypertension

III. **Screening**
   A. Universal screening should be performed at 24 to 28 weeks. However, screening is done at the first prenatal visit if there is a high degree of

suspicion of type 2 diabetes (eg, obesity, personal history of GDM, glycosuria, or family history of diabetes). Women with a history of GDM have a 33 to 50% risk of recurrence.
B. Evaluation of any woman who has a random serum glucose value above 200 mg/dL or a fasting serum glucose value >126 mg/dL is unnecessary, because these findings alone are diagnostic of diabetes, if confirmed on a subsequent day.
C. Screening is done with a 50-g oral glucose challenge test. A 50-g oral glucose load is given without regard to the time elapsed since the last meal and plasma or serum glucose is measured one hour later; a value >130 is considered abnormal.
D. Women with an abnormal value are then given a 100-g, three hour oral glucose tolerance test (GTT).

IV. **Diagnostic testing**
   A. **Three hour oral GTT.** GDM is present if two or more of the following serum glucose values are met or exceeded:

Criteria for Gestational Diabetes with Three Hour Oral Glucose Tolerance Test	
Fasting	>95 mg/dL
1 hour	>180 mg/dL
2 hour	>155 mg/dL
3 hour	>140 mg/dL
Any two or more abnormal results are diagnostic of gestational diabetes.	

   B. **One abnormal GTT value.** Women with one abnormal value on the oral GTT are more likely to deliver a macrosomic infant than women without GDM. Treatment of women with one abnormal GTT value decreases the risk of a macrosomic infant.

V. **Pregestational diabetes.** Previously unrecognized type 1 or type 2 diabetes may be diagnosed as GDM during pregnancy. Postpartum documentation of persistent glucose intolerance suggests one of these diagnoses.
   A. Fasting hyperglycemia at diagnosis of GDM is associated with an increased risk of congenital anomalies (4.8 versus 1.5% in nondiabetic women).
   B. Clues to the presence of type 1 diabetes include:
      1. GDM in lean women
      2. Diabetic ketoacidosis during pregnancy
      3. Severe hyperglycemia during pregnancy requiring large doses of insulin
      4. Postpartum hyperglycemia

VI. **Treatment and course of gestational diabetes mellitus**
   A. Identifying women with GDM is important because appropriate therapy can decrease fetal and maternal morbidity, particularly macrosomia. Treatment consists of dietary therapy, self blood glucose monitoring, and insulin if target blood glucose values are not met with diet alone.
   B. Treatment of GDM results in a significantly lower rate of perinatal death, shoulder dystocia, bone fracture, and nerve palsy, and a lower frequency of macrosomia (10 versus 21%).

VII. **Nutritional therapy**
   A. Calorie allotment is approximately:
      1. 30 kcal per kg current weight per day in pregnant women who are BMI 22 to 27.

2. 24 kcal per kg current weight per day in overweight pregnant women (BMI 27 to 29).
3. 12 to 15 kcal per kg current weight per day for morbidly obese pregnant women (BMI >30).
4. 40 kcal per kg current weight per day in pregnant women who are less than BMI 22.

B. Carbohydrate intake is restricted to 35 to 40% of calories, with the remainder divided between protein (about 20%) and fat (about 40%).

VIII. **Glucose monitoring**
A. **Timing and frequency.** Blood glucose should be measured upon awakening and one hour after each meal.
B. **Glucose goal.** Insulin should be initiated if blood glucose concentrations reach the following values on two or more occasions within a two-week interval despite dietary therapy:
1. Fasting blood glucose concentration >90 mg/dL.
2. One-hour postprandial blood glucose concentration >120 mg/dL.
C. **Glycosylated hemoglobin (HbA1c)** is a helpful ancillary test in assessing glycemic control during pregnancy. HbA1c should be measured every four weeks.

IX. **Medical therapy.** If normoglycemia cannot be maintained by nutritional therapy, then insulin should be initiated.
A. **Insulin.** 15% of women with GDM are placed on insulin because target glucose levels are exceeded despite dietary therapy.
B. The dose of insulin ranges from 50 to 90 units to achieve glucose control.
   1. **If fasting blood glucose concentration is high**, intermediate-acting NPH insulin is given before bedtime. The initial dose is 0.2 U/kg body weight.
   2. **If postprandial blood glucose concentrations are high**, regular insulin or insulin lispro should be given before meals at a dose calculated to be 1.5 U per 10 grams carbohydrate in the breakfast meal and 1 U per 10 grams carbohydrate in the lunch and dinner meals.
   3. **If both preprandial and postprandial blood glucoses are high**, then a four injection per day regimen should be started. Total dosage should be 0.7 U/kg up to week 18, 0.8 U/kg for weeks 18 to 26, 0.9 U/kg for weeks 26 to 36, and 1.0 U/kg for weeks 36 to term.
   4. The insulin is divided as 45% NPH insulin (30% before breakfast and 15% before bedtime) and 55% as preprandial regular insulin (22% before breakfast, 16.5% before lunch, and 16.5% before dinner).
C. **Acute hypoglycemia** is treated with 10 to 20 g of carbohydrate. One unit of rapid-acting insulin lowers blood glucose by 25 mg/dL.

X. **Peripartum management.** Insulin can usually be withheld during labor delivery; an infusion of normal saline is usually sufficient to maintain normoglycemia. Maternal blood glucose should be maintained between 70 and 90 mg/dL.

References: See page 208.

Management of Diabetes Mellitus in Pregnancy

Management of diabetes mellitus in pregnancy has the goals of achieving and maintaining excellent glycemic control and intervention for maternal medical complications. Monitoring of and intervention for fetal and obstetrical complications (eg, congenital anomalies, preeclampsia, macrosomia) is essential.

I. **First trimester**
A. **First prenatal visit.** Pregestational diabetes can be categorized as "vascular disease present" or "vascular disease absent" because

placental dysfunction and aggravation of maternal end-organ disease are more common in women with vasculopathy.

B. Testing. Routine prenatal laboratory evaluations are performed. Treatment of asymptomatic bacteriuria is important because there is a three- to five-fold greater propensity for asymptomatic bacteriuria in diabetic women.

1. **Glycosylated hemoglobin concentration** is obtained for counseling regarding the risks of miscarriage and congenital malformations.
2. **Quantification of urinary proteinuria** should be performed using the urinary protein-to-creatinine ratio on a random urine sample.
3. **Thyrotropin (TSH) and free thyroxine (T4).** The incidence of thyroid dysfunction in type I diabetes is 40%.
4. **Electrocardiogram.** Ischemic heart disease should be screened for.
5. **Dilated eye examination** by an ophthalmologist to detect retinopathy.
6. **First trimester ultrasound examination** should be obtained to document viability and to assist in estimation of gestational age.

Initial prenatal laboratory examination

Blood type and antibody screen
Rhesus type
Hematocrit or hemoglobin
Blood glucose
Creatinine
Free T4, TSH
Hemoglobin A1c
PAP smear
Rubella status (immune or nonimmune)
Syphilis screen
Urinalysis
Urinary protein-to-creatinine ratio
Hepatitis B surface antigen
HIV counseling and testing
Chlamydia
Electrocardiogram
Eye examination
Ultrasound

C. Management
1. Women receiving angiotensin converting enzyme (ACE) inhibitors or receptor blockers (ARBs) for hypertension or nephropathy should be taken off these medications prior to pregnancy because of teratogenicity.
2. Blood pressure should be maintained at 110 to 129 /65 to 79 mmHg in diabetic women with known vascular disease. Antihypertensive therapy is withheld when mild hypertension occurs in pregnant women without vasculopathy because of lack of proven benefit. Severe hypertension is treated to prevent maternal stroke.
D. Second prenatal visit is scheduled about one week after the first. Self-monitored blood glucose values and results from the ophthalmologic and laboratory examination (eg, renal function, glycosylated hemoglobin, thyroid function) are reviewed.
E. Risk of congenital anomalies. A high risk of major congenital malformations and miscarriage is associated with increasing first trimester glycosylated hemoglobin values. A value >1% above the upper limit of the normal range is associated with an increased risk of congenital anomalies.

F. Aneuploidy testing with full integrated test. The full integrated test consists of ultrasound measurement of nuchal translucency thickness combined with a pregnancy-associated plasma protein-A at 10 to 13 weeks.

Frequency of Testing During Pregnancy in Women with Type I Diabetes	
Test	**Frequency**
Hemoglobin A1c	Every 4-6 weeks
Blood glucose	Home measurements 4-8 times daily; during weekly/biweekly visits in physician's office
Urine ketones	During period of illness; when any blood glucose value is $\geq$200 mg/dL
Urinalysis	Weekly/biweekly office visits
Serum creatinine	Each trimester
Thyroid function tests	Baseline measurements of serum-free T4 and TSH
Eye examination	Baseline and then every 3 months

II. Second trimester

A. After the first two prenatal visits, which are scheduled about one week apart, women are seen every two to four weeks through the second trimester.

B. **Quadruple markers** should be obtained at 15 to 18 weeks, measuring alpha-fetoprotein (AFP), unconjugated estriol (uE3), hCG, and inhibin A. The prevalence of NTDs is higher in women with pregestational diabetes mellitus. NTDs occur in 2% of diabetic pregnancies versus 0.1 to 0.2% of the general population. The median maternal serum AFP (MSAFP) level is also 15% lower than in nondiabetic women. For these reasons, a lower threshold MSAFP value (eg, approximately 1.5 MoM) is used in diabetic women.

 1. Levels of MSAFP, unconjugated estriol (uE3), and inhibin A are significantly reduced in women with diabetes, thereby mimicking the pattern suggestive of Down syndrome.

C. **Ultrasound examination** is obtained for the usual obstetric indications. In addition, a level II ultrasound examination is done at approximately 18 weeks of gestation in pregnancies complicated by pregestational diabetes because of the increased prevalence of congenital anomalies. Biometric measurements are obtained to confirm or revise the estimated date of confinement.

D. The ultrasound examination should include a fetal survey with a four-chamber view of the heart and visualization of the outflow tracts. Congenital heart disease occurs more frequently in the offspring of diabetic women.

III. Third trimester

A. In the third trimester, diabetic gravida are typically seen every one to two weeks until 32 weeks of gestation and then weekly until delivery.

 1. Continued close monitoring of maternal blood glucose levels

 2. Avoidance of intrauterine fetal demise

3. Monitoring for obstetrical or medical complications necessitating premature delivery
   4. Detection of fetal macrosomia
B. Insulin resistance due to the hormones produced by the placenta increases most rapidly during the third trimester, changes in insulin dose are common at this time.
C. **Fetal surveillance.** Antepartum monitoring using fetal movement counting, biophysical profile, nonstress test (NST), and/or contraction stress test is initiated at 32 to 34 weeks of gestation.
D. **Antepartum surveillance** begins with weekly NSTs at 32 weeks of gestation when there is suboptimal glycemic control (glycosylated hemoglobin values >7%) and at 34 to 35 weeks with good control (glycosylated hemoglobin <7%), increasing the frequency of testing to two times per week from 36 weeks until delivery.
E. **Assessment of fetal growth.** A sonogram is performed at 38 weeks of gestation to estimate fetal weight, reevaluate cardiac morphology, and assist with delivery plans. Maternal diabetes can impair, but more commonly accelerates, fetal growth. Ultrasound examination should be done at 28 to 30 weeks to assess fetal growth.
F. **Growth restriction.** If there is evidence of intrauterine growth restriction, which is uncommon but often related to preeclampsia or preexisting maternal vasculopathy, tests of fetal well-being are initiated.
G. **Large for gestational age infants.** A large for gestational age (LGA) infant is defined as a fetal weight >4.0 to 4.5 kg or birth weight above the 90th%ile for gestational age. Maternal diabetes mellitus may double the incidence of LGA infants.
   1. LGA fetuses are at increased risk for a prolonged second stage of labor, shoulder dystocia, operative delivery, birth trauma, and perinatal death. Maternal diabetes mellitus increases the likelihood of shoulder dystocia two- to six-fold.
   2. Cesarean delivery is recommended for estimated fetal weight over 4500 g.
H. **Preeclampsia.** The incidences of hypertension and preeclampsia are increased in pregnant women with diabetes. The incidence of preeclampsia in diabetic women with and without vascular disease are 17 and 8%, respectively.
I. **Polyhydramnios.** Diabetic pregnancy is a common etiology of polyhydramnios. Intervention is unnecessary because polyhydramnios related to diabetes is usually mild.
J. **Preterm labor.** Women with pregestational diabetes have higher rates of both indicated preterm delivery (22%) and spontaneous preterm delivery (16%).
   1. Tocolytic therapy should consist of nifedipine or magnesium sulfate. Well-controlled diabetes mellitus is not a contraindication to beta-adrenergic receptor agonist therapy, as long as glucose and potassium concentrations are followed carefully and regulated.
   2. Women with poorly controlled diabetes mellitus should not receive beta-adrenergic receptor agonists, which can cause severe hyperglycemia.
   3. **Betamethasone** administration to reduce neonatal complications associated with preterm birth should be done cautiously. Transient hyperglycemia can be severe in the diabetic. The hyperglycemic effect begins 12 hours after the first dose and lasts for five days.

IV. **Delivery**
A. **Fetal lung maturity.** Respiratory distress syndrome (hyaline membrane disease) is more likely to develop in infants of diabetic mothers delivered early than in infants of nondiabetic mothers. Maternal diabetes delays fetal lung maturation.
   1. Fetal lung maturity should be assessed with the saturated phosphatidylcholine (SPC) in amniotic fluid. An SPC $\geq$1000 mg/dL is required before electively delivering a diabetic woman prior to 39 completed weeks.

2. RDS usually does not occur in any infant of a diabetic mother delivered at or beyond 39 weeks of gestation; assessment of fetal lung maturity is not required at this gestational age.

B. Timing of delivery. Preterm delivery is generally performed only for the usual obstetric indications (eg, preeclampsia, fetal growth restriction, abruption, premature labor with or without premature rupture of membranes) or for worsening maternal renal or retinal disease.

C. Labor should be induced at term (ie, between 39 and 40 completed weeks of gestation).

D. In women with an unfavorable cervix, induction can be safely delayed until 40 and 0/7 weeks in women with excellent glycemic control, no vascular disease or preeclampsia, normal fetal growth, reassuring antepartum fetal surveillance, and no history of stillbirth. If these criteria for continued pregnancy are not met or the patient is not compliant, induction is warranted before the cervix is favorable with cervical ripening agents.

E. Route of delivery. Prophylactic cesarean delivery may be considered to prevent brachial plexus injury when the estimated fetal weight is >4500 g in a woman with diabetes.

F. Labor and delivery. Peripartum maintenance of maternal euglycemia is essential and generally requires hourly capillary glucose determinations and intravenous insulin infusion if hyperglycemia is present.

V. Postpartum. Insulin requirements drop sharply after delivery and should be recalculated based on serial blood glucose determinations.

VI. Obstetrical management of gestational diabetes. Women with GDM may have poor metabolic control and macrosomic fetuses, which may affect the preferred mode of delivery and neonatal outcome.

A. Fetal surveillance and timing of delivery. Women with gestational diabetes who can maintain normal blood sugars (fasting <105 mg/dL and two-hour postprandial <120 mg/dL) on a diabetic diet and have no other pregnancy complications do not appear to be at increased risk of stillbirth and probably do not require fetal surveillance.

B. Women with good glycemic control and no other complications of pregnancy ideally will deliver at 39 to 40 weeks of gestation. If early delivery is indicated, lung maturity should be assessed by amniocentesis if delivery could be safely postponed in the absence of fetal pulmonary maturity.

C. Intrapartum blood glucose control. The maternal blood glucose concentration should be maintained between 70 and 90 mg/dL. Insulin is rarely needed during labor, and a normal saline infusion is usually sufficient to maintain normoglycemia.

D. Postpartum follow-up. At 6 to 12 weeks postpartum, women who had gestational diabetes should be tested for type 2 diabetes.

References: See page 208.

Glycemic Control in Type 1 and Type 2 Diabetes Mellitus During Pregnancy

Diabetes in pregnancy can be classified as pregestational diabetes if the diabetes was diagnosed before pregnancy, or gestational diabetesif the diabetes was diagnosed during pregnancy. Maintenance of maternal blood glucose at or near normal decreases the occurrence of miscarriage, congenital anomalies, macrosomia, fetal death, and neonatal morbidity.

I. Assessing glycemic control

A. Glycosylated hemoglobin values provide an assessment of the degree of chronic glycemic control, reflecting the mean blood glucose concentration during the preceding six to eight weeks. An A1C level of 6% correlates with an average glucose concentration of 120 mg/dL and each 1% increase in A1C reflects a 30 mg/dL increase in average glucose concentration.

1. A1C should be measured every four to six weeks. The goal is to achieve a value at or near the normal range (<6.1%) without inducing hypoglycemia. The normal range of glucose concentration and A1C for pregnant women is lower than that for nonpregnant individuals since both average blood glucose concentration and A1C values fall by about 20% in nondiabetic pregnant women. The goal is to achieve A1C levels at, or ideally below, the normal range in nonpregnant individuals.

B. **Glucose monitoring.** Self-glucose testing should be done before and after meals, at bedtime, and occasionally during the night if nocturnal hypoglycemia is suspected. Peak postprandial glucose concentration occurs 60 to 90 minutes after eating.

II. **Target blood glucose values**. Blood glucose goals in pregnant diabetic women are:

A. Fasting blood glucose concentration of 55 to 65 mg/dL.

B. One-hour postprandial blood glucose concentration less than 120 mg/dL.

III. **Nutritional therapy**

A. **Calorie requirements** during pregnancy are increased by about 300 kcal above basal daily needs in nonpregnant women. Recommended caloric intake:

1. 30 to 35 kcal per kg current weight per day in pregnant women who are BMI 22 to 27.

2. 24 kcal per kg current weight per day in overweight pregnant women (BMI 27 to 29).

3. 12 to 15 kcal per kg current weight per day for obese pregnant women (BMI >30).

4. 30 to 40 kcal per kg current weight per day in pregnant women who are less than BMI 22.

IV. **Insulin drug therapy**

A. Most women with type 1 diabetes require at least three injections of insulin per day. A two-injection regimen can cause nocturnal hypoglycemia if the action of evening-meal dose of intermediate-acting insulin is maximal in the middle of the night.

B. Women with type 2 diabetes may achieve good glycemic control with diet alone. Those who do not, or are on oral anti-hyperglycemic agents, should be treated with insulin for blood glucose control during pregnancy. During the first trimester, insulin requirements are similar in women with type 1 and type 2 diabetes; however, in the second half of pregnancy, insulin requirements increase proportionately more in women with type 2 than type 1 diabetes; the respective insulin doses in the third trimester are 1.6 and 1.2 U/kg per day for type 2 and type 1 diabetes, respectively.

C. **Lispro and aspart insulin analogs** both improve postprandial excursions compared to human regular insulin and are associated with lower risk of delayed postprandial hypoglycemia.

D. **Human NPH insulin** should be used as part of a multiple injection regimen in pregnant women, and women who were taking glargine prior to pregnancy should be changed to NPH. A combination of lispro or aspart insulin and NPH insulin is recommended for therapy in pregnancy.

E. **Regimen.** After an early rise in insulin requirements between weeks 3 and 7, there is a significant decline between weeks 7 and 15 (hypoglycemia may occur), followed by a rise during the remainder of pregnancy, especially between weeks 28 and 32.

F. The average insulin requirement in pregnant women with type 1 diabetes is 0.7 units/kg in the first trimester, increasing to 0.8 U/kg for weeks 13 to 28, 0.9 U/kg for weeks 29 to 34, and 1.0 U/kg for weeks 35 to term.

    G. Meal related insulin lispro and aspart doses are 50% of the insulin requirement. This dose is 0.15 times their pregnant weight in kilograms (12 units of lispro or aspart before meals). The other 50% of insulin should cover basal needs. The dose is calculated as 0.45 times weight in kilograms (12 units of NPH three times a day).

V. Intrapartum management

    A. Spontaneous labor

        1. Insulin is required during the latent phase of labor, and can be given subcutaneously or by intravenous infusion with a goal of maintaining glucose between 70 and 90 mg/dL. Insulin infusion consists of 15 units of regular insulin in 150 mL of normal saline at a rate of 2-3 units/hour.

        2. Normal saline may be sufficient to maintain euglycemia when labor is anticipated.

        3. During active labor, insulin resistance rapidly decreases and insulin requirements fall rapidly. Thus, continuing insulin often causes hypoglycemia. To prevent this, glucose should be infused at a rate of 2.55 mg/kg per min. Capillary blood glucose should be measured hourly.

        4. Glucose, values of 120 mg/dL or greater require rapid-acting insulin subcutaneously or regular insulin intravenously until the blood glucose value falls to 70 to 90 mg/dL. At this time, the insulin dose is titrated to maintain normoglycemia while glucose is infused at a rate of 2.55 mg/kg per min.

    B. Cesarean delivery. The bedtime NPH insulin dose may be given on the morning of surgery and every eight hours thereafter if surgery is delayed.

    C. Induction of labor. Women with type 1 and 2 diabetes who receive labor induction should receive either no morning insulin or a small dose of NPH insulin. Blood glucose monitoring and glucose and insulin infusion are managed as described above for spontaneous labor.

Low-dosage Constant Insulin Infusion for the Intrapartum Period		
Blood Glucose (mg/100 mL)	**Insulin Dosage (U/h)**	**Fluids (125 mL/h)**
<100	0	5% dextrose solution
100-140	1.0	5% dextrose/solution
141-180	1.5	Normal saline
181-220	2.0	Normal saline
>220	2.5	Normal saline

Dilution is 15 U of regular insulin in 150 mL of normal saline, with 25 mL flushed through line, administered intravenously.

VI. Postpartum management. Insulin requirements drop sharply after delivery, and the new mother may not require insulin for 24 to 72 hours. Insulin requirements should be recalculated at this time at 0.6 units/kg per day based upon postpartum weight. Postpartum calorie requirements are 25 kcal/kg per day, and somewhat higher (27 kcal/kg per day) in lactating women.

References: See page 208.

Group B Streptococcal Infection in Pregnancy

Group B streptococcus (GBS; Streptococcus agalactiae), a Gram positive coccus, is an important cause of infection in neonates, causing sepsis, pneumonia, and meningitis. GBS infection is acquired in utero or during passage through the vagina. Vaginal colonization with GBS during pregnancy may lead to premature birth, and GBS is a frequent cause of maternal urinary tract infection, chorioamnionitis, postpartum endometritis, and bacteremia.

I. **Clinical evaluation**
   A. The primary risk factor for GBS infection is maternal GBS genitourinary or gastrointestinal colonization.
   B. The rate of transmission from colonized mothers to infants is approximately 50%. However, only 1 to 2% of all colonized infants develop early-onset GBS disease.
   C. **Maternal obstetrical factors associated with neonatal GBS disease:**
      1. Delivery at less than 37 weeks of gestation
      2. Premature rupture of membranes
      3. Rupture of membranes for 18 or more hours before delivery
      4. Chorioamnionitis
      5. Temperature >38°C during labor
      6. Sustained intrapartum fetal tachycardia
      7. Prior delivery of an infant with GBS disease
   D. **Manifestations of early-onset GBS disease.** Early-onset disease results in bacteremia, generalized sepsis, pneumonia, or meningitis. The clinical signs usually are apparent in the first hours of life.
II. **2002 CDC guidelines for intrapartum antibiotic prophylaxis:**
   A. All pregnant women should be screened for GBS colonization with swabs of both the lower vagina and rectum at 35 to 37 weeks of gestation. Patients are excluded from screening if they had GBS bacteriuria earlier in the pregnancy or if they gave birth to a previous infant with invasive GBS disease. These latter patients should receive intrapartum antibiotic prophylaxis regardless of the colonization status.
   B. **Intrapartum antibiotic prophylaxis is recommended for the following:**
      1. Pregnant women with a positive screening culture unless a planned Cesarean section is performed in the absence of labor or rupture of membranes
      2. Pregnant women who gave birth to a previous infant with invasive GBS disease
      3. Pregnant women with documented GBS bacteriuria during the current pregnancy
      4. Pregnant women whose culture status is unknown (culture not performed or result not available) and who also have delivery at <37 weeks of gestation, amniotic membrane rupture for ≥18 hours, or intrapartum temperature >100.4°F (>38°C)
   C. **Intrapartum antibiotic prophylaxis is not recommended for the following patients:**
      1. Positive GBS screening culture in a previous pregnancy (unless the infant had invasive GBS disease or the screening culture is also positive in the current pregnancy)
      2. Patient who undergoes a planned Cesarean section without labor or rupture of membranes
      3. Pregnant women with negative GBS screening cultures at 35 to 37 weeks of gestation even if they have one or more of the above intrapartum risk factors
   D. **Recommended IAP regimen**
      1. **Penicillin G** (5 million units IV initial dose, then 2.5 million units IV Q4h) is recommended for most patients.

2. **In women with non-immediate-type penicillin-allergy**, cefazolin (Ancef, 2 g initial dose, then 1 g Q8h) is recommended.
3. **Patients at high risk for anaphylaxis to penicillins** are treated with clindamycin (900 mg IV Q8h) or erythromycin (500 mg IV Q6h) as long as their GBS isolate is documented to be susceptible to both clindamycin and erythromycin.
4. **For patients at high risk for anaphylaxis and a GBS resistant isolate** (or with unknown susceptibility) to clindamycin or erythromycin, vancomycin (1 g Q12h) should be given.
5. Antibiotic therapy is continued from hospital admission through delivery.

E. **Approach to threatened preterm delivery at <37 weeks of gestation:** A patient with negative GBS cultures (after 35 weeks of gestation) should not be treated during threatened labor. If GBS cultures have not been performed, these specimens should be obtained and penicillin G administered as above; if cultures are negative at 48 hours, penicillin can be discontinued. If such a patient has not delivered within four weeks, cultures should be repeated.

F. **If screening cultures taken at the time of threatened delivery or previously performed (after 35 weeks of gestation) are positive**, penicillin should be continued for at least 48 hours unless delivery supervenes. Patients who have been treated for >48 hours and have not delivered should receive IAP as above when delivery occurs.

References: See page 208.

Premature Rupture of Membranes

Premature rupture of the membranes (PROM) refers to rupture of membranes prior to the onset of labor or regular uterine contractions. It can occur at term or prior to term, in which case it is designated preterm premature rupture of the membranes (PPROM). The frequencies of term, preterm, and midtrimester PROM are 8, 1 to 3, and less than 1% of pregnancies, respectively.

The incidence of this disorder to be 7-12%. In pregnancies of less than 37 weeks of gestation, preterm birth (and its sequelae) and infection are the major concerns after PROM.

I. **Pathophysiology**
   A. **Premature rupture of membranes** is defined as rupture of membranes prior to the onset of labor.
   B. **Preterm premature rupture of membranes** is defined as rupture of membranes prior to term.
   C. **Prolonged rupture of membranes** consists of rupture of membranes for more than 24 hours.
   D. **The latent period** is the time interval from rupture of membranes to the onset of regular contractions or labor.
   E. Many cases of preterm PROM are caused by idiopathic weakening of the membranes, many of which are caused by subclinical infection. Other causes of PROM include hydramnios, incompetent cervix, abruptio placentae, and amniocentesis.
   F. At term, about 8% of patients will present with ruptured membranes prior to the onset of labor.

II. **Maternal and neonatal complications**
   A. Labor usually follows shortly after the occurrence of PROM. Ninety% of term patients and 50% of preterm patients go into labor within 24 hours after rupture.
   B. Patients who do not go into labor immediately are at increasing risk of infection as the duration of rupture increases. Chorioamnionitis, endometritis, sepsis, and neonatal infections may occur.

    C. Perinatal risks with preterm PROM are primarily complications from immaturity, including respiratory distress syndrome, intraventricular hemorrhage, patent ductus arteriosus, and necrotizing enterocolitis.

    D. Premature gestational age is a more significant cause of neonatal morbidity than is the duration of membrane rupture.

III. **Diagnosis of premature rupture of membranes**

    A. Diagnosis is based on history, physical examination, and laboratory testing. The patient's history alone is correct in 90% of patients. Urinary leakage or excess vaginal discharge is sometimes mistaken for PROM.

    B. **Sterile speculum exam** is the first step in confirming the suspicion of PROM. Digital examination should be avoided because it increases the risk of infection.

        1. The general appearance of the cervix should be assessed visually, and prolapse of the umbilical cord or a fetal extremity should be excluded. Cultures for group B streptococcus, gonorrhea, and chlamydia are obtained.

        2. A pool of fluid in the posterior vaginal fornix supports the diagnosis of PROM.

        3. The presence of amniotic fluid is confirmed by nitrazine testing for an alkaline pH. Amniotic fluid causes nitrazine paper to turn dark blue because the pH is above 6.0-6.5. Nitrazine may be false-positive with contamination from blood, semen, or vaginitis.

        4. If pooling and nitrazine are both non-confirmatory, a swab from the posterior fornix should be smeared on a slide, allowed to dry, and examined under a microscope for "ferning," indicating amniotic fluid.

        5. **Ultrasound examination** for oligohydramnios is useful to confirm the diagnosis, but oligohydramnios may be caused by other disorders besides PROM.

    C. **Laboratory diagnosis**

        1. **Alpha-fetoprotein** (AFP) is present at high concentrations in amniotic fluid, but not in vaginal secretions, urine, or semen.

        2. **Ultrasonography** may be of value in the diagnosis of PROM. The finding of anhydramnios or severe oligohydramnios combined with a characteristic history is highly suggestive, but not diagnostic, of rupture of membranes.

        3. **Gestational age assessment** should be calculated. Ultrasonography on admission is useful for determining presentation, residual amniotic fluid volume, fetal size and anatomic survey, and fetal well-being.

        4. **Assessment of fetal well-being.** Fetal well-being is generally assessed via an external fetal monitor. A reactive nonstress test is reassuring. Patients with nonreassuring fetal heart rate testing should be delivered or further evaluated.

IV. **Assessment of premature rupture of membranes**

    A. The gestational age must be carefully assessed. Menstrual history, prenatal exams, and previous sonograms are reviewed. An ultrasound examination should be performed.

    B. The patient should be evaluated for the presence of chorioamnionitis [fever (over 38°C), leukocytosis, maternal and fetal tachycardia, uterine tenderness, foul-smelling vaginal discharge].

    C. The patient should be evaluated for labor, and a sterile speculum examination should assess cervical change.

    D. The fetus should be evaluated with heart rate monitoring because PROM increases the risk of umbilical cord prolapse and fetal distress caused by oligohydramnios.

V. **Management of premature rupture of membranes**

    A. **Management of term patients**

        1. At 36 weeks and beyond, management of PROM consists of delivery. Patients in active labor should be allowed to progress.

        2. Patients with chorioamnionitis, who are not in labor, should be immediately induced with oxytocin (Pitocin).

3. Patients who are not yet in active labor (in the absence of fetal distress, meconium, or clinical infection) may be discharged for 48 hours, and labor usually follows. If labor has not begun within a reasonable time after rupture of membranes, induction with oxytocin (Pitocin) is appropriate. Use of prostaglandin E2 is safe for cervical ripening.

B. Management of Preterm Premature Rupture of Membranes

1. Women with PPROM should be hospitalized until delivery. Expeditious delivery is indicated for abruptio placentae, intrauterine infection, or evidence of fetal compromise (eg, repetitive FHR decelerations or an unstable fetal presentation that poses a risk of cord prolapse). Pregnancies >32 weeks of gestation with documented fetal lung maturity will achieve better outcomes with immediate delivery than with expectant management.

2. **Group beta-hemolytic streptococcal (GBS) status** should be determined and intrapartum antibiotic prophylaxis considered for pregnant women whose GBS culture status is unknown (culture not performed or result not available) and who also are likely to deliver before 37 weeks of gestation, have amniotic membranes that have been ruptured for ≥18 hours, or have an intrapartum temperature >100.4°F.

3. Patients are typically kept at modified bedrest and frequently assessed for evidence of infection or labor.

4. **Tocolytics** can be given to allow administration of antenatal corticosteroids and antibiotics.

5. **Fetal surveillance** consists of kick counts, nonstress tests, biophysical profiles (BPP). Abnormalities of these tests are predictive of fetal infection and umbilical cord compression related to oligohydramnios.

6. **Fetal lung maturity.** Antenatal corticosteroid administration is recommended for pregnancies complicated by PPROM at less than 32 weeks of gestation, as long as there is no clinical evidence of chorioamnionitis. A single course of corticosteroids should be administered. In more advanced gestations, fetal lung maturity tests may be performed via amniocentesis or on amniotic fluid samples aspirated from the vagina.

7. All patients with PPROM should be delivered at >32 weeks after confirmation of fetal lung maturity or a course of corticosteroids.

8. When there is confirmed fetal lung maturation at or beyond 32 weeks of gestation, the risks of expectant management often exceed those of delivery. Women with PPROM who are >32 weeks of gestation with a mature fetal lung profile are best managed by prompt induction of labor. Antibiotic prophylaxis for possible GBS colonization should be given during labor in the absence of a documented, recent negative GBS culture.

9. **Contraindications to expectant management.** Women are not candidates for expectant management if they have advanced labor, intrauterine infection, significant vaginal bleeding, or nonreassuring fetal testing.

10. **Antibiotic prophylaxis**
   a. Antibiotic therapy is important in the management of patients with PPROM.
   b. Ampicillin (1 or 2 g IV every 6 hours for 24 hours, then 500 mg PO every 6 hours until delivery) plus erythromycin or azithromycin is recommended.
      (1) Azithromycin (Zithromax, 1 g orally as a single dose) may be substituted for erythromycin because of improved oral absorption, a broader spectrum of antibacterial properties, and better tolerance.
      (2) Women with bacterial vaginosis should be treated with metronidazole (250 mg PO three times daily for seven days).

Sample Antibiotic Regimens Used for Prophylaxis in Women with PPROM	
Antibiotic	**Dose**
Ampicillin	1 or 2 g IV every 6 hours for 24 hours, then 500 mg PO every 6 hours until delivery
Ampicillin Gentamicin Clindamycin Amoxicillin plus clavulanic acid (Augmentin)	2 g IV every 6 hours for 4 doses and 90 mg IV initially, then 60 mg IV every 8 hours for three doses and 900 mg IV every 8 hours for three doses, followed by 500 mg PO TID for 7 days
Erythromycin base	333 mg PO every 8 hours until delivery
Piperacillin	3 g IV every 6 hours for 3 days
Ampicillin-sulbactam (Unasyn)	3 g every 6 hours for 7 days
Ampicillin	2 g IV every 6 hours for 7 days
Ampicillin-sulbactam Amoxicillin-clavulante	1.5 g IV every 6 hours for 72 hours, followed by 500 mg PO every 8 hours until delivery

References: See page 208.

Preterm Labor and Delivery

Preterm birth (PTB) is defined as a birth that before 37 completed weeks (less than 259 days) of gestation. A very preterm birth is defined as less than 32 weeks, and an extremely preterm birth is a birth at less than 28 weeks. Preterm birth is the leading cause of infant mortality. 12.7% of births are preterm and 2% are less than 32 weeks.

I. **Pathogenesis**. 70 to 80% of PTBs occur spontaneously: preterm labor (PTL) accounts for 40 to 50% of all PTBs and preterm premature rupture of membranes (PPROM) accounts for 20 to 30%. The remaining 20 to 30% of PTBs are due to intervention for maternal or fetal problems.
II. **Clinical manifestations and diagnosis**
   A. 30% of preterm labors spontaneously resolve. 50% of patients hospitalized for PTL deliver at term.
   B. Signs and symptoms of early PTL include menstrual-like cramping, constant low back ache, mild uterine contractions at infrequent and/or irregular intervals, and bloody show.
   C. The diagnosis of PTL is generally based upon clinical criteria of regular painful uterine contractions accompanied by cervical dilation and/or effacement. Specific criteria include persistent uterine contractions (four every 20 minutes or eight every 60 minutes) with documented cervical change or cervical effacement of at least 80%, or cervical dilatation >2 cm.

Risk Factors for Preterm Labor	
Previous preterm delivery Low socioeconomic status Non-white race Maternal age <18 years or >40 years Preterm premature rupture of the membranes Multiple gestation Maternal history of one or more spontaneous second-trimester abortions Maternal complications --Maternal behaviors --Smoking --Illicit drug use --Alcohol use --Lack of prenatal care Uterine causes --Myomata (particularly submucosal or subplacental) --Uterine septum --Bicornuate uterus --Cervical incompetence --Exposure to diethylstilbestrol (DES)	Infectious causes --Chorioamnionitis --Bacterial vaginosis --Asymptomatic bacteriuria --Acute pyelonephritis --Cervical/vaginal colonization Fetal causes --Intrauterine fetal death --Intrauterine growth retardation --Congenital anomalies Abnormal placentation Presence of a retained intrauterine device

D. Digital cervical examination has limited reproducibility between examiners; therefore, evaluation of the cervix via transvaginal ultrasound is useful to confirm the diagnosis. Sonographic measurement of cervical length is a more sensitive indicator of a patient's risk for PTB than cervical dilatation. A short cervix has been variously defined as a cervical length <2.0 cm.

III. **Initial evaluation**
   A. Initial evaluation should address the following issues
      1. The presence and frequency of uterine contractions
      2. Uterine bleeding
      3. Fetal membrane rupture
      4. Gestational age
      5. Fetal well-being
   B. Uterine contractions and fetal well-being are evaluated using an electronic fetal heart rate and contraction monitor.
   C. **Physical examination**. The uterus is examined to assess firmness, tenderness, fetal size, and fetal position. A sterile speculum examination is performed to rule out ruptured membranes, to visually examine the vagina and cervix, and to obtain specimens for laboratory testing. A digital examination to assess cervical dilatation and effacement is performed after placenta previa and PPROM have been excluded (by history and physical, laboratory, and ultrasound examinations, as indicated).
   D. **Laboratory tests**
      1. **Urine culture**, since bacteriuria and pyelonephritis are associated with PTB.
      2. **Rectovaginal group B streptococcal culture**, to determine need for antibiotic prophylaxis.
      3. **Tests for gonorrhea and chlamydia.** Testing for gonorrhea and chlamydia may be omitted if previously performed, the results were negative, and the patient is not at high risk for sexually transmitted infections.
      4. **Fetal fibronectin (fFN).** A swab for fFN should be obtained for all patients, but only send the swab to the laboratory if the cervical length is 20 to 30 mm
      5. **Drug testing** is indicated in patients with risk factors for drug abuse because cocaine use is associated with placental abruption.

     6. Imaging. Ultrasound examination should be performed to measure cervical length.

Preterm Labor, Threatened or Actual

IV. Initial assessment to determine whether patient is experiencing preterm labor
  A. Assess for the following:
    1. Uterine activity
    2. Rupture of membranes
    3. Vaginal bleeding
    4. Presentation
    5. Cervical dilation and effacement
    6. Station
  B. Reassess estimate of gestational age
V. Search for a precipitating factor/cause
VI. Consider specific management strategies, which may include the following:
  A. Intravenous tocolytic therapy (decision should be influenced by gestational age, cause of preterm labor and contraindications)
  B. Corticosteroid therapy (eg, betamethasone, in a dosage of 12 mg IM every 24 hours for a total of two doses)
  C. Antibiotic therapy if specific infectious agent is identified or if preterm premature rupture of the membranes

---

VII. **Triage based upon cervical length**
  A. **Cervical length >30 mm**
    1. These women are at low risk of PTB, regardless of fFN result; therefore, fFN swabs do not need to be sent to the laboratory. These patients should be discharged home after an observational period of four to six hours during which fetal well-being (eg, reactive nonstress test) should be confirmed, and the presence of abruption or infection should be excluded. The assessment should confirm that the cervix is not dilating or effacing.
    2. Follow-up in one to two weeks is arranged and the patient is given instructions to call if she experiences additional signs or symptoms of PTL, or has other pregnancy concerns (eg, bleeding, PROM, decreased fetal activity).
  B. **Cervical length 20 to 30 mm.** PTB is more likely in women with cervices 20 to 30 mm than in women with longer cervices, but most women in this group do not deliver preterm. Therefore, the swab should be sent for fFN testing in this subgroup of women. If the test is positive (>50 ng/mL), the pregnancy should be managed to prevent PTB.
  C. **Cervical length <20 mm.** These women are at high risk of PTB regardless of fFN result. Therefore, their swabs should not be sent for fFN testing. Prevention of PTB is indicated.
VIII. **Management of women with preterm labor**
  A. Women diagnosed with PTL at less than 34 weeks of gestation should be hospitalized, and the following treatments should be initiated:
    1. Antenatal glucocorticoids to reduce neonatal morbidity and mortality associated with PTB.
    2. Antibiotics for GBS chemoprophylaxis.
    3. Tocolytic drugs for 48 hours to delay delivery so that glucocorticoids given to the mother can achieve their maximum effect.
    4. Antibiotics to women with positive urine culture results or positive tests for gonorrhea or chlamydia.

IX. **Inhibition of acute preterm labor**
  A. **Goals of treatment of preterm labor**
    1. Delay delivery by at least 48 hours so that glucocorticoids given to the mother can achieve their maximum effect. Predelivery admin-

istration of glucocorticoids reduces the risk of neonatal death, respiratory distress syndrome, intraventricular hemorrhage, and necrotizing enterocolitis in premature neonates.

2. Provide time to transport the mother to a facility that can provide neonatal care if the patient delivers preterm.

3. Prolong pregnancy when there are underlying, self-limited conditions that can cause labor (such as pyelonephritis) and are unlikely to cause recurrent PTL.

B. Lower and upper limits of gestational age. The lowest gestational age for which inhibition of PTL should be considered is fifteen weeks gestational age since it defines a point at which early pregnancy loss is less commonly attributable to karyotypic abnormality.

C. Thirty-four weeks of gestation defines the threshold at which perinatal morbidity and mortality are felt to be too low to justify the potential complications associated with the inhibition of labor.

D. **Contraindications to inhibition of labor**
1. Intrauterine fetal demise
2. Lethal fetal anomaly
3. Nonreassuring fetal status
4. Severe fetal growth restriction
5. Severe preeclampsia or eclampsia
6. Maternal hemorrhage with hemodynamic instability
7. Chorioamnionitis

E. **Bedrest, hydration, and sedation** is recommended even though there is no high quality evidence of the efficacy of bedrest for prevention or treatment of PTL.

F. **Beta-adrenergic receptor agonists**
1. **Mechanism of action.** Terbutaline causes myometrial relaxation by binding with beta-2 adrenergic receptors and increasing intracellular adenyl cyclase, resulting in diminished myometrial contractility. Target cells eventually become desensitized to the effect of beta-adrenergic receptor agonists, thereby limiting efficacy because of tachyphylaxis.

2. Efficacy
   a. Beta-adrenergic receptor agonists decreased the number of women giving birth within 48 hours (RR 0.63 and possibly within seven days (RR 0.67).

3. Maternal side effects include tachycardia, palpitations, and lower blood pressure.
   a. Common symptoms include tremor (39%), palpitations (18%), shortness of breath (15%), and chest discomfort (10%).
   b. Pulmonary edema is uncommon, occurring in 0.3% of patients.
   c. Beta-adrenergic receptor agonists effects, include hypokalemia (39%), hyperglycemia (30%), and lipolysis. Myocardial ischemia is a rare complication.

4. **Fetal side effects,** such as fetal tachycardia. Neonatal hypoglycemia may result from fetal hyperinsulinemia due to prolonged maternal hyperglycemia.

5. **Contraindications.** Labor inhibition with a beta-adrenergic receptor agonist is relatively contraindicated among women with cardiac disease, poorly controlled hyperthyroidism or diabetes mellitus.

6. **Dose**
   a. Terbutaline is the most commonly used beta-adrenergic receptor agonist for labor inhibition. It is typically administered as a continuous intravenous infusion. The infusion is started at 2.5 to 5 mcg/min; this can be increased by 2.5 to 5 mcg/min every 20 to 30 minutes to a maximum of 25 mcg/min, or until the contractions have abated. At this point, the infusion is reduced by decrements of 2.5 to 5 mcg/min to the lowest dose that maintains uterine quiescence.

   b. Terbutaline can also be given subcutaneously by intermittent injection. 0.25 mg can be administered every 20 to 30 minutes for up to four doses or until tocolysis is achieved. Once labor is inhibited, 0.25 mg can be administered every three to four hours until the uterus is quiescent for 24 hours.

G. Monitoring.
   1. During beta-adrenergic receptor agonist administration, cumulative fluid intake, urine output, shortness of breath, chest pain or tachycardia should be monitored. The drug be withheld if the maternal heart rate exceeds 120 beats/min.
   2. Glucose and potassium concentrations should be monitored every four to six hours during parenteral drug administration, since hyperglycemia and hypokalemia commonly occur. Significant hypokalemia should be treated to minimize risk of arrhythmias.

H. Magnesium sulfate
   1. Mechanism of action. Magnesium competes with calcium at the level of the plasma membrane voltage-gated channels, reducing myometrial contractility.
   2. Efficacy. Compared to no treatment or placebo, magnesium sulfate therapy did not significantly reduce the risk of birth within 48 hours (RR 0.57). In comparative trials, magnesium sulfate was neither more nor less effective than other tocolytics.
   3. Maternal side effects. Magnesium sulfate causes fewer minor maternal side effects than beta-adrenergic agonists, but the risk of major adverse risk events is comparable. Rapid infusion causes diaphoresis, flushing, and warmth. Nausea, vomiting, headache, visual disturbances, and palpitations can also occur. Dyspnea or chest pain may be symptoms of pulmonary edema, which is a rare complication.
      a. Magnesium toxicity: loss of deep tendon reflexes occurs at 9.6 to 12.0 mg/dL, respiratory paralysis at 12.0 to 18.0 mg/dL, and cardiac arrest at 24 to 30 mg/dL. Symptoms will resolve after the magnesium infusion is stopped. Calcium gluconate (1 g intravenously over 5 to 10 minutes) should be administered only to counteract life-threatening symptoms of magnesium toxicity (such as cardiorespiratory compromise).
      b. Magnesium therapy also results in a transient reduction of serum calcium concentration due to rapid suppression of parathyroid hormone release. Rarely, the hypocalcemia becomes symptomatic (myoclonus, delirium, ECG abnormalities).
   4. Contraindications. Magnesium sulfate tocolysis is contraindicated in women with myasthenia gravis. It also should not be used in women with known myocardial compromise or cardiac conduction defects because of its antiinotropic effects.
      a. Magnesium is eliminated by the kidneys. Thus, women with impaired renal function will have an exaggerated rise in serum magnesium and may develop magnesium toxicity.
   5. Dose. Magnesium sulfate is usually administered as a 4 to 6 g intravenous load over 20 minutes, followed by a continuous infusion of 2 to 4 g/hour.
   6. Monitoring. Since magnesium sulfate is excreted by the kidneys, dosing should be reduced in renal insufficiency (creatinine >1.0 mg/dL).Women with renal insufficiency should receive a standard loading dose, but a reduced maintenance dose (1 g per hour or no maintenance dose if the serum creatinine is >2.5 mg/dL) with monitoring of the serum magnesium every six hours.

I. Calcium channel blockers
   1. Mechanism of action. Calcium channel blockers directly block the influx of calcium ions through the cell membrane, resulting in myometrial relaxation.

2. Efficacy
a. Compared to other tocolytics, calcium channel blockers did not significantly reduce the risk of birth within 48 hours of initiation of treatment (RR 0.80), but did reduce the risk of birth within seven days (RR 0.76).
b. Comparing treatment of PTL with nifedipine versus beta-adrenergic receptor agonists (terbutaline). Nifedipine was more effective than beta-adrenergic receptor agonists for delaying delivery at least 48 hours (OR 1.52).

3. Maternal side effects.
Nifedipine is a peripheral vasodilator, thus it may cause symptoms such as nausea, flushing, headache, dizziness, and palpitations.

4. Contraindications.
Calcium channel blockers should be used with caution in women with left ventricular dysfunction or congestive heart failure.

5. Dose.
Administer an initial loading dose of 30 mg orally, followed by an additional 20 mg orally in 90 minutes. The half-life of nifedipine is 2-3 hours and the duration of action is up to six hours.

Tocolytic Therapy for the Management of Preterm Labor

Medication	Mechanism of action	Dosage
Nifedipine (Procardia)	Calcium channel blocker	30 mg orally, followed by 20 mg orally in 90 minutes, followed by 20 mg orally every four to eight hours.
Terbutaline (Bricanyl)	Beta$_2$-adrenergic receptor agonist sympathomimetic; decreases free intracellular calcium ions	2.5 to 5 µg/min; increased by 2.5 to 5 µg/min every 20 to 30 minutes to a maximum of 25 µg/min, or until the contractions have abated. 0.25 mg subcutaneously every 20 to 30 minutes for up to four doses or until tocolysis is achieved. 0.25 mg every 3 to 4 hours.
Indomethacin (Indocin)	Prostaglandin inhibitor	50- to 100-mg rectal suppository, then 25 to 50 mg orally every six hours

Complications Associated With the Use of Tocolytic Agents

Beta-adrenergic agents
- Hypokalemia
- Hyperglycemia
- Hypotension
- Pulmonary edema
- Arrhythmias
- Cardiac insufficiency
- Myocardial ischemia
- Maternal death

Indomethacin (Indocin)
- Renal failure
- Hepatitis
- Gastrointestinal bleeding

Nifedipine (Procardia)
- Transient hypotension

J. Cyclooxygenase inhibitors

1. Mechanism of action.
Cyclooxygenase (COX) is the enzyme responsible for conversion of arachidonic acid to prostaglandins, which are critical in parturition.

2. Efficacy
a. Indomethacin, a nonspecific COX inhibitor, is the most commonly used tocolytic of this class. COX inhibition showed a

trend in reduction in risk of delivery within 48 hours of initiation of treatment (RR 0.20) and within seven days (RR 0.41).
   b. Indomethacin is significantly more effective than placebo in inhibition of PTL during a 24-hour course of therapy.
3. **Maternal side effects**, including nausea, esophageal reflux, gastritis, and emesis, are seen in 4% of patients treated with indomethacin for PTL. Platelet dysfunction may occur.
4. **Fetal side effects.** The primary fetal concerns with use of indomethacin, and other COX inhibitors (eg, sulindac), are constriction of the ductus arteriosus and oligohydramnios.
   a. **Ductus arteriosus**. Premature narrowing or closure of the ductus arteriosus can lead to pulmonary hypertension, tricuspid regurgitation, and persistent fetal circulation. Several cases of premature ductal closure have been reported in pregnancies in which the duration of indomethacin exposure exceeded 48 hours.
   b. **Oligohydramnios.** Indomethacin causes a reduction in amniotic fluid volume. Fetal urine output is reduced.
   c. **Other.** Neonatal complications associated with In-utero indomethacin exposure include bronchopulmonary dysplasia, necrotizing enterocolitis, patent ductus arteriosus, and intraventricular hemorrhage.
5. **Contraindications.** Maternal contraindications to COX inhibitors include platelet dysfunction or bleeding disorder, hepatic dysfunction, gastrointestinal ulcerative disease, renal dysfunction, and asthma.
6. **Dose.** Indomethacin is given as a 50 to 100 mg loading dose, followed by 25 mg orally every four to six hours.
7. **Monitoring.** If indomethacin is continued for longer than 48 hours, sonographic evaluation for oligohydramnios and narrowing of the fetal ductus arteriosus is indicated. Evidence of oligohydramnios or ductal constriction should prompt discontinuation of this therapy.

X. **Recommendations**
   A. Nifedipine is the initial choice for tocolysis because of oral administration, low frequency of side effects, and efficacy in reducing neonatal morbidity.
   B. Beta-adrenergic receptor agonists are also effective agents for initial treatment of PTL, but have a high rate of side effects.
   C. For second line treatment of PTL in pregnancies under 32 weeks of gestation, indomethacin should be intitiated. These agents should be avoided in gestations over 32 weeks and should be used with caution if needed for more than 72 hours because of concern about premature narrowing or closure of the ductus arteriosus. For second line therapy of pregnancies at 32 to 34 weeks of gestation, beta-adrenergic receptor agonists are recommended.

References: See page 208.

Bleeding in the Second Half of Pregnancy

Bleeding in the second half of pregnancy occurs in 4% of all pregnancies. In 50% of cases, vaginal bleeding is secondary to placental abruption or placenta previa.

I. **Clinical evaluation of bleeding second half of pregnancy**
   A. **History** of trauma or pain and the amount and character of the bleeding should be assessed.
   B. **Physical examination**
      1. Vital signs and pulse pressure are measured. Hypotension and tachycardia are signs of serious hypovolemia.
      2. Fetal heart rate pattern and uterine activity are assessed.

3. Ultrasound examination of the uterus, placenta and fetus should be completed.
4. Speculum and digital pelvic examination should not be done until placenta previa has been excluded.

C. **Laboratory Evaluation**
1. **Hemoglobin** and hematocrit.
2. **INR, partial thromboplastin time, platelet count, fibrinogen level, and fibrin split products** are checked when placental abruption is suspected or if there has been significant hemorrhage.
3. **A red-top tube** of blood is used to perform a bedside clot test.
4. **Blood type** and cross-match.
5. **Urinalysis** for hematuria and proteinuria.
6. The **Apt test** is used to distinguish maternal or fetal source of bleeding. (Vaginal blood is mixed with an equal part 0.25% sodium hydroxide. Fetal blood remains red; maternal blood turns brown.)
7. **Kleihauer-Betke test** of maternal blood is used to quantify fetal to maternal hemorrhage.

II. **Placental abruption (abruptio placentae)** is defined as complete or partial placental separation from the decidua basalis after 20 weeks gestation.

A. Placental abruption occurs in 1 in 100 deliveries.

B. **Factors associated with placental abruption**
1. Preeclampsia and hypertensive disorders
2. History of placental abruption
3. High multiparity
4. Increasing maternal age
5. Trauma
6. Cigarette smoking
7. Illicit drug use (especially cocaine)
8. Excessive alcohol consumption
9. Preterm premature rupture of the membranes
10. Rapid uterine decompression after delivery of the first fetus in a twin gestation or rupture of membranes with polyhydramnios
11. Uterine leiomyomas

C. **Diagnosis of placental abruption**
1. Abruption is characterized by vaginal bleeding, abdominal pain, uterine tenderness, and uterine contractions.
   a. Vaginal bleeding is visible in 80%; bleeding is concealed in 20%.
   b. Pain is usually of sudden onset, constant, and localized to the uterus and lower back.
   c. Localized or generalized uterine tenderness and increased uterine tone are found with severe placental abruption.
   d. An increase in uterine size may occur with placental abruption when the bleeding is concealed. Concealed bleeding may be detected by serial measurements of abdominal girth and fundal height.
   e. Amniotic fluid may be bloody.
   f. Fetal monitoring may detect distress.
   g. Placental abruption may cause preterm labor.
2. **Uterine contractions** by tocodynamometry is the most sensitive indicator of abruption.
3. **Laboratory findings** include proteinuria and a consumptive coagulopathy, characterized by decreased fibrinogen, prothrombin, factors V and VIII, and platelets. Fibrin split products are elevated.
4. **Ultrasonography** has a sensitivity in detecting placental abruption of only 15%.

D. **Management of placental abruption**
1. **Mild placental abruption**
   a. If maternal stability and reassuring fetal surveillance are assured and the fetus is immature, close expectant observation with fetal monitoring is justified.

      b. Maternal hematologic parameters are monitored and abnormalities corrected.

      c. Tocolysis with magnesium sulfate is initiated if the fetus is immature.

  2. Moderate to severe placental abruption

    a. Shock is aggressively managed.

    b. Coagulopathy

      (1) Blood is transfused to replace blood loss.

      (2) Clotting factors may be replaced using cryoprecipitate or fresh-frozen plasma. One unit of fresh-frozen plasma increases fibrinogen by 10 mg/dL. Cryoprecipitate contains 250 mg fibrinogen/unit; 4 gm (15-20 U) is an effective dose.

      (3) Platelet transfusion is indicated if the platelet count is <50,000/mcL. One unit of platelets raises the platelet count 5000-10,000/mcL; 4 to 6 U is the smallest useful dose.

    c. Oxygen should be administered and urine output monitored with a Foley catheter.

    d. Vaginal delivery is expedited in all but the mildest cases once the mother has been stabilized. Amniotomy and oxytocin (Pitocin) augmentation may be used. Cesarean section is indicated for fetal distress, severe abruption, or failed trial of labor.

III. Placenta previa occurs when any part of the placenta implants in the lower uterine segment. It is associated with a risk of serious maternal hemorrhage. Placenta previa occurs in 1 in 200 pregnancies. Ninety% of placenta previas diagnosed in the second trimester resolve spontaneously.

  A. Total placenta previa occurs when the internal cervical os is completely covered by placenta.

  B. Partial placenta previa occurs when part of the cervical os is covered by placenta.

  C. Marginal placenta previa occurs when the placental edge is located within 2 cm of the cervical os.

  D. Clinical evaluation

    1. Placenta previa presents with a sudden onset of painless vaginal bleeding in the second or third trimester. The peak incidence occurs at 34 weeks. The initial bleeding usually resolves spontaneously and then recurs later in pregnancy.

    2. One fourth of patients present with bleeding and uterine contractions.

  E. Ultrasonography is accurate in diagnosing placenta previa.

  F. Management of placenta previa

    1. In a pregnancy >36 weeks with documented fetal lung maturity, the neonate should be immediately delivered by cesarean section.

    2. Low vertical uterine incision is probably safer in patients with an anterior placenta. Incisions through the placenta should be avoided.

    3. If severe hemorrhage jeopardizes the mother or fetus, cesarean section is indicated regardless of gestational age.

    4. Expectant management is appropriate for immature fetuses if bleeding is not excessive, maternal physical activity can be restricted, intercourse and douching can be prohibited, and the hemoglobin can be maintained at >10 mg/dL.

    5. Rh immunoglobulin is administered to Rh-negative-unsensitized patients.

    6. Delivery is indicated once fetal lung maturity has been documented.

    7. Tocolysis with magnesium sulfate may be used for immature fetuses.

IV. Cervical bleeding

  A. Cytologic sampling is necessary.

  B. Bleeding can be controlled with cauterization or packing.

  C. Bacterial and viral cultures are sometimes diagnostic.

V. **Cervical polyps**
   A. Bleeding is usually self-limited.
   B. Trauma should be avoided.
   C. Polypectomy may control bleeding and yield a histologic diagnosis.
VI. **Bloody show** is a frequent benign cause of late third trimester bleeding. It is characterized by blood-tinged mucus associated with cervical change.

References: See page 208.

Preeclampsia

Preeclampsia is defined as the new onset of hypertension and proteinuria after 20 weeks of gestation in a previously normotensive woman. Preeclampsia is classified as mild or severe. Eclampsia is defined as the development of seizures in a woman with gestational hypertension or preeclampsia.

I. **Clinical evaluation**
   A. **Chronic hypertension** is defined as systolic pressure $\geq$140 mmHg, diastolic pressure >90 mmHg, or both, that antedates pregnancy, is present before the 20th week of pregnancy, or persists longer than 12 weeks postpartum.
   B. **Preeclampsia superimposed upon chronic hypertension** occurs when a patient with preexisting hypertension develops proteinuria after 20 weeks of gestation. Women with both preexisting hypertension and proteinuria are considered preeclamptic if there is an exacerbation of blood pressure to the severe range (systolic $\geq$160 mmHg or diastolic >110 mmHg) in the last half of pregnancy.
   C. **Gestational hypertension** is defined as hypertension without protein-uria (or other signs of preeclampsia) developing in the latter part of pregnancy. Some women with gestational hypertension will develop preeclampsia later in the pregnancy.
II. **Incidence.** Hypertension occurs in 10 to 20% of pregnancies.
   A. Preeclampsia occurs in 5 to 8% of pregnancies. The disease is mild in 75% of cases, and severe in 25%. Ten% of preeclampsia occurs in pregnancies less than 34 weeks of gestation.
   B. Preexisting hypertension complicates about 3% of pregnancies.
   C. Gestational hypertension complicates about 6% of pregnancies.
III. **Risk factors for preeclampsia**
   A. Past obstetrical history of preeclampsia is a strong risk factor for preeclampsia in a future pregnancy. In women who had mild preeclampsia during the first pregnancy, the incidence of preeclampsia in a second pregnancy is 5 to 7%.
   B. First pregnancy increases the risk for developing preeclampsia (RR 2.91). A family history of preeclampsia is associated with an increase in risk (RR 2.90).
   C. Pregestational diabetes increases risk of preeclampsia (RR 3.56).
   D. Multiple gestation increases the risk of preeclampsia; for twin pregnan-cies the relative risk is 2.93.
   E. Obesity increases the risk of preeclampsia.
   F. Preexisting hypertension, renal disease, and collagen vascular dis-ease are risk factors.
   G. The antiphospholipid syndrome has been associated with preeclampsia, fetal loss, and maternal thrombosis.
   H. Advanced maternal age is an independent risk factor for preeclampsia (maternal age >40 RR 1.96).
   I. A prolonged interval between pregnancies appears to increase the risk of developing preeclampsia.
   J. Women who smoke cigarettes have a lower risk of preeclampsia than nonsmokers.

IV. **Clinical manifestations**
   A. Hypertension, proteinuria, and edema in pregnancy is usually caused by preeclampsia, particularly in a primigravida. These findings typically develop in the latter part of the third trimester and progress until delivery.
   B. The occurrence of preeclampsia before 20 weeks of gestation is unusual and may be suggestive of a molar pregnancy. The possibility of illicit drug use or withdrawal or chromosomal aneuploidy in the fetus should also be considered.
   C. **Pregnancy related hypertension** is defined as a systolic blood pressure >140 mmHg or diastolic blood pressure >90 mmHg in a woman who was normotensive prior to 20 weeks of gestation. Hypertension is usually the earliest clinical finding of preeclampsia. The blood pressure (BP) may rise in the second trimester, but usually does not reach the hypertensive range (>140/90 mmHg) until the third trimester, often after the 37th week of gestation. In some cases, however, preeclampsia develops suddenly in a previously normotensive woman or early in pregnancy.
   D. **Proteinuria** (>0.3 g protein in a 24-hour urine specimen or persistent 1+ on dipstick) must be present with hypertension to diagnose preeclampsia.
   E. **Hyperuricemia and hypocalciuria** also occur.
   F. **Edema.** Most pregnant women have edema. However, sudden and rapid weight gain (eg, >5 pounds/week) and facial edema may occur in women who develop preeclampsia.
   G. **Hematologic changes.** The most common coagulation abnormality in preeclampsia is thrombocytopenia. Microangiopathic hemolysis may also occur and is detected by examination of a blood smear for schistocytes and helmet cells or elevation in the serum lactate dehydrogenase concentration.
   H. **Liver.** Glomerular and hepatic injury may be caused by vasospasm and precipitation of fibrin in both organs. The clinical manifestations of liver involvement include right upper quadrant or epigastric pain, elevated transaminases and subcapsular hemorrhage or hepatic rupture, which may represent HELLP syndrome (Hemolysis, Elevated Liver function tests, Low Platelets).
   I. **Central nervous system and eye** manifestations of preeclampsia include headache, blurred vision, scotomata, and, rarely, cortical blindness. Seizures in a preeclamptic woman signify a change in diagnosis to eclampsia. One in 400 mildly preeclamptic and 2% of severely preeclamptic women will develop eclamptic seizures. Stroke is a rare complication of severe preeclampsia/eclampsia.
   J. **Pulmonary edema.** Elevated pulmonary vascular hydrostatic pressure (PCWP) may produce pulmonary edema in some women.
   K. **Fetus and placenta.** Placental hypoperfusion may cause fetal growth restriction and oligohydramnios. Abruptio placenta is infrequent (<1%) with mild preeclampsia, but occurs in 3% of severe disease.
   L. **Iatrogenic preterm delivery** is a secondary result of fetal or maternal complications.
V. **Diagnosis**
   A. **Diagnosis of preeclampsia** is based upon hypertension and proteinuria developing after 20 weeks of gestation in a woman who was previously normotensive. Hypertension should be documented on two occasions.
   B. **Screening for proteinuria.** Testing is performed by dipping a test strip into a urine specimen. Women with proteinuria on dipstick should undergo quantitative measurement of protein excretion (urine protein to creatine ratio or 24-hour urine protein excretion).

Diagnosis of Preeclampsia

Systolic blood pressure $\geq$140 mm Hg
or
Diastolic blood pressure $\geq$ 90 mm Hg
AND
A random urine protein determination of 1+ on dipstick or 30 mg/dL or proteinuria of 0.3 g or greater in a 24-hour urine specimen

Criteria for Gestational Hypertension

Systolic blood pressure $\geq$140 mm Hg
Diastolic blood pressure $\geq$90 mm Hg
AND no proteinuria
Developing AFTER the 20th week of gestation in women known to be normotensive before pregnancy

Criteria for Severe Preeclampsia

New onset proteinuria hypertension and at least one of the following:
Symptoms of central nervous system dysfunction: Blurred vision, scotomata, altered mental status, severe headache
Symptoms of liver capsule distention: Right upper quadrant or epigastric pain
Hepatocellular injury: Serum transaminase concentration at least twice normal
Severe blood pressure elevation: Systolic blood pressure $\geq$160 mm Hg or diastolic $\geq$110 mm Hg on two occasions at least six hours apart
Thrombocytopenia: <100,000 platelets per mm^3
Proteinuria: Over 5 grams in 24 hours or 3+ or more on two random samples four hours apart
Oliguria <500 mL in 24 hours
Intrauterine fetal growth restriction
Pulmonary edema or cyanosis
Cerebrovascular accident
Coagulopathy

VI. **Laboratory evaluation**
   A. **Hematocrit.** Hemoconcentration supports the diagnosis of preeclampsia, but hemolysis can decrease the hematocrit.
   B. **Platelet count.** Thrombocytopenia is a criterion of severe disease.
   C. **Quantification of protein excretion.** Proteinuria is defined as excretion of 300 mg or more in 24 hours or at least 1+ protein on dipstick of two urine specimens collected at least four hours apart; 3+ or greater or 5 g or more per day is a criterion of severe disease.
   D. **Serum creatinine concentration.** An elevated or rising level suggests severe disease.
   E. **Serum alanine and aspartate aminotransferase concentrations (ALT and AST).** Elevated or rising levels suggest hepatic dysfunction indicative of severe disease.
   F. **Lactate dehydrogenase (LDH).** Microangiopathic hemolysis is suggested by an elevated LDH level and red cell fragmentation (schistocytes or helmet cells) on peripheral blood smear. Microangiopathic hemolysis is present in severe disease of HELLP syndrome (Hemolysis, Elevated Liver function tests, Low Platelets).
   G. **Serum uric acid** is often elevated in preeclampsia.

H. Fetal well-being is evaluated by a nonstress test or biophysical profile. The fetus is examined by ultrasound to evaluate growth and amniotic fluid volume.

I. Coagulation function tests. The prothrombin time, activated partial thromboplastin time, and fibrinogen concentration are usually normal if there is no thrombocytopenia or liver dysfunction, and therefore do not need to be monitored routinely.

VII. Management of preeclampsia. The definitive treatment of preeclampsia is delivery to prevent development of maternal or fetal complications from disease progression. Patients at term are delivered, but preterm delivery is not always in the best interests of the fetus. As a result, a more conservative approach is often considered in selected women remote from term. Maternal end-organ dysfunction and nonreassuring tests of fetal well-being may be indications for delivery at any gestational age.

A. Mild preeclampsia. At term, women are induced if there are no contraindications to vaginal birth.

B. Women who are at least 37 weeks of gestation with a favorable cervix (Bishop score >6) should be induced. Delivery should be accomplished by 40 weeks of gestation for all preeclamptic women. Cervical ripening agents should be considered in women with unfavorable cervices.

C. Women with mild disease remote from term can be managed expectantly to enable further fetal growth and maturation.

D. Inpatient versus outpatient care. Hospitalization is useful for making initial assessments. After the initial diagnostic evaluation, outpatient care is a cost-effective option for some women with mild preeclampsia.

   1. Outpatients should be able to comply with frequent maternal and fetal evaluations (every one to three days) and have ready access to medical care. Restricted activity is recommended. If signs or symptoms of disease progression occur, hospitalization and delivery may be indicated.

   2. Patients should be told to call if they develop severe or persistent headache, visual changes, right upper quadrant or epigastric pain, nausea or vomiting, shortness of breath, or decreased urine output. Decreased fetal movement, vaginal bleeding, abdominal pain, rupture of membranes, or uterine contractions should be reported immediately.

Fetal Assessment in Preeclampsia	
Mild preeclampsia	Daily fetal movement counting Ultrasound examination for estimation of fetal weight and amniotic fluid determination at diagnosis. Repeat in three weeks if the initial examination is normal, twice weekly if there is evidence of fetal growth restriction or oligohydramnios. Nonstress test and/or biophysical profile once or twice weekly. Testing should be repeated immediately if there is an abrupt change in maternal condition.
Severe preeclampsia	Daily nonstress testing and/or biophysical profile

E. Laboratory evaluation should include platelet count, serum creatinine, serum ALT and AST. These tests should be repeated once or twice weekly in women with mild preeclampsia.

F. A rising hematocrit indicates hemoconcentration, which suggests contraction of intravascular volume and progression to more severe disease, while a falling hematocrit may be a sign of hemolysis. An elevated serum LDH concentration is also a sign of hemolysis, and a marker of severe disease or HELLP syndrome. Hemolysis can be confirmed by observation of schistocytes and helmet cells on a blood smear.

G. **Quantification of protein excretion** can be performed using a 24-hour collection or protein-to creatinine ratio on a random specimen to determine whether the threshold for severe preeclampsia (5 g/24 hours) has been reached.

H. **Treatment of hypertension.** Antihypertensive therapy should be initiated at systolic pressures between 150 and 160 mm Hg and diastolic blood pressures between 100 and 105 mm Hg. Target blood pressures are 130 to 150 mm Hg systolic and 80 to 100 mm Hg diastolic.

1. Intravenous labetalol is recommended for acute therapy because it is effective and generally safe in pregnancy. Begin with 20 mg intravenously followed at 10 minute intervals by doses of 20 to 80 mg up to a maximum total cumulative dose of 300 mg. A constant infusion of 1 to 2 mg/min can be used. The oral dosage is 100 mg twice daily orally, maximum dose 2400 mg/day.

I. **Assessment of fetal well-being.** Daily fetal movement counts and twice weekly fetal nonstress testing with assessment of amniotic fluid volume, or biophysical profile are recommended.

J. **Assessment of fetal growth.** Early fetal growth restriction may be the first manifestation of preeclampsia or a sign of severe preeclampsia. A sonographic estimation of fetal weight should be performed to look for growth restriction and oligohydramnios at the time of diagnosis of preeclampsia and then repeated serially. Doppler velocimetry is useful for assessing fetal status if fetal growth restriction is present.

K. **Antenatal corticosteroids** (betamethasone) should be administered to promote fetal lung maturity for women less than 34 weeks of gestation since preterm delivery is common (two doses of 12 mg given intramuscularly 24 hours apart).

L. Indications for delivery. Women with mild preeclampsia should be delivered by 40 weeks of gestation. Progression to eclampsia is also an indication for delivery.

1. Severe preeclampsia is generally regarded as an indication for delivery, regardless of gestational age, to minimize the risk of development of maternal and fetal complications. Prolonged antepartum management at a tertiary care setting or in consultation with a maternal-fetal medicine specialist may be considered in selected women under 32 to 34 weeks of gestation. However, women who develop severe preeclampsia at or beyond 32 to 34 weeks of gestation should be delivered.

2. The decision to expedite delivery in the setting of severe preeclampsia does not mandate immediate cesarean birth. Cervical ripening agents may be used prior to induction if the cervix is not favorable.

Indications for Delivery in Preeclampsia	
Maternal indications	Gestational age >38 weeks of gestation Platelet count <100,000 cells per mm^3 Deteriorating liver function Progressive deterioration in renal function Abruptio placentae Persistent severe headaches or visual changes Persistent severe epigastric pain, nausea, or vomiting
Fetal indications	Severe fetal growth restriction Nonreassuring results from fetal testing Oligohydramnios

VIII. Intrapartum monitoring. Close, continuous maternal-fetal monitoring is indicated to identify worsening hypertension, deteriorating maternal hepatic, renal, cardiopulmonary, or hematologic function, and uteroplacental insufficiency or abruptio placentae (often manifested by nonreassuring fetal heart rate tracings and/or vaginal bleeding).

    A. A low platelet count may preclude neuraxial anesthesia, which is associated with an increased risk of spinal hematoma in this setting.

    B. Invasive hemodynamic monitoring can be useful in patients with severe cardiac disease, severe renal disease, oliguria, refractory hypertension, or pulmonary edema.

IX. Anticonvulsant therapy is started during labor and is continued for 24 hours postpartum. Magnesium sulfate is the drug of choice for the prevention of eclampsia.

    A. Indications for treatment

        1. Severe preeclampsia. Anticonvulsant therapy should be administered to prevent a first seizure in women with severe preeclampsia. Progression to eclampsia is significantly lower with magnesium (0.3 versus 3.2%).

        2. Mild preeclampsia. Anticonvulsant therapy is also used for prevention of seizures in women with mild preeclampsia.

        3. Intrapartum magnesium sulfate seizure prophylaxis should be administered for preeclampsia, but not for nonproteinuric gestational hypertension.

    B. Magnesium is usually initiated at the onset of labor or induction or prior to cesarean delivery. A loading dose of 6 g is given intravenously over 15 to 20 minutes followed by 2 g per hour as a continuous infusion.

        1. Magnesium sulfate is excreted by the kidneys; therefore, dosing should be adjusted in renal insufficiency (creatinine >1.0 mg/dL). Such women should receive a standard loading dose, but a reduced maintenance dose (1 g per hour or no maintenance dose if creatinine is >2.5 mg/dL) and close monitoring of serum magnesium level every six hours.

        2. Magnesium sulfate is contraindicated in myasthenia gravis since it can precipitate a severe myasthenic crisis. Use of magnesium sulfate with calcium channel blockers may result in hypotension.

        3. The maintenance phase is given only if a patellar reflex is present (loss of reflexes being the first manifestation of symptomatic hypermagnesemia), respirations exceed 12 per minute, and the urine output exceeds 100 mL per four hours. Following serum magnesium levels is not required if clinical status is closely monitored for signs of magnesium toxicity.

        4. Magnesium sulfate is usually continued for 24 hours postpartum. In women who have only mild preeclampsia, 12 hours may be adequate. In severe preeclampsia or eclampsia, anticonvulsant drugs are continued for 24 to 48 hours postpartum, when the risk of recurrent seizures is low.

5. **Complications.** Rapid infusion of magnesium sulfate causes diaphoresis, flushing, and warmth. Nausea, vomiting, headache, muscle weakness, visual disturbances, and palpitations can also occur. Dyspnea or chest pain may be symptoms of pulmonary edema, a rare side effect of magnesium sulfate administration.

6. **Magnesium toxicity** is related to serum concentration: loss of deep tendon reflexes occurs at 9.6 to 12.0 mg/dL, respiratory paralysis at 12.0 to 18.0 mg/dL, and cardiac arrest at 24 to 30 mg/dL. Calcium gluconate (1 g intravenously over 5 to 10 minutes) should be administered only to counteract life-threatening symptoms of magnesium toxicity (such as cardiorespiratory compromise).

7. **Hypocalcemia.** Magnesium therapy also results in a transient reduction of total and ionized serum calcium concentration due to rapid suppression of parathyroid hormone release. Rarely, the hypocalcemia becomes symptomatic (myoclonus, delirium, ECG abnormalities). Cessation of magnesium therapy will restore normal serum calcium levels. However, calcium administration may be required if symptoms are present (calcium gluconate 1 g intravenously over 5 to 10 minutes).

X. **Postpartum course.** Hypertension and proteinuria due to preeclampsia resolves postpartum, within a few days, but sometimes taking a few weeks. Severe hypertension should be treated; some patients will have to be discharged on antihypertensive medications that can be discontinued when blood pressure returns to normal. Elevated blood pressures that remain 12 weeks postpartum are probably not caused by preeclampsia and may require long-term treatment.

References: See page 208.

Eclampsia

Eclampsia is defined as the occurrence of one or more generalized convulsions and/or coma in the setting of preeclampsia and in the absence of other neurologic conditions. The manifestations appear anytime from the second trimester to the puerperium. Seizures are only one of several clinical manifestation of severe preeclampsia. Preeclampsia/eclampsia is a common cause of maternal death, along with thromboembolic disease and hemorrhage.

I. **Incidence and epidemiology**
   A. An eclamptic seizure occurs in 0.5% of mildly preeclamptic pregnancies and 2% of severe preeclamptics. The incidence of eclampsia is 4 to 5 cases per 10,000 live births.
   B. Eclampsia is more common in nonwhite, nulliparous women from lower socioeconomic backgrounds. Peak incidence is in the teenage years and low twenties, but there is also an increased incidence in women over 35 years of age. Risk factors are similar to those for preeclampsia.
   C. **Timing in pregnancy.** Eclampsia prior to 20 weeks of gestation is rare and should raise the possibility of an underlying molar pregnancy or antiphospholipid syndrome.
   D. One-half of all cases of eclampsia occur prior to term, with more than one-fifth occurring before 31 weeks of gestation. One-third of cases occur at term, developing intrapartum or within 48 hours of delivery. Late postpartum eclampsia accounts for the remainder (13 to 16%).
II. **Pathogenesis of seizures.** Proposed etiologies of seizures in women with eclampsia include (1) cerebral vasospasm with local ischemia/infarction and cytotoxic (intracellular) edema and (2) hypertensive encephalopathy with hyperperfusion, vasogenic (extracellular) edema, and endothelial damage.

III. Clinical manifestations and diagnosis

   A. Maternal. Eclamptic seizures are almost always self-limiting and usually last for 60-75 seconds (seldom longer than 3 minutes). Persistent frontal or occipital headache, blurred vision, photophobia, right upper quadrant or epigastric pain, and altered mental status may occur before the seizure.

   B. The diagnosis of preeclampsia/eclampsia may not be suspected prior to the development of seizures in women with relative hypertension and no proteinuria. However, 15 to 22% of eclamptic women have no evidence of proteinuria prior to their seizure, 25 to 33% have no edema, and 16% have no hypertension.

   C. Women with typical eclamptic seizures who do not have focal neurologic deficits or prolonged coma do not require either electroencephalographic or cerebral imaging studies. If cerebral imaging is performed, MRI is the optimal study.

   D. Fetal bradycardia lasting at least three to five minutes is a common finding during and immediately after an eclamptic seizure, and does not necessitate emergent cesarean delivery. Stabilizing the mother by administering anticonvulsant drugs and oxygen and treating severe hypertension can help the fetus recover in-utero from the effects of maternal hypoxia, hypercarbia, and uterine hyperstimulation.

   E. Resolution of maternal seizure activity is associated with compensatory tachycardia and loss of variability, sometimes associated with transient fetal heart rate decelerations which typically resolve within 20 to 30 minutes. However, if the fetal heart rate tracing remains nonreassuring for more than 10 to 15 minutes with no improvement despite maternal and fetal resuscitative interventions, then occult abruption and delivery should be considered.

IV. Differential diagnosis. Eclamptic seizures are clinically and electro-encephalographically indistinguishable from other generalized tonic-clonic seizures.

   A. Differential diagnosis of seizures in pregnancy
   1. Cerebrovascular accident (hemorrhage, arterial or venous thrombosis).
   2. Hypertensive disease (hypertensive encephalopathy, pheochromocytoma).
   3. Space-occupying lesions of the central nervous system (brain tumor, abscess).
   4. Metabolic disorders (hypoglycemia, uremia, inappropriate antidiuretic hormone secretion resulting in water intoxication).
   5. Infection (meningitis, encephalitis).
   6. Thrombotic thrombocytopenic purpura or thrombophilia.
   7. Idiopathic epilepsy.
   8. Use of methamphetamine, cocaine.
   9. Cerebral vasculitis.
   10. Reversible posterior leukoencephalopathy syndrome.
   11. Postdural puncture syndrome.

V. Management

   A. If the seizure is witnessed, maintenance of airway patency and prevention of aspiration should be the first responsibilities of management. The gravida should be rolled onto her left side. Supplemental oxygen (8 to 10 L/min) via a face mask is recommended.
   1. Maintenance of maternal vital functions to prevent hypoxia
   2. Control of convulsions and blood pressure
   3. Prevention of recurrent seizures
   4. Evaluation for prompt delivery

   B. The definitive treatment of eclampsia is delivery, irrespective of gestational age, to reduce the risk of maternal morbidity and mortality.

   C. Control of convulsions. The drug of choice is intravenous magnesium sulfate. A benzodiazepine is another option. Phenytoin can also be used, but is less effective in preventing recurrent seizures. Prevention of recurrent convulsions is more important than stopping the initial convulsion because it is usually of short duration.

1. **Magnesium sulfate** (6 g intravenously over 15 minutes) is administered to stop the convulsion. An alternative dose/route is magnesium sulfate 5 g intramuscularly into each buttock. A diazepam gel for rectal administration is available (0.2 mg/kg). Magnesium sulfate is contraindicated in myasthenia gravis because it can cause myasthenic crisis. Use of magnesium sulfate with calcium channel blockers may cause hypotension.

2. **Diazepam**(0.1 to 0.3 mg/kg IV over 60 seconds, max cumulative dose of 20 mg) achieves anticonvulsant levels within one minute, and will control seizures in >80% within five minutes. Benzodiazepines should be avoided because of profound depressant effects on the fetus and mother.

D. **Treatment of hypertension.** Cerebrovascular accident accounts for 15-20% of deaths from eclampsia. Antihypertensive therapy is recommended for diastolic pressures of >105 to 110 mmHg and systolic blood pressures of 160 mmHg.

1. **Labetalol (Trandate).** 10 or 20 mg intravenously followed by doubling the dose at 10 minute intervals up to 80 mg for a maximum total cumulative dose of 220 to 230 mg. Goal is a systolic of 140-155 mmHg and diastolic of 90-105 mmHg.

E. **Prevention of subsequent seizures.** Magnesium sulfate is the drug of choice for prevention of recurrent eclamptic seizures.

1. **Maintenance magnesium dose**after the initial 6 g loading dose is 2 to 3 g/hour intravenous infusion. The maintenance phase is given only if a patellar reflex is present, respirations are >12 per minute, and urine output >100 mL in four hours.

2. **Recurrent convulsions** occurring in patients on maintenance magnesium sulfate therapy can be treated with an additional bolus of 2 grams of magnesium sulfate over 15 to 20 minutes. If two boluses of magnesium sulfate do not control seizures, lorazepam (Ativan) 0.02 to 0.03 mg/kg intravenously is administered. If seizures continue, additional doses of lorazepam (up to a cumulative dose of 0.1 mg/kg) should be infused at a max 2 mg/minute. Other options include amobarbital (250 mg IV over 3 to 5 minutes), phenytoin or paralysis with intubation and mechanical ventilation.

F. **Delivery.** Eclampsia is usually an absolute contraindication to expectant management. The definitive treatment for eclampsia is delivery.

1. Cesarean delivery is a reasonable option for women with severe preeclampsia/eclampsia remote from term (eg, <28 to 32 weeks gestation) with an unfavorable cervix and not in labor.

2. Cervical ripening agents can be used to improve the Bishop score; however, long inductions should be avoided (eg, 24 hours).

G. **Postpartum course.** Seizures due to eclampsia always resolve postpartum, generally within a few hours to days. Anticonvulsant drugs are continued for 24 to 48 hours postpartum.

References: See page 208.

Herpes Simplex Virus Infections in Pregnancy

Herpes simplex virus (HSV) is a major source of morbidity and mortality for newborns infected with HSV. HSV-2 is primarily responsible for genital HSV disease. Spread is principally through sexual contact. The incidence is 22%. The majority of cases are asymptomatic or symptoms are unrecognized. HSV-1 infection generally involves the mucosal surfaces of the mouth, pharynx, lips and eyes, but the virus can also be recovered from genital lesions.

I. **Clinical presentation**
   A. **Primary genital episode genital HSV** is characterized by multiple painful vesicles in clusters. They may be associated with pruritus, dysuria, vaginal discharge, and tender regional adenopathy. Fever, malaise, and myalgia often occur one to two days prior to the appearance of lesions. The lesions may last four to five days prior to crusting. The skin will reepithelialize in about 10 days. Viral shedding may last for 10 to 12 days after reepithelialization.
   B. **Nonprimary first-episode genital HSV** refers to patients with preexisting antibodies to one of the two types of virus who acquire the other virus and develop genital lesions. Nonprimary disease is less severe with fewer systemic symptoms, and less local pain.
   C. **Recurrent HSV episodes** are characterized by local pain or paresthesia followed by vesicular lesions. Lesions are generally fewer in number and often unilateral but may be painful.

II. **Diagnosis**
   A. PCR to detect HSV DNA from lesions or genital secretions is recommended for diagnosis. The gold standard for diagnosis of acute HSV infection is viral culture. Although the highest yield is from vesicular fluid of skin lesions, cultures may be obtained from the eyes, mouth, cerebral spinal fluid, rectum, urine, and blood.

Clinical Designation of Genital Herpes Simplex Virus Infection
Primary genital HSV infection Antibodies to both HSV-1 and HSV-2 are absent at the time the patient acquires genital HSV due to HSV-1 or HSV-2
Nonprimary first episode genital HSV infection Acquisition of genital HSV-1 with pre-existing antibodies to HSV-2 or acquisition of genital HSV-2 with pre-existed antibodies rto HSV-1
Recurrent genital HSV infection Reactivation of genital HSV in which the HSV type recovered from the lesion is the same type as antibodies in the serum

III. **Maternal treatment**
   A. **Primary infection.** Acyclovir therapy (200 mg PO five times per day or 400 mg PO TID for 7 to 14 days) is recommended. Acyclovir is safe in pregnancy. Acyclovir should be administered to pregnant women experiencing a first episode of HSV during pregnancy to reduce the duration of active lesions. Suppressive therapy (400 mg PO BID) for the remainder of pregnancy should also be considered.
   B. **Recurrent Infection.** Women with one or more HSV recurrence during pregnancy benefit from suppression given at 36 weeks of gestation through delivery.
   C. **Cesarean delivery** should be offered to women who have active lesions or symptoms of vulvar pain or burning at the time of delivery in those with a history of genital herpes. However, delivery by cesarean birth does not prevent all infections. Approximately 20 to 30% of HSV-infected infants are born by cesarean. Prophylactic cesarean delivery is not recommended for women with recurrent HSV and no evidence of active lesions at the time of delivery. Lesions which have crusted fully are considered healed and not active.
   D. **Prevention**
      1. Nongenital invasive procedures (eg, amniocentesis) should be delayed if there is evidence of systemic disease. Use of fetal scalp electrodes should be avoided among women who are known to have recurrent HSV, and who are in labor.

2. Mothers with active lesions should cover their lesions, and hands should be washed before touching the baby. Breastfeeding is not contraindicated as long as there are no breast lesions.

References: See page 208.

Dystocia and Augmentation of Labor

I. Normal labor
A. First stage of labor
1. The first stage of labor consists of the period from the onset of labor until complete cervical dilation (10 cm). This stage is divided into the latent phase and the active phase.
2. Latent phase
a. During the latent phase, uterine contractions are infrequent and irregular and result in only modest discomfort. They result in gradual effacement and dilation of the cervix.
b. A prolonged latent phase is one that exceeds 20 hours in the nullipara or one that exceeds 14 hours in the multipara.
3. Active phase
a. The active phase of labor occurs when the cervix reaches 3-4 cm of dilatation.
b. The active phase of labor is characterized by an increased rate of cervical dilation and by descent of the presenting fetal part.
B. Second stage of labor
1. **The second stage of labor** consists of the period from complete cervical dilation (10 cm) until delivery of the infant. This stage is usually brief, averaging 20 minutes for parous women and 50 minutes for nulliparous women.
2. The duration of the second stage of labor is unrelated to perinatal outcome in the absence of a nonreassuring fetal heart rate pattern as long as progress occurs.

II. Abnormal labor
A. **Dystocia** is defined as difficult labor or childbirth resulting from abnormalities of the cervix and uterus, the fetus, the maternal pelvis, or a combination of these factors.
B. **Cephalopelvic disproportion** is a disparity between the size of the maternal pelvis and the fetal head that precludes vaginal delivery. This condition can rarely be diagnosed in advance.
C. **Slower-than-normal (protraction disorders) or complete cessation of progress (arrest disorder)** are disorders that can be diagnosed only after the parturient has entered the active phase of labor.

III. Assessment of labor abnormalities
A. Labor abnormalities caused by inadequate uterine contractility (powers). The minimal uterine contractile pattern of women in spontaneous labor consists of 3 to 5 contractions in a 10-minute period.
B. Labor abnormalities caused by fetal characteristics (passenger)
1. Assessment of the fetus consists of estimating fetal weight and position. Estimations of fetal size, even those obtained by ultrasonography, are frequently inaccurate.
2. In the first stage of labor, the diagnosis of dystocia can not be made unless the active phase of labor and adequate uterine contractile forces have been present.
3. Fetal anomalies such as hydrocephaly, encephalocele, and soft tissue tumors may obstruct labor. Fetal imaging should be considered when malpresentation or anomalies are suspected based on vaginal or abdominal examination or when the presenting fetal part is persistently high.
C. Labor abnormalities due to the pelvic passage (passage)
1. Inefficient uterine action should be corrected before attributing dystocia to a pelvic problem.

2. The bony pelvis is very rarely the factor that limits vaginal delivery of a fetus in cephalic presentation. Radiographic pelvimetry is of limited value in managing most cephalic presentations.
3. Clinical pelvimetry can only be useful to qualitatively identify the general architectural features of the pelvis.

IV. Augmentation of labor

A. Uterine hypocontractility should be augmented only after both the maternal pelvis and fetal presentation have been assessed.
B. Contraindications to augmentation include placenta or vasa previa, umbilical cord prolapse, prior classical uterine incision, pelvic structural deformities, and invasive cervical cancer.
C. Oxytocin (Pitocin)
   1. The goal of oxytocin administration is to stimulate uterine activity that is sufficient to produce cervical change and fetal descent while avoiding uterine hyperstimulation and fetal compromise.
   2. **Minimally effective uterine activity** is 3 contractions per 10 minutes averaging >25 mm Hg above baseline. A maximum of 5 contractions in a 10-minute period with resultant cervical dilatation is considered adequate.
   3. **Hyperstimulation** is characterized by more than five contractions in 10 minutes, contractions lasting 2 minutes or more, or contractions of normal duration occurring within 1 minute of each other.
   4. Oxytocin is administered when a patient is progressing slowly through the latent phase of labor or has a protraction or an arrest disorder of labor, or when a hypotonic uterine contraction pattern is identified.
   5. A pelvic examination should be performed before initiation of oxytocin infusion.
   6. Oxytocin is usually diluted 10 units in 1 liter of normal saline IVPB.

Labor Stimulation with Oxytocin (Pitocin)			
Starting Dose (mU/min)	**Incremental Increase (mU/min)**	**Dosage Interval (min)**	**Maximum Dose (mU/min)**
6	6	15	40

   7. **Management of oxytocin-induced hyperstimulation**
      a. The most common adverse effect of hyperstimulation is fetal heart rate deceleration associated with uterine hyperstimulation. Stopping or decreasing the dose of oxytocin may correct the abnormal pattern.
      b. Additional measures may include changing the patient to the lateral decubitus position and administering oxygen or more intravenous fluid.
      c. If oxytocin-induced uterine hyperstimulation does not respond to conservative measures, intravenous terbutaline (0.125-0.25 mg) or magnesium sulfate (2-6 g in 10-20% dilution) may be used to stop uterine contractions.

References: See page 208.

Fetal Macrosomia

Excessive birth weight is associated with an increased risk of maternal and neonatal injury. Macrosomia is defined as a fetus with an estimated weight of more than 4,500 grams, regardless of gestational age.

I. **Diagnosis of macrosomia**
   A. Clinical estimates of fetal weight based on Leopold's maneuvers or fundal height measurements are often inaccurate.
   B. Diagnosis of macrosomia requires ultrasound evaluation; however, estimation of fetal weight based on ultrasound is associated with a large margin of error.
   C. Maternal weight, height, previous obstetric history, fundal height, and the presence of gestational diabetes should be evaluated.

II. **Factors influencing fetal weight**
   A. **Gestational age.** Post-term pregnancy is a risk factor for macrosomia. At 42 weeks and beyond, 2.5% of fetuses weigh more than 4,500 g. Ten to twenty% of macrosomic infants are post-term fetuses.
   B. **Maternal weight.** Heavy women have a greater risk of giving birth to excessively large infants. Fifteen to 35% of women who deliver macrosomic fetuses weigh 90 kg or more.
   C. **Multiparity.** Macrosomic infants are 2-3 times more likely to be born to parous women.
   D. **Macrosomia in a prior infant.** The risk of delivering an infant weighing more than 4,500 g is increased if a prior infant weighed more than 4,000 g.
   E. **Maternal diabetes**
      1. Maternal diabetes increases the risk of fetal macrosomia and shoulder dystocia.
      2. Cesarean delivery is indicated when the estimated fetal weight exceeds 4,500 g.

III. **Morbidity and mortality**
   A. **Abnormalities of labor.** Macrosomic fetuses have a higher incidence of labor abnormalities and instrumental deliveries.
   B. **Maternal morbidity.** Macrosomic fetuses have a two- to threefold increased rate of cesarean delivery.
   C. **Birth injury**
      1. The incidence of birth injuries occurring during delivery of a macrosomic infant is much greater with vaginal than with cesarean birth. The most common injury is brachial plexus palsy, often caused by shoulder dystocia.
      2. The incidence of shoulder dystocia in infants weighing more than 4,500 g is 8-20%. Macrosomic infants also may sustain fractures of the clavicle or humerus.

IV. **Management of delivery**
   A. If the estimated fetal weight is >4500 gm in the nondiabetic or >4000 gm in the diabetic patient, delivery by cesarean section is indicated.
   B. **Management of shoulder dystocia**
      1. If a shoulder dystocia occurs, an assistant should provide suprapubic pressure to dislodge the impacted anterior fetal shoulder from the symphysis. McRoberts maneuver (extreme hip flexion) should be done simultaneously.
      2. If the shoulder remains impacted anteriorly, an ample episiotomy should be cut and the posterior arm delivered.
      3. In almost all instances, one or both of these procedures will result in successful delivery. The Zavanelli maneuver consists of replacement of the fetal lead into the vaginal canal and delivery by emergency cesarean section.
      4. Fundal pressure is not recommended because it often results in further impaction of the shoulder against the symphysis.

References: See page 208.

Shoulder Dystocia

Shoulder dystocia, defined as failure of the shoulders to deliver following the head, is an obstetric emergency. The incidence varies from 0.6% to 1.4% of all vaginal deliveries. Up to 30% of shoulder dystocias can result in brachial plexus injury; many fewer sustain serious asphyxia or death. Most commonly, size discrepancy secondary to fetal macrosomia is associated with difficult shoulder delivery. Causal factors of macrosomia include maternal diabetes, postdates gestation, and obesity. The fetus of the diabetic gravida may also have disproportionately large shoulders and body size compared with the head.

I. Prediction

A. The diagnosis of shoulder dystocia is made after delivery of the head. The "turtle" sign is the retraction of the chin against the perineum or retraction of the head into the birth canal. This sign demonstrates that the shoulder girdle is resisting entry into the pelvic inlet, and possibly impaction of the anterior shoulder.

B. Macrosomia has the strongest association. ACOG defines macrosomia as an estimated fetal weight (EFW) >4500 g.

C. Risk factors for macrosomia include maternal birth weight, prior macrosomia, preexisting diabetes, obesity, multiparity, advanced maternal age, and a prior shoulder dystocia. The recurrence rate has been reported to be 13.8%, nearly seven times the primary rate. Shoulder dystocia occurs in 5.1% of obese women. In the antepartum period, risk factors include gestational diabetes, excessive weight gain, short stature, macrosomia, and postterm pregnancy. Intrapartum factors include prolonged second stage of labor, abnormal first stage, arrest disorders, and instrumental (especially midforceps) delivery. Many shoulder dystocias will occur in the absence of any risk factors.

II. Management

A. Shoulder dystocia is a medical and possibly surgical emergency. Two assistants should be called for if not already present, as well as an anesthesiologist and pediatrician. A generous episiotomy should be cut. The following sequence is suggested:

1. **McRoberts maneuver:** The legs are removed from the lithotomy position and flexed at the hips, with flexion of the knees against the abdomen. Two assistants are required. This maneuver may be performed prophylactically in anticipation of a difficult delivery.

2. **Suprapubic pressure:** An assistant is requested to apply pressure downward, above the symphysis pubis. This can be done in a lateral direction to help dislodge the anterior shoulder from behind the pubic symphysis. It can also be performed in anticipation of a difficult delivery. Fundal pressure may increase the likelihood of uterine rupture and is contraindicated.

3. **Rotational maneuvers:** The Woods' corkscrew maneuver consists of placing two fingers against the anterior aspect of the posterior shoulder. Gentle upward rotational pressure is applied so that the posterior shoulder girdle rotates anteriorly, allowing it to be delivered first. The Rubin maneuver is the reverse of Woods's maneuver. Two fingers are placed against the posterior aspect of the posterior (or anterior) shoulder and forward pressure applied. This results in adduction of the shoulders and displacement of the anterior shoulder from behind the symphysis pubis.

4. **Posterior arm release:** The operator places a hand into the posterior vagina along the infant's back. The posterior arm is identified and followed to the elbow. The elbow is then swept across the chest, keeping the elbow flexed. The fetal forearm or hand is then grasped and the posterior arm delivered, followed by the anterior shoulder. If the fetus still remains undelivered, vaginal delivery

should be abandoned and the Zavanelli maneuver performed followed by cesarean delivery.
5. **Zavanelli maneuver:** The fetal head is replaced into the womb. Tocolysis is recommended to produce uterine relaxation. The maneuver consists of rotation of the head to occiput anterior. The head is then flexed and pushed back into the vagina, followed abdominal delivery. Immediate preparations should be made for cesarean delivery.
6. If cephalic replacement fails, an emergency symphysiotomy should be performed. The urethra should be laterally displaced to minimize the risk of lower urinary tract injury.
B. The McRoberts maneuver alone will successfully alleviate the shoulder dystocia in 42% to 79% of cases. For those requiring additional maneuvers, vaginal delivery can be expected in more than 90%. Finally, favorable results have been reported for the Zavanelli maneuver in up to 90%.

References: See page 208.

Postdates Pregnancy

A term gestation is defined as one completed in 38 to 42 weeks. Pregnancy is considered prolonged or postdates when it exceeds 294 days or 42 weeks from the first day of the last menstrual period (LMP). About 10% of those pregnancies are postdates. The incidence of patients reaching the 42nd week is 3-12%.

I. Morbidity and mortality
 A. The rate of maternal, fetal, and neonatal complications increases with gestational age. The cesarean delivery rate more than doubles when passing the 42nd week compared with 40 weeks because of cephalopelvic disproportion resulting from larger infants and by fetal intolerance of labor.
 B. Neonatal complications from postdates pregnancies include placental insufficiency, birth trauma from macrosomia, meconium aspiration syndrome, and oligohydramnios.

II. Diagnosis
 A. The accurate diagnosis of postdates pregnancy can be made only by proper dating. The estimated date of confinement (EDC) is most accurately determined early in pregnancy. An EDC can be calculated by subtracting 3 months from the first day of the last menses and adding 7 days (Naegele's rule). Other clinical parameters that should be consistent with the EDC include maternal perception of fetal movements (quickening) at about 16 to 20 weeks; first auscultation of fetal heart tones with Doppler ultrasound by 12 weeks; uterine size at early examination (first trimester) consistent with dates; and, at 20 weeks, a fundal height 20 cm above the symphysis pubis or at the umbilicus.

Clinical Estimates of Gestational Age	
Parameter	**Gestational age (weeks)**
Positive urine hCG	5
Fetal heart tones by Doppler	11 to 12

Quickening
    Primigravida
    Multigravida
	
	20
	16

Fundal height at umbilicus	20

B. In patients without reliable clinical data, ultrasound is beneficial. Ultrasonography is most accurate in early gestation. The crown-rump length becomes less accurate after 12 weeks in determining gestational age because the fetus begins to curve.

III. Management of the postdates pregnancy

A. A postdates patient with a favorable cervix should receive induction of labor. Only 8.2% of pregnancies at 42 weeks have a ripe cervix (Bishop score >6). Induction at 41 weeks with cervical ripening lowers the cesarean delivery rate.

B. **Placement of a balloon catheter** immediately followed by vaginal or intracervical prostaglandin E2 administration is recommended. Oxytocin, if required, can be started six hours after the last prostaglandin dose.

C. **Stripping of membranes**, starting at 38 weeks and repeated weekly may be an effective method of inducing labor in post-term women with a favorable cervix. Stripping of membranes is performed by placing a finger in the cervical os and circling 3 times in the plane between the fetal head and cervix.

D. **Expectant management with antenatal surveillance**
   1. Begin testing near the end of the 41st week of pregnancy. Antepartum testing consists of the nonstress test (NST) combined with the amniotic fluid index (AFI) twice weekly. The false-negative rate is 6.1/1000 (stillbirth within 1 week of a reassuring test) with twice weekly NSTs.
   2. The AFI involves measuring the deepest vertical fluid pocket in each uterine quadrant and summing the four together. Less than 5 cm is considered oligohydramnios, 5 to 8 cm borderline, and >8 cm normal.

E. **Fetal movement counting (kick counts).** Fetal movement has been correlated with fetal health. It consist of having the mother lie on her side and count fetal movements. Perception of 10 distinct movements in a period of up to 2 hours is considered reassuring. After 10 movements have been perceived, the count may be discontinued.

F. **Delivery** is indicated if the amniotic fluid index is <5 cm, a nonreactive non-stress test is identified, or if decelerations are identified on the nonstress test.

G. **Intrapartum management**
   1. **Meconium staining** is more common in postdates pregnancies. If oligohydramnios is present, amnioinfusion dilutes meconium and decreases the number of infants with meconium below the vocal cords. Instillation of normal saline through an intrauterine pressure catheter may reduce variable decelerations.
   2. **Macrosomia** should be suspected in all postdates gestations. Fetal weight should be estimated prior to labor in all postdates pregnancies. Ultrasonographic weight predictions generally fall within 20% of the actual birth weight.
   3. **Management of suspected macrosomia.** The pediatrician and anesthesiologist should be notified so that they can prepare for delivery. Cesarean delivery should be considered in patients with an estimated fetal weight >4500 g and a marginal pelvis, or someone with a previous difficult vaginal delivery with a similarly sized or larger infant.
   4. Intrapartum asphyxia is also more common in the postdates pregnancy. Therefore, close observation of the fetal heart rate tracing is necessary during labor. Variable decelerations representing cord compression are frequently seen in postdates pregnancies.
   5. Cord compression can be treated with amnioinfusion, which can reduce variable decelerations. Late decelerations are more direct evidence of fetal hypoxia. If intermittent, late decelerations are managed conservatively with positioning and oxygen. If persistent late decelerations are associated with decreased variability or an

elevated baseline fetal heart rate, immediate evaluation or delivery is indicated. This additional evaluation can include observation for fetal heart acceleration following fetal scalp or acoustic stimulation, or a fetal scalp pH.

References: See page 208.

Induction of Labor

Induction of labor refers to stimulation of uterine contractions prior to the onset of spontaneous labor. Between 1990 and 1998, the rate of labor induction doubled from 10 to 20%.

I. **Indications for labor induction:**
   A. Preeclampsia/eclampsia, and other hypertensive diseases
   B. Maternal diabetes mellitus
   C. Prelabor rupture of membranes
   D. Chorioamnionitis
   E. Intrauterine fetal growth restriction (IUGR)
   F. Isoimmunization
   G. In-utero fetal demise
   H. Postterm pregnancy

II. **Absolute contraindications to labor induction:**
   A. Prior classical uterine incision
   B. Active genital herpes infection
   C. Placenta or vasa previa
   D. Umbilical cord prolapse
   E. Fetal malpresentation, such as transverse lie

II. **Requirements for induction**
   A. Prior to undertaking labor induction, assessments of gestational age, fetal size and presentation, clinical pelvimetry, and cervical examination should be performed. Fetal maturity should be evaluated, and amniocentesis for fetal lung maturity may be needed prior to induction.
   B. **Clinical criteria that confirm term gestation:**
      1. Fetal heart tones documented for 30 weeks by Doppler.
      2. Thirty-six weeks have elapsed since a serum or urine human chorionic gonadotropin (hCG) pregnancy test was positive.
      3. Ultrasound measurement of the crown-rump length at 6 to 11 weeks of gestation or biparietal diameter/femur length at 12 to 20 weeks of gestation support a clinically determined gestational age equal to or >39 weeks.
   C. **Assessment of cervical ripeness**
      1. A cervical examination should be performed before initiating attempts at labor induction.
      2. The modified Bishop scoring system is most commonly used to assess the cervix. A score is calculated based upon the station of the presenting part and cervical dilatation, effacement, consistency, and position.

Modified Bishop Scoring System				
	0	**1**	**2**	**3**
Dilation, cm	Closed	1-2	3-4	5-6
Effacement, percent	0-30	40-50	60-70	>80
Station*	-3	-2	-1, 0	+1, +2

	0	1	2	3
Cervical consistency	Firm	Medium	Soft	
Position of the cervix	Posterior	Midposition	Anterior	
* Based on a -3 to +3 scale.				

3. The likelihood of a vaginal delivery after labor induction is similar to that after spontaneous onset of labor if the Bishop score is >8.

III. Induction of labor with oxytocin

A. The uterine response to exogenous oxytocin administration is periodic uterine contractions.

B. **Oxytocin regimen (Pitocin)**
   1. Oxytocin is given intravenously. Oxytocin is diluted by placing 10 units in 1000 mL of normal saline, yielding an oxytocin concentration of 10 mU/mL. Begin at 6 mU/min and increase by 6 mU/min every 15 minutes.
   2. Active management of labor regimens use a high-dose oxytocin infusion with short incremental time intervals.

High Dose Oxytocin Regimen

Begin oxytocin 6 mU per minute intravenously
Increase dose by 6 mU per minute every 15 minutes
Maximum dose: 40 mU per minute
Maximum total dose administered during labor: 10 U Maximum duration of administration: six hours

3. The dose of maximum oxytocin is usually 40 mU/min. The dose is typically increased until contractions occur at two to three minute intervals.

IV. Cervical ripening agents

A. A ripening process should be considered prior to use of oxytocin use when the cervix is unfavorable.

B. **Mechanical methods**
   1. **Membrane stripping** is a widely utilized technique, which causes release of either prostaglandin F2-alpha from the decidua and adjacent membranes or prostaglandin E2 from the cervix. Weekly membrane stripping beginning at 38 weeks of gestation results in delivery within a shorter period of time (8.6 versus 15 days).
   2. **Amniotomy** is an effective method of labor induction when performed in women with partially dilated and effaced cervices. Caution should be exercised to ensure that the fetal vertex is well-applied to the cervix and the umbilical cord or other fetal part is not presenting.
   3. **Foley catheter.** An uninflated Foley catheter can be passed through an undilated cervix and then inflated. This technique is as effective as prostaglandin E2 gel. The use of extra-amniotic saline infusion with a balloon catheter or a double balloon catheter (Atad ripener) also appears to be effective for cervical ripening.

C. **Prostaglandins**
   1. Local administration of prostaglandins to the vagina or the endocervix is the route of choice because of fewer side effects and acceptable clinical response. Uncommon side effects include fever, chills, vomiting, and diarrhea.
   2. **Prepidil** contains 0.5 mg of dinoprostone in 2.5 mL of gel for intracervical administration. The dose can be repeated in 6 to 12 hours if there is inadequate cervical change and minimal uterine activity following the first

dose. The maximum cumulative dose is 1.5 mg (ie, 3 doses) within a 24-hour period. The time interval between the final dose and initiation of oxytocin should be 6 to 12 hours because of the potential for uterine hyperstimulation with concurrent oxytocin and prostaglandin administration.

3. **Cervidil** is a vaginal insert containing 10 mg of dinoprostone in a timed-release formulation. The vaginal insert administers the medication at 0.3 mg/h and should be left in place for 12 hours. Oxytocin may be initiated 30 to 60 minutes after removal of the insert.

4. An advantage of the vaginal insert over the gel formulation is that the insert can be removed in cases of uterine hyperstimulation or abnormalities of the fetal heart rate tracing.

V. **Complications of labor induction**

  A. **Hyperstimulation and tachysystole** may occur with use of prostaglandin compounds or oxytocin. Hyperstimulation is defined as uterine contractions lasting at least two minutes or five or more uterine contractions in 10 minutes. Tachysystole is defined as six or more contractions in 20 minutes.

  B. **Prostaglandin E2 (PGE2) preparations** have up to a 5% rate of uterine hyperstimulation. Fetal heart rate abnormalities can occur, but usually resolve upon removal of the drug. Rarely hyperstimulation or tachysystole can cause uterine rupture. Removing the PGE2 vaginal insert will usually help reverse the effects of the hyperstimulation and tachysystole. Cervical and vaginal lavage after local application of prostaglandin compounds is not helpful.

  C. If oxytocin is being infused, it should be discontinued to achieve a reassuring fetal heart rate pattern. Placing the woman in the left lateral position, administering oxygen, and increasing intravenous fluids may also be of benefit. Terbutaline 0.25 mg subcutaneously (a tocolytic) may be given.

References: See page 208.

Postpartum Hemorrhage

Obstetric hemorrhage remains a leading causes of maternal mortality. Postpartum hemorrhage is defined as the loss of more than 500 mL of blood following delivery. However, the average blood loss in an uncomplicated vaginal delivery is about 500 mL, with 5% losing more than 1,000 mL.

I. **Clinical evaluation of postpartum hemorrhage**

  A. **Uterine atony** is the most common cause of postpartum hemorrhage. Conditions associated with uterine atony include an overdistended uterus (eg, polyhydramnios, multiple gestation), rapid or prolonged labor, macrosomia, high parity, and chorioamnionitis.

  B. **Conditions associated with bleeding from trauma** include forceps delivery, macrosomia, precipitous labor and delivery, and episiotomy.

  C. **Conditions associated with bleeding from coagulopathy and thrombocytopenia** include abruptio placentae, amniotic fluid embolism, preeclampsia, coagulation disorders, autoimmune thrombocytopenia, and anticoagulants.

  D. **Uterine rupture** is associated with previous uterine surgery, internal podalic version, breech extraction, multiple gestation, and abnormal fetal presentation. High parity is a risk factor for both uterine atony and rupture.

  E. **Uterine inversion** is detected by abdominal vaginal examination, which will reveal a uterus with an unusual shape after delivery.

II. **Management of postpartum hemorrhage**

  A. **Following delivery** of the placenta, the uterus should be palpated to determine whether atony is present. If atony is present, vigorous fundal massage should be administered. If bleeding continues despite uterine massage, it can often be controlled with bimanual uterine compression.

  B. **Genital tract lacerations** should be suspected in patients who have a firm uterus, but who continue to bleed. The cervix and vagina should be inspected to rule out lacerations. If no laceration is found but bleeding is still profuse, the uterus should be manually examined to exclude rupture.

C. **The placenta and uterus should be examined** for retained placental fragments. Placenta accreta is usually manifest by failure of spontaneous placental separation.

D. **Bleeding from non-genital areas** (venous puncture sites) suggests coagulopathy. Laboratory tests that confirm coagulopathy include INR, partial thromboplastin time, platelet count, fibrinogen, fibrin split products, and a clot retraction test.

E. **Medical management of postpartum hemorrhage**
   1. **Oxytocin (Pitocin)** is usually given routinely immediately after delivery to stimulate uterine firmness and diminish blood loss. 20 units of oxytocin in 1,000 mL of normal saline or Ringer's lactate is administered at 100 drops/minute. Oxytocin should not be given as a rapid bolus injection because of the potential for circulatory collapse.
   2. **Methylergonovine (Methergine)** 0.2 mg can be given IM if uterine massage and oxytocin are not effective in correcting uterine atony and provided there is no hypertension.
   3. **15-methyl prostaglandin F2-alpha (Hemabate)**, one ampule (0.25 mg), can be given IM, with repeat injections every 20min, up to 4 doses can be given if hypertension is present; it is contraindicated in asthma.

Treatment of Postpartum Hemorrhage Secondary to Uterine Atony	
Drug	**Protocol**
Oxytocin	20 U in 1,000 mL of lactated Ringer's as IV infusion
Methylergonovine (Methergine)	0.2 mg IM
Prostaglandin (15 methyl PGF2-alpha [Hemabate, Prostin/15M])	0.25 mg as IM every 15-00 minutes as necessary

F. **Volume replacement**
   1. Patients with postpartum hemorrhage that is refractory to medical therapy require a second large-bore IV catheter. If the patient has had a major blood group determination and has a negative indirect Coombs test, type-specific blood may be given without waiting for a complete cross-match. Lactated Ringer's solution or normal saline is generously infused until blood can be replaced. Replacement consists of 3 mL of crystalloid solution per 1 mL of blood lost.
   2. A Foley catheter is placed, and urine output is maintained at >30 mL/h.

G. **Surgical management of postpartum hemorrhage**. If medical therapy fails, ligation of the uterine or uteroovarian artery, infundibulopelvic vessels, or hypogastric arteries, or hysterectomy may be indicated.

H. **Management of uterine inversion**
   1. The inverted uterus should be immediately repositioned vaginally. Blood and/or fluids should be administered. If the placenta is still attached, it should not be removed until the uterus has been repositioned.
   2. Uterine relaxation can be achieved with a halogenated anesthetic agent. Terbutaline is also useful for relaxing the uterus.
   3. Following successful uterine repositioning and placental separation, oxytocin (Pitocin) is given to contract the uterus.

References: See page 208.

Postpartum Endometritis

Endometritis is an infection that begins in the decidua, and then extends into the myometrium (endomyometritis) and parametrium. Postpartum endometritis is a common cause of postpartum fever, which is defined as an oral temperature of $\geq$38.0 degrees Celsius (100.4 degrees Fahrenheit) on any two of the first 10 days postpartum, exclusive of the first 24 hours. The first 24 hours are excluded because low grade fever during this period is common and often resolves spontaneously.

I. **Microbiology**. Postpartum endometritis is typically a polymicrobial infection caused by two to three aerobes and anaerobes from the genital tract.
   A. Sexually transmitted infections, such as Neisseria gonorrhoeae and Chlamydia trachomatis, are uncommon causes of postpartum endometritis, but more frequent causes of endometritis unrelated to pregnancy.

II. **Risk factors**. Cesarean delivery is the most important risk factor for postpartum endometritis. The rates of endometritis after nonelective cesarean, elective cesarean, and vaginal delivery are about 30, 7, and <3%, respectively.
   A. Additional risk factors for postpartum endometritis include:
      1. Prolonged labor
      2. Prolonged rupture of membranes
      3. Multiple cervical examinations
      4. Internal fetal or uterine monitoring
      5. Large amount of meconium in amniotic fluid
      6. Manual removal of the placenta
      7. Low socioeconomic status
      8. Maternal diabetes mellitus or severe anemia
      9. Preterm birth
      10. Bacterial vaginosis
      11. Operative vaginal delivery
      12. Postterm pregnancy
      13. Colonization with group B streptococcus
   B. Bacterial vaginosis is most important in the setting of cesarean delivery. The odds of developing postcesarean endometritis associated with bacterial vaginosis are 5.8.

III. **Clinical manifestations and diagnosis**
   A. Clinical findings. The diagnosis of postpartum endometritis is largely based upon the findings of fever and uterine tenderness occurring in a postpartum woman. Other signs and symptoms include foul lochia, chills, and lower abdominal pain. The uterus may be soft and subinvoluted, which can lead to excessive uterine bleeding. Sepsis is an unusual presentation.
   B. Most cases develop within the first week after delivery, but 15% present between one and six weeks postpartum. Delayed presentation may manifest as late postpartum hemorrhage.
   C. Clostridium sordellii, streptococci, and staphylococci can lead to endometritis with toxic shock syndrome.
   D. Differential diagnosis of postpartum fever:
      1. Surgical site infection (cesarean delivery incision, episiotomy incision, perineal lacerations)
      2. Mastitis or breast abscess
      3. Urinary tract infection
      4. Complications of anesthesia, such as aspiration pneumonia.
      5. Deep vein thrombosis and pulmonary embolism.
      6. Disorders unrelated to pregnancy, such as appendicitis and viral syndrome, should also be considered.

IV. **Laboratory**. An elevated white blood cell count supports the diagnosis, but can be a normal finding in postpartum women. However, a rising neutrophil count associated with elevated numbers of bands is suggestive of an infectious process.
   A. **Cultures.** Testing for gonorrhea and chlamydia should be obtained if not previously performed, if prior results were positive, or the patient is at high risk for sexually transmitted infections. General endometrial cultures are not performed routinely.

    B. Bacteremia occurs in 10 to 20% of patients. Blood cultures can be useful in guiding antimicrobial treatment if the patient fails to respond to empiric therapy.

    C. Imaging studies are used to search for other causes of an initial postpartum fever (eg, pneumonia, deep vein thrombosis, or pulmonary embolus) or persistent postpartum fever (eg, abscess, ovarian vein thrombosis, septic pelvic thrombophlebitis) in patients refractory to 48 to 72 hours of antimicrobial therapy.

Type and Frequency of Bacterial Isolates in Postpartum Endometritis*

Isolate	Frequency (percent)
Gram positive	
Group B streptococci	8
Enterococci	7
S. epidermidis	9
Lactobacilli	4
Diphtheroids	2
S. Aureus	1
Gram negative	
G. vaginalis	15
E. Coli	6
Enterobacterium spp.	2
P. mirabilis	2
Others	3
Anaerobic	
S. bivius	11
Other Bacteroides spp.	9
Peptococci-peptostreptocci	22
Mycoplasma	
U. urealyticum	39
M. hominis	11
O. trachomatis	2

V. Treatment

    A. Broad spectrum parenteral antibiotics with coverage for beta-lactamase producing anaerobes should be initiated.

    B. Clindamycin (900 mg every eight hours) plus gentamicin (1.5 mg/kg every eight hours for patients with normal renal function) is an effective regimen. cure rates are 90 to 97%. Extended interval dosing of gentamicin (5 mg/kg every 24 hours) is as efficacious as the thrice daily dosing.

    C. Antibiotic regimens that are also effective include cefotetan, cefoxitin, ceftizoxime, cefotaxime, piperacillin with or without tazobactam, and ampicillin/sulbactam.

    D. **Duration.** Treatment should be continued until the patient is clinically improved and afebrile for 24 to 48 hours. Oral antibiotics after parenteral treatment is not required. However, if bacteremia was present, oral antibiotic therapy should be continued to complete a seven-day course.

Antibiotic Regimens for Endometritis

Clindamycin (900 mg IV Q 8 hours) plus gentamicin (1.5 mg/kg IV Q 8 hours)
Ampicillin-sulbactam (Unasyn) 3 grams IV Q 6 hours
Ticarcillin-clavulanate (Timentin)3.1 grams IV Q 4 hours
Cefoxitin (Mefoxin) 2 grams IV Q 6 hours
Ceftriaxone (Rocephin) 2 grams IV Q 24 hours plus metronidazole 500 mg PO or IV Q 8 hours*
Levofloxacin (Levaquin) 500 mg IV Q 24 hours plus metronidazole 500 mg PO or IV Q 8 hours*

---

* Should not be given to breastfeeding mothers
If chlamydia infection is suspected, azithromycin 1 gram PO for one dose should be added to the regimen

---

VI. Prevention
   A. Antibiotic prophylaxis at cesarean delivery significantly reduces the prevalence of postcesarean delivery endometritis, for both elective and nonelective procedures. A single dose of cefazolin (Ancef) 2 g IV or ampicillin is given just after cord clamping.

References: See page 208.

Postpartum Fever Workup

History: Postpartum fever is >100.4 F (38 degrees C) on 2 occasions >6h apart after the first postpartum day (during the first 10 days postpartum), or >101 on the first postpartum day. Dysuria, abdominal pain, distention, breast pain, calf pain.
Predisposing Factors: Cesarean section, prolonged labor, premature rupture of membranes, internal monitors, multiple vaginal exams, meconium, manual placenta extraction, anemia, poor nutrition.
Physical Examination: Temperature, throat, chest, lung exams; breasts, abdomen. Costovertebral angle tenderness, uterine tenderness, phlebitis, calf tenderness; wound exam. Speculum exam.
Differential Diagnosis: UTI, upper respiratory infection, atelectasis, pneumonia, wound infection, mastitis, episiotomy abscess; uterine infection, deep vein thrombosis, pyelonephritis, pelvic abscess.
Labs: CBC, SMA7, blood C&S x 2, catheter UA, C&S. Gonococcus culture, chlamydia; wound C&S, CXR.

References

References may be obtained at www.ccspublishing.com/ccs

Index

Order Form

Current Clinical Strategies books can also be purchased at all medical bookstores

Title	Book	CD
Treatment Guidelines in Medicine, 2006 Edition	$19.95	$36.95
Psychiatry History Taking, Third Edition	$12.95	$28.95
Psychiatry, 2008 Edition	$12.95	$28.95
Pediatric Drug Reference, 2004 Edition	$9.95	$28.95
Anesthesiology, 2008 Edition	$16.95	$28.95
Medicine, 2007 Edition	$16.95	$28.95
Pediatric Treatment Guidelines, 2007 Edition	$19.95	$29.95
Physician's Drug Manual, 2005 Edition	$9.95	$28.95
Surgery, Sixth Edition	$12.95	$28.95
Gynecology and Obstetrics, 2008 Edition	$16.95	$30.95
Pediatrics, 2007 Edition	$12.95	$28.95
Family Medicine, 2008 Edition	$26.95	$46.95
History and Physical Examination in Medicine, Tenth Edition	$14.95	$28.95
Outpatient and Primary Care Medicine, 2008 Edition	$16.95	$28.95
Critical Care Medicine, 2007 Edition	$16.95	$32.95
Handbook of Psychiatric Drugs, 2008 Edition	$14.95	$28.95
Pediatric History and Physical Examination, Fourth Edition	$12.95	$28.95
Current Clinical Strategies CD-ROM Collection for Palm, Pocket PC, Windows, and Macintosh		$59.95

CD-ROMs are compatible with Palm, Pocket PC, Windows and Macintosh.

Quantity	Title	Amount